Contents

Contents

Evidence-Based Anaesthesia and Intensive Care

Edited by

Ann Møller and Tom Pedersen

Co-ordinating Editors, Cochrane Anaesthesia Review Group, Rigshospitalet, Blegdamsvej
Copenhagen, Denmark

Project co ordinator

Jane Cracknell

Co-ordinator & Managing Editor, Cochrane Anaesthesia Review Group, Rigshospitalet,
Blegdamsvej, Copenhagen, Denmark

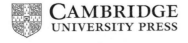

CAMBRIDGE
UNIVERSITY PRESS

CAMBRIDGE UNIVERSITY PRESS
Cambridge, New York, Melbourne, Madrid, Cape Town, Singapore, São Paulo

Cambridge University Press
The Edinburgh Building, Cambridge CB2 2RU, UK
Published in the United States of America by Cambridge University Press, New York

www.cambridge.org
Information on this title: www.cambridge.org/9780521690526

First published 2006

Printed in the United Kingdom at the University Press, Cambridge

A catalogue record for this publication is available from the British Library

Library of Congress Cataloguing in Publication data

ISBN-13 978-0-521-69052-6 paperback
ISBN-10 0-521-69052-0 paperback

Cambridge University Press has no responsibility for the persistence or accuracy of URLs for external or
third-party Internet websites referred to in this publication, and does not guarantee that any content on such
websites is, or will remain, accurate or appropriate.

Every effort has been made in preparing this publication to provide accurate and up-to-date information
which is in accord with accepted standards and practice at the time of publication. Although case histories
are drawn from actual cases, every effort has been made to disguise the identities of the individuals
involved. Nevertheless, the authors, editors and publishers can make no warranties that the information contained herein is totally free from error, not least because clinical standards are constantly changing through
research and regulation. The authors, editors and publishers therefore disclaim all liability for direct or conse-
quential damages resulting from the use of material contained in this publication. Readers are strongly
advised to pay careful attention to information provided by the manufacturer of any drugs or equipment that
they plan to use.

Foreword

George Hall

Evidence-based medicine has become the new religion for many in the healthcare professions. It is greeted by the believers as the answer to all their clinical problems while the sceptics view this new upstart with grave suspicion and delight in finding discrepancies between the conclusions of evidence-based medicine and large randomised controlled trials. Like many new ideas in medicine, evidence-based practice has matured over the past decade so that a more balanced view of the strengths and weaknesses of this technique is now possible. Ann Møller and Tom Pedersen are authorities in evidence-based medicine as applied to anaesthesia and in this book have assembled a group of distinguished authors.

The first part of the book describes the underlying principles used in evidence-based medicine with a critical evaluation of potential errors and pitfalls. The teaching of evidence-based medicine is a particularly important topic as it is used increasingly in undergraduate medicine. There remains fierce debate over its role in education. The second part of the book explores the use of evidence-based anaesthesia. Many key topics in the specialty are covered and the authors have published extensively in their areas of expertise. Thus this book not only covers the theoretical basis of the subject but also provides practical help for the anaesthesiologist. Unfortunately for the editors and the authors I have no doubt that a second edition will be essential in only a few years time. The "evidence" is always evolving and older studies are found to be no longer relevant to modern anaesthesia.

Ann Møller and Tom Pedersen are to be congratulated on this tome. Although I am unconvinced by all the arguments for, and analysis of, evidence-based medicine I have little doubt that the book will be a *sine qua non* for all departments of anaesthesiology and for many anaesthesiologists.

George M Hall
Chairman and Professor of Anaesthesia,
St George's Hospital Medical School
London, UK

Contributors

Dr. R Peter Alston, MD, FRCA
Consultant in Anaesthesia
Critical Care and Pain Medicine
Royal Infirmary of Edinburgh
51 Little France Crescent
Edinburgh, EH16 4SA, Scotland, UK
peter.alston@ed.ac.uk

Dr. J Mark Ansermino, MD, MSc(Epid), MBBCh
MSc (Med Inform) FRCPC
Director of Research
British Columbia's Children's Hospital
Department Anesthesia
4480 Oak Street
Vancouver, V6H 3V4, Canada
anserminos@yahoo.ca

Dr. Jane Ballantyne
Associate Professor of Anesthesia and
Chief, Division of Pain Medicine
Department of Anaesthesia, Clinics 309
Massachusetts General Hospital
15 Parkman Street WACC 333
Boston, MA 02114, USA
jballantyne@partners.org

Dr. Timothy Canty
Pain Management Fellow
Arnold Pain Management Center
Beth Israel Deaconess Medical Center
330 Brookline Avenue
Boston, MA 02115, USA
tcanty@partners.org

Dr. John Carlisle, MRCP FRCA
Consultant Anaesthetist
Department of Anaesthetics
NHS Torbay Hospital
Lawes Bridge, Torquay
Devon, TQ2 7AA, UK
john.carlisle@nhs.net

Dr. Divya Chander, MD, PhD
Department of Anesthesia and
Perioperative Care
University of California
521 Parnassus Avenue C450
San Francisco, CA 94143-0648, USA

Dr. Robyn Chirnside
Specialist Anaesthetist
Anaesthesia and Intensive Care
Dunedin Hospital
Great King Street
Private Bag 192
Dunedin, Otago, New Zealand
rchirnside@xtra.co.nz

Dr. Peter Choi, MD, MSc(Epid), FRCPC
Assistant Professor, Clinical Research
Director
Department of Anesthesia
Vancouver Hospital
University of British Columbia
910 West 10th Avenue
Room 3200
Vancouver, BC V5Z 4E3, Canada
petert.choi@vch.ca

Prof. Adrian Gelb, MB, ChB, DA, FRCPC
Professor of Anesthesia and
Perioperative Care
University of California
521 Parnassus Avenue C450
San Francisco, CA 94143-0648, USA
gelba@anesthesia.ucsf.edu

Prof. Stephen Halpern, MD, MSc, FRCPC
Professor of Anaesthesia
University of Toronto
Director of Obstetrical Anaesthesia
Sunnybrook and Women's College Health
Sciences Centre
76 Grenville Street
Toronto, ON, Canada
stephen.halpern@sw.ca

Dr. Helen Handoll
Senior Lecturer, School of Health and
Social Care,
University of Teesside
The James Cook University Hospital
Marton Road, Middlesbrough
TS4 3BW, UK
h.handoll@tees.ac.uk

Dr. Christof Havel
Resident Internal Medicine
Department of Emergency Medicine 6D,
Vienna General Hospital/Medical
University of Vienna
Währinger Gürtel 18–20
Vienna A-1090, Austria
christof.havel@meduinwein.ac.at

Dr. Harald Herkner
Associate Professor of Emergency Medicine
Specialist Internal Medicine, Intensive Care
Medicine
Editor, Cochrane Anaesthesia Review Group
Department of Emergency Medicine
6D, Vienna General Hospital/Medical

University of Vienna
Währinger Gürtel 18–20
Vienna A-1090, Austria
harald.herkner@meduniwien.ac.at

Dr. Ruth Hutchinson, MB, BChir (Cantab),
FRCA, DRCOG
Retired Consultant Anaesthetist
Harare Central Hospital
Harare, Zimbabwe
rhutchinson@healthnet.zw

Dr. Steven Knight, FRCA
Consultant in Anaesthesia and
Intensive Care Medicine
Wythenshawe Hospital
Southmoor Road, Wythenshawe
Manchester, MZ3 9LT, UK
srknight@ntlworld.com

Dr. Kate Leslie, MBBS, MD, MEpi, FANZCA
Staff Anaesthetist and Head of Research
Department of Anaesthesia and Pain
Management
Royal Melbourne Hospital, Australia
Honorary Associate Professor
Department of Pharmacology
University of Melbourne
Melbourne, VIC 3004, Australia
kate.leslie@mh.org.au

Dr. Ann Møller, MD
Co-ordinating Editor
The Cochrane Anaesthesia Review Group
Department of Anaesthesiology
Consultant Anaesthetist
Herlev University Hospital
2730 Herlev, Denmark
doctcamm@yahoo.com
annmo@herlevhosp.kbhamt.dk

Dr. Neil S Morton
Consultant in Paediatric Anaesthesia and
Pain Management

Royal Hospital for Sick Children
Glasgow, G3 8SJ, Scotland, UK
neil.morton@yorkhill.scot.nhs.uk

Prof. Paul Myles, MBBS, MPH, MD, FCARCSI,
FANZCA
Professor and Director
Department of Anaesthesia and
Perioperative Medicine
Alfred Hospital and Monash University
Commercial Road
Melbourne, VIC 3004, Australia
p.myles@alfred.org.au

Dr. Mina Nishimori
Research Fellow,
Pain Center
Department of Anesthesia and Critical Care
Massachusetts General Hospital
101 Merrimac Street Suite 610
Boston, MA 02114, USA
mnishimori@partners.org

Prof. Nathan Pace, MD, MStat
Professor of Anesthesiology
Department of Anaesthesiology
University of Utah
3C444 SOM, Salt Lake City
Utah 84132, USA
n.l.pace@m.cc.utah.edu

Dr. Tom Pedersen, MD, DMSc
Co-ordinating Editor
The Cochrane Anaesthesia Review Group
Director of Centre of Head-Orthopaedics
University of Copenhagen
Rigshospitalet
Blegdamsvej 9
Copenhagen 2100, Denmark
doctp@yahoo.com

Dr. Stephen Priestley
Director of Emergency Medicine
Sunshine Hospital

176 Furlong Road
St Albans, Melbourne, VIC 3021, Australia
stephen.priestley@wh.org.au

Dr. Michael Ragg
Consultant Emergency Physician
Medicine
Geelong Hospital
Ryrie Street
Geelong, VIC 3220, Australia
mragg@barwonhealth.org.au

Dr. Andrew Smith, FRCA, MRCP
Consultant Anaesthetist
Department of Anaesthetics
Royal Lancaster Infirmary, UK
Ashton Road
Honorary Professor Institute for Health
Research
Lancaster, University, UK
andrew.f.smith@mbht.nhs.uk

Dr. Maurizio Solca
Consultant Anaesthetist,
Head, Anaesthesia and Intensive Care
Medicine
Presidio Ospedaliero A. Uboldo di
Cernusco sul Naviglio
Azienda Ospedaliera Ospedale di Circolo di
Melegnano
Ospedale A. Uboldo
Via Uboldo 21
I-20063 Cernusco sul Naviglio MI, Italy
maurizio.solca@rcm.inet.it

Nete Villebro, RN, MI
Education Consultant,
Cochrane Anaesthesia Review Group
Consumer Co-ordinator
Department of Anaesthesiology
H:S Bispebjerg University Hospital
Bispebjerg Bakke 23
2400 Copenhagen NV, Denmark
villebro@yahoo.com

Dr. Janet Wale, PhD
Health Consumer Representative
Cochrane Consumer Network
Perth, Australia
socrates@q-net.net.au

Dr. Kevin Walker, MBChB, FRCA
Specialist Registrar in Anaesthesia,
Department of Anaesthetics
Royal Lancaster Infirmary
Ashton Road
Lancaster, LA1 4RP, UK
kwalker@doctors.org.uk

Dr. Mathew Zacharias, FRCA, PhD
Specialist Anaesthetist and Clinical
Senior Lecturer
Department of Anaesthesia and
Intensive Care
Dunedin Hospital and Dunedin School of
Medicine, Dunedin
Great King Street
Private Bag 192
Dunedin, Otago, New Zealand
mathew.zacharias@stonebow.otago.ac.nz,
mzach@xtra.co.nz

Introducing evidence-based anaesthesia

Ann Møller[1] and Tom Pedersen[2]

[1]The Cochrane Anaesthesia Review Group, Department of Anaesthesiology, Herlev University Hospital, Herlev, Denmark
[2]The Cochrane Anaesthesia Review Group, Centre of Head-Orthopaedics, University of Copenhagen, Rigshospitalet, Copenhagen, Denmark

Every year, more than two million new papers are published in scientific medical journals. To keep updated even in a small field or speciality takes an ever-increasing amount of time. The main purpose of evidence-based medicine (EBM) is to aid busy clinicians in making decisions based on scientific evidence. The goal of EBM is to produce systematic reviews and clinical guidelines that summarise scientific knowledge about a topic in a single publication that preferably is updated regularly.

So why should you read (and buy) this book? Because today's clinical anaesthesiologists are faced with an ever-increasing amount of work and new challenges. We have to handle our patients in both a safe and high-quality manner and at the same time adopt new scientific developments. On top of this, we have to teach our skills to those who will succeed us: the trainees. All in all, time is short and our duties are many.

The aim of this book is to meet the needs of health professionals in anaesthesiology as medicine moves to be evidence-based. Our aim is that this book should be a tool to understand the basic and advanced use of evidence-based methodology. It should integrate the results from research articles into useful, clinically orientated summaries of diagnosis, treatment and patient management in anaesthesiology and critical care medicine. Hopefully this book will become both a resource for clinical decision-making, and for decisions concerning the implementation of new technologies or interventions. This book is aimed at practising clinicians, trainees, other health professionals, medical students, teachers in evidence-based anaesthesia and EBM and, last but not least, politicians, managers and decision-makers. The chapters make clear what we know, what we think we know and what we do not know.

The book has been organised into two parts. The first 12 chapters provide the basics of EBM. They introduce EBM, critical appraisal and meta-analysis to identify and/or minimise bias. Other chapters explore clinical and statistical heterogeneity, how papers can be read and their results interpreted. Integrating the principles of EBM into daily practice is an important but often difficult task. Although we are faced with obstacles caused by lack of knowledge, skills and resources, many tools exist to help us teach and learn EBM. This book attempts to provide, you, the reader with the highlights of educational programmes in EBM, which have been shown to change the behaviour of clinicians; improve critical appraisal skills and the implementation of EBM in the clinical workplace.

Established educational activities, such as journal clubs, can be modified in such a manner as to place EBM at their core. Strategies to disseminate evidence, such as educational programmes, clinical decision support systems and audit, can be useful tools for changing the practice of our colleagues.

The final 14 chapters of this book detail how to practise EBM in preoperative evaluation, regional and general anaesthesia, fluid therapy and the use of antiemetics; and how to use EBM in the subspecialities in anaesthesia, postoperative pain therapy, critical care and emergency medicine. These chapters deal with a selection of topics, which currently are of practical and scientific importance to clinicians.

We hope that this book will provide an exciting agenda for research and clinical work in the field of evidence-based anaesthesia.

2

How to define the questions

Ann Møller

The Cochrane Anaesthesia Review Group, Department of Anaesthesiology, Herlev University Hospital, Herlev, Denmark

The practice of evidence-based medicine (EBM) begins with the formulation of a clinical question. Defining the clinical question forces you to think about what you really want to know. Clinical questions consist of three parts: the patient or population, the interventions to be compared and the clinically relevant outcomes. The clinical question can be about a single patient, or any group of patients. It can be narrow and thus specific, or it can be wide and sensitive. The intervention can be compared to nothing, to a placebo or to any other relevant intervention or interventions. The outcomes should be clinically relevant; all important outcomes should be considered. Spending time on the question helps the researcher focus on what is important. A well-defined question is a good starting point for finding relevant literature.

Introduction

In our practice, we come across clinical questions many times a day. These clinical questions may arise from several sources: the patient asking for information; your colleagues seeking advice; or from you, simply asking yourself what to do in a clinical situation. The question will often start off as open ended and poorly defined, such as: is propofol better than sevoflurane?

If you want to use an evidence-based approach to finding the answer to your question, your question needs to be well defined. The question can be about diagnosis, prognosis or management. The purpose of this chapter is to describe a strategy for formulating answerable clinical questions. That strategy can help you make conscientious, explicit and judicious use of the current best evidence for making decisions about the care of an individual patient, or a group of patients.

Formulating the question

A well-defined clinical question has three core elements:
1 The patient/population/problem

Key words: clinical question, systematic reviews, outcomes.

2 The interventions/exposures considered

3 The relevant outcomes

Formulating the clinical questions has several purposes. The process of formulating the question helps you consider what you really want to know; several choices have to be made within this process. Once the question has been formulated, it will be a great aid in the process of searching and evaluating the results (as described later in this book).

The formulation of the clinical question is the starting point; whether you intend to use EBM in the handling of an individual patient, if you are writing a clinical guideline for the department you work in, or you are preparing a systematic review.

The patient/population/problem

The patient population can be described from basic factors such as age, sex, race and educational status, or by the presence or absence of a clinical condition such as obesity, chronic heart disease or the need for a specific surgical procedure. Other factors used to describe the patient could be whether they are outpatients or inpatients; whether they live in urban or rural surroundings. The list is endless.

When choosing the patient population, one must be aware that a very narrow and well-defined population description will provide a very precise result (i.e. if a result can be found). An example of this could be: male patients aged between 50 and 70 years, with coronary heart disease scheduled for colorectal cancer surgery. This detailed description is likely to produce very specific results, but only for the narrow group in question. If the next patient is not like the first (i.e. is older, younger or a woman), problems may arise when trying to extrapolate the result.

On the contrary, choosing a wider group of patients will probably yield more results, and these results will cover a much larger group of patients. An example could be: all patients scheduled for knee arthroscopy. This group will include athletic, fit people in their 20s as well as older people with multiple co-existing diseases. With a broader group, there is always the risk that some subgroups of patients will react differently to the intervention. However, the results are much easier to extrapolate. The decision whether to use a narrow or broad question has to be placed within sound clinical judgement on the composition of the patient group.

When performing a systematic review, the approach could be to include a wide group of patients and if plausible, plan some subgroup analysis in advance if there is a suspicion that some groups will be different from the others (e.g. children, ASA3+, etc.).

The interventions/exposures considered

The intervention is something we consider "doing" to the patient. It could be a medication, surgical procedure or lifestyle counselling. An intervention could also be anaesthesia, intensive care, ventilatory support or fast tracking. The exposure could be a toxin, tobacco smoke, or any other substance or incident that "happened" to the patient. The handling would be the same, except usually we find no randomised controlled trials (RCTs) dealing with exposure.

It is important when trying to focus our clinical question to consider which interventions we would offer the patient. If the hospital cannot offer a specific treatment, we may not need to look for it. On the other hand, if the literature search finds that a specific treatment does have a beneficial effect, we may after all wish to consider it to be introduced.

A treatment can be compared to another treatment (surgical versus medical treatment, or comparison of two different surgical methods), to placebo (mostly pharmaceutical trials) or to no treatment.

If feasible, more than two interventions can be compared. Again, this depends on the purpose of the search and how generalised or specific we wish the results to be.

A thorough description of the interventions will help the researcher find relevant papers and appraise their quality.

The relevant outcomes

The definition of, and dealing with, relevant outcomes are described elsewhere in this book (Chapter 6).

However, clinically relevant outcomes are outcomes that the patients feel, function or survive. Other relevant outcomes are for example: costs, length of stay in hospital or intensive care unit and ease of practice. When comparing different interventions it is important to take all relevant outcomes into consideration: even when information on these specific outcomes is likely not to be found.

As in the other part of the question, it is important to define the outcome measures carefully. This will often be a source of heterogeneity between trials. A straight definition will help overcome this problem.

Practice points

1 The formulation of the clinical question helps focus the question. It is the basis of literature search and helps the researcher appraise the papers critically.

2 A clinical question consists of three parts:
   The patient/population/problem
   The interventions/exposures considered
   The relevant outcomes

3 A narrow question yields specific results that are hard to extrapolate. A broad question yields sensitive results that are easier to extrapolate, but carries the risk of overlooking differences in subgroups.

Conclusion

Spending time and energy, formulating the clinical question before undertaking the literature search, and appraisal, is likely to improve the outcome of the process. By concentrating on the problem, one can "straighten" the search and make the critical appraisal more focused.

SUGGESTED READING

1 Sackett DL, Straus SE, Glasziou P, Richardson WS, Rosenberg W, Haynes RB. *Evidence Based Medicine*. Churchill Livingstone: London, 2005.
2 Chalmers I (ed.) et al. *Systematic Reviews. BMJ Publishing Group,* London 2002.
3 Higgins J, Green S. (eds). *Cochrane Handbook for Systematic Reviews of Interventions 4.2.5*. The Cochrane Library. Chichester, UK: John Wiley & Sons Ltd, 2005.

3

Developing a search strategy, locating studies and electronic databases

Tom Pedersen

The Cochrane Anaesthesia Review Group, Centre of Head-Orthopaedics, University of Copenhagen, Rigshospitalet, Copenhagen, Denmark

This chapter shows how to conduct a comprehensive, objective and reproducible search for studies. It can be the most time-consuming and challenging task in preparing a clinical question for a project or a systematic review. Yet it is also one of the most important. Identifying all relevant studies, and documenting the search for studies with sufficient detail so that it can be reproduced, is after all, largely what distinguishes a systematic review from a traditional narrative review in evidence-based medicine. This chapter explains how, and where, the reviewers should look for studies that may be eligible for inclusion in *The Cochrane Library*, MEDLINE, EMBASE and other relevant databases that identify appropriate MeSH terms (Medical Subjects Headings). Although currently it is necessary to search multiple sources to identify relevant published studies, it is envisioned that the *Cochrane Central Register of Controlled Trials* (CENTRAL) in *The Cochrane Library* will become a comprehensive source for published studies, thus reducing the searching burden for authors. Identifying ongoing studies, however, will continue to remain a challenge until a comprehensive, searchable, ongoing trial register is produced to track, organise, and disseminate reports for ongoing studies, as CENTRAL in *The Cochrane Library* does for reports of studies that have been published.

Introduction

How do you find studies that meet your review's inclusion criteria?

You could do a very quick search of one electronic database and find a couple of relevant articles that meet your review's inclusion criteria. At the other extreme you could try to find every single study that has ever been done which addresses your review's question. As you might expect, there are problems with both these approaches. If you do not look very hard, the studies you do find are unlikely to

Key words: Search Strategy, *The Cochrane Library*, MEDLINE, EMBASE, CENTRAL.

be representative of all the studies done on the subject. The reasons for this are explained in detail in Chapter 8 (section "Publication bias"). For the moment, you just need to know that studies with dramatic results are much easier to find than studies that do not have dramatic findings. Another problem with only looking for a few studies is that you end up with less information. This can limit the precision of the results of your review, and restrict the conclusions you can make. However, is it feasible to find absolutely every relevant study that has ever been done? It is certainly not easy and might not be possible in most reviews. Many studies are never published, and those that are, may not be indexed in places, such as MEDLINE, that you would normally look. At some point, the effort required to find more studies becomes too much, but there is relatively little evidence on exactly when we need to stop searching. So, for now, most people adopt a pragmatic approach: look as far and as wide as possible, taking care to look in such a way that we take account of what we know about the biases in finding studies.

Search strategy for the identification of studies

Databases should include: *The Cochrane Library*, MEDLINE, EMBASE and all other relevant databases that identify appropriate MeSH terms and include the optimally sensitive. A common problem with search terms is inadequate indexing in MEDLINE and other databases. For example, random allocation was first introduced as a descriptor term in 1978; randomised controlled trial (RCT) was not introduced as a descriptor term until 1990 and did not appear as a publication type until 1991. All efforts should be made to search conference proceedings of important meetings and abstracts and contact experts in the field in order to identify unpublished research and trials still underway. Any speciality journals that have been hand searched should be identified and referenced. The name of the journal should be entered in full. Your search strategy must be reproducible, and not limited by language or publication status.

How to develop a search strategy?

It is always necessary to strike a balance between comprehensiveness and precision when developing a search strategy. Increasingly the comprehensiveness of a search entails reducing its precision and retrieving more non-relevant articles. Developing a search strategy is an iterative process in which the terms that are used are modified, based on what has already been retrieved. There are diminishing returns for search efforts; after a certain stage, each additional unit of time invested in searching returns fewer references that are relevant to the review. Consequently there comes a point when the rewards of further searching may not be worth the effort required to identify the additional references. The decision as to how much time and effort to invest in the search process depends on the question the review addresses, and the resources that are available to the reviewer.

CENTRAL serves as the most comprehensive source of records related to controlled trials. As of January 2006, the register contained 463 763 citations to reports of trials and other studies potentially relevant to Cochrane Reviews. CENTRAL includes citations to reports of controlled trials that might not indexed in MEDLINE, EMBASE or other bibliographic databases; citations published in many languages; and citations that are available only in conference proceedings or other sources that are difficult to access [1].

Boolean operators: "OR" and "AND"

An electronic search strategy should generally have three sets of terms: (1) terms to search for the health condition of interest; (2) terms to search for the intervention(s) evaluated and (3) terms to search for the types of study design to be included (typically randomised trials). The exception to this is CENTRAL, which aims to contain only reports with study designs possibly relevant for inclusion in Cochrane Reviews, so searches of CENTRAL should be based on health condition and intervention only. A good approach to developing an electronic search strategy is to begin with multiple terms that describe the health condition of interest and join these together with the Boolean "OR" operator. This means you will retrieve articles containing at least one of these search terms. You can do likewise for a second set of terms related to the intervention(s) and for a third set of terms related to the appropriate study design.

These three sets of terms can then be joined together with the "AND" operator. This final step of joining the three sets with the "AND" operator limits the retrieved set to articles of the appropriate study design that address both the health condition of interest and the intervention(s) to be evaluated. A note of caution about this approach is warranted however: if an article does not contain at least one term from each of the three sets, it will not be identified. For example, if an index term has not been added to the record for the intervention or the intervention is not mentioned in the title and abstract, the article would be missed. A possible remedy is to omit one of the three sets of terms and decide which records to check on the basis of the number retrieved and the time available to check them. An example of Boolean operators is given in Table 3.1.

In the pulse oximetry review [2] the objective was to assess the effect of perioperative monitoring with pulse oximetry and to clearly identify the adverse outcomes that might be prevented or improved by the use of pulse oximetry. We searched MEDLINE (1966 to January 2005) using the following search strategy (Table 3.2).

It is helpful to approach an information specialist for help in suggesting suitable terms for the health condition and intervention. (We consulted the Cochrane Anaesthesia Review Group's Trials Search Co-ordinator.) In general, both controlled

Table 3.1. Example of search strategy for identifying reports of studies about propofol and sevoflurane in relation to postoperative nausea and vomiting (PONV) and complications in *The Cochrane Library*

Search strategy in text words

#1 propofol

#2 sevoflurane

#3 #1 OR #2

#4 PONV

#5 Complications

#6 #4 AND #5

#7 #3 AND #6

Search results: 1 Cochrane Review and 54 records in CENTRAL. For more information see: http://www.mrw.interscience.wiley.com/cochrane/cochrane_search_fs.html

Table 3.2. Search History in MEDLINE to identify perioperative adverse outcomes using pulse oximetry

#23 #6 and #13 and #20 and #21 and #22 (184 records)

#22 #14 or #15 or #16 or #17 (16 572 records)

#21 #7 or #8 or #9 or #10 or #11 or #12 (3 063 655 records)

#20 #18 or #19 (1 584 938 records)

#19 #1 or #2 or #3 or #4 or #5 (1 582 123 records)

#18 explode "Postoperative-Complications" in MIME, MJME (94 776 records)

#17 spo2 (900 records)

#16 desaturation* (4116 records)

#15 anox?em* (6408 records)

#14 hypox?em* (9665 records)

#13 an?esth* (279 578 records)

#12 blind* (132 561 records)

#11 mask* (28 347 records)

#10 control* (1 670 827 records)

#9 trial* (306 176 records)

#8 compar* (1 583 124 records)

#7 random* (290 202 records)

#6 pulse near ox?met* (3161 records)

#5 surg* (1 484 592 records)

#4 intra?op* (60 436 records)

#3 post?op* (350 479 records)

#2 peri?op* (26 679 records)

#1 operation (133 660 records)

vocabulary terms and text words (i.e. those found in the title or abstract) should be used. You should assume that earlier articles are harder to identify. For example, abstracts are not included in MEDLINE for most articles published before 1976 and, so, text word searches will only apply to titles. In addition, few MEDLINE indexing terms relating to study design were available before the 1990s. In designing a search strategy, it may be helpful to look at published papers on the same topic and check the controlled vocabulary terms and text words. Although a research question may address particular populations, settings or outcomes, these concepts are often not well indexed with controlled vocabulary terms and generally do not lend themselves well to searching.

The Cochrane highly sensitive search strategy for MEDLINE [3] was developed specifically with the needs of Cochrane Reviews in mind. The earliest version of this search strategy was developed in 1994 and subsequent versions have been developed, each with a different syntax, specific to the version of MEDLINE being searched.

We applied the first phase of the pulse oximetry strategy to search MEDLINE for all years from 1966 to 2005. We downloaded, printed out and classified the results of our search as definite or possible randomised or quasi-randomised trials, or not using the information in the title and abstract. If no abstract was available, our decision was based on the title alone. Because identification relies solely on the titles and, where available, the abstracts, some relevant articles may not be identified. Therefore, it may still be worthwhile for authors to search MEDLINE using the Cochrane highly sensitive search strategy and to obtain and check the full reports of possibly relevant citations.

> **Developing a logical approach to searching**
> In developing your search strategy, there are a few principles. Your search should:
>   (i)   be sensitive: trying to find as many studies as possible;
>   (ii) minimise bias;
>   (iii) be efficient.

Search strategies in the Cochrane Anaesthesia Review Group for the identification of studies

Published RCTs and clinical-controlled trials (CCTs) of interventions within the scope of the Cochrane Anaesthesia Review Group (CARG) (http://www.carg.dk) are identified by systematically handsearching specialist journals, relevant conference proceedings and abstracts, and by systematically searching electronic databases such as the Cochrane Register of Controlled Trials (CENTRAL), MEDLINE and EMBASE. We encourage authors to design search strategies specifically for their own review. In Table 3.3 is shown the specific search strategy used for CARG's specialised register.

Table 3.3. The specific search strategy used for CARG's specialised register is quoted below

Electronic searches

MeSH terms
1 Anaesthesia
2 Anaesthetics
3 Analgesia
4 Analgesics
5 Critical care
6 Critical illness
7 Emergency treatment
8 Emergency medical services
9 Emergency medicine
10 Intensive care
11 Fluid therapy
12 Perioperative care
13 Preoperative care
14 Postoperative complications
15 Postoperative period

Key and text words
1 ANAESTHE*
2 ANALGESI*
3 Prehospital
4 Critical care
5 Intensive care
6 Emergency (treatment or medical services or medicine)
7 Recovery room
8 Fluid therapy

Locating studies

Systematic reviews of the effects of health care interventions generally focus on reports from RCTs, when such data are available, because of the general acceptance that this study design will lead to the most reliable estimates of effects. A comprehensive search for relevant RCTs, which seeks to minimise bias, is one of the essential steps in doing a systematic review, and one of the factors that distinguishes a systematic review from a traditional review.

A quick search of, for example, MEDLINE is generally not considered adequate. Studies have shown that only 30–80% of all known published RCTs were identifiable using MEDLINE (depending on the area or specific question). Even if relevant records are in MEDLINE, it can be difficult to easily retrieve them. A comprehensive search is important not only for ensuring that as many studies as possible are identified but also to minimise selection bias for those that are found. Relying exclusively on a MEDLINE search may retrieve a set of reports unrepresentative of all reports that would have been identified through a comprehensive search of several sources. For example, the majority of the journals indexed in MEDLINE are published in English. If studies showing an intervention to be effective are more likely to be published in English, then any summary of only the English language reports retrieved through a MEDLINE search may result in an overestimate of effectiveness due to a language bias [4–7]. In addition, the results of many studies are never published, and most of these probably remain unknown. If studies showing an intervention to be effective are more likely to be published, then any summary of only the published reports may result in an overestimate of effectiveness due to a publication bias [8–15].

Electronic databases

Where to look for studies?

A search for relevant studies generally begins with health-related electronic bibliographic databases. Searches of electronic databases are generally the easiest and least time-consuming way to identify an initial set of relevant reports. Some electronic bibliographic databases, such as MEDLINE and EMBASE, include abstracts for the majority of recent records. Often a researcher can determine an article's relevance to a review based on the abstract, and can thereby avoid retrieving the full journal article, if the reported study is clearly not eligible for inclusion. Another advantage of these databases is that they can be searched electronically, for either words in the title and abstract, or using standardised subject-related indexing terms that have been assigned to the record. For example, the MEDLINE indexing term RANDOMISED-CONTROLLED-TRIAL (Publication Type) was introduced in 1991 and allows a user to search for articles describing individual randomised trials.

Hundreds of electronic bibliographic databases exist. Some databases, such as MEDLINE/PubMed and EMBASE, cover all areas of health care and index journals published from around the world. Other databases, such as the Australasian Medical Index, the Chinese Biomedical Literature Database, the Latin American Caribbean Health Sciences Literature (LILACS), and the Japan Information Centre of Science and Technology File on Science, Technology and Medicine (JICST-E) index journals published in specific regions of the world. Others, such as the Cumulative Index of Nursing and Allied Health (CINAHL) and AIDSLINE, focus on specific areas of health. The Cochrane Collaboration has been developing an electronic database of reports of controlled trials (CENTRAL) that is now the best single source of information about records that relate to studies, which might be eligible for inclusion in Cochrane Reviews. Details of other databases that might contain eligible records are available in the Gale Directory of Online, Portable and Internet databases (http://www. dialog.com). The three electronic bibliographic databases generally considered as the richest sources of trials – CENTRAL, MEDLINE, EMBASE – are described in more detail below.

CENTRAL

This register is part of *The Cochrane Library*. The idea behind this register is that it should be a central place to put all the reports of controlled trials identified through the work of The Cochrane Collaboration. This means that it contains the results of searching MEDLINE, EMBASE, some other databases and a long list of journals, books and conference proceedings. Many of the reports of studies on the register have been included because they might be reports of trials, based on reading the title and abstract (if there was one). The content of CENTRAL changes all the time, as does the indexing of entries and retrieval methods. Guidance on searching CENTRAL has been prepared as part of the CENTRAL Management Plan (http://www.cochrane.us/central.htm). Many of the records in CENTRAL have been identified through systematic searches of MEDLINE and EMBASE.

MEDLINE and EMBASE

Index Medicus (published by the US National Library of Medicine, NLM) and Excerpta Medica (published by Elsevier) are indexes of healthcare journals that are available in electronic form as MEDLINE and EMBASE, respectively. MEDLINE indexes about 4600 journals. PubMed is a free, online MEDLINE database that also includes up-to-date citations not yet indexed (http://www.ncbi.nlm.nih.gov). EMBASE, which is often considered the European counterpart to MEDLINE, indexes nearly 4000 journals from over 70 countries.

The overlap in journals covered by MEDLINE and EMBASE has been estimated to be approximately 34% [16]. The actual degree of reference overlap depends on the topic, with reported overlap values in particular areas ranging from 10% to 75% [17–20]. Studies comparing searches of the two databases have generally concluded that a comprehensive search requires that both databases be searched. Although MEDLINE and EMBASE searches tend not to identify the same sets of references, they have been found to return similar numbers of relevant references.

MEDLINE and EMBASE can be searched using standardised subject terms assigned by indexers employed by the publishing organisation. Using the appropriate standardised subject terms, a simple search strategy can quickly identify articles pertinent to the topic of interest. This approach works well if the goal is to identify a few good articles on a topic or to identify one particular article. However, when searching for studies for a systematic review the precision with which subject terms are applied to references should be viewed with healthy scepticism. Authors may not describe their methods or objectives well, indexers are not always expert in the subject area of the article that they are indexing, and indexers make mistakes, like all people. In addition, the available indexing terms might not correspond to the terms the searcher wishes to use. The controlled vocabulary search terms for MEDLINE and EMBASE are not identical. Search strategies need to be customised for each database. One way to begin to identify controlled vocabulary terms for a particular database is to retrieve articles from that database, which meet the inclusion criteria for the review and to note common text words and the terms the indexers had applied to the articles, which could then be used for a full search.

Assuming that search results from each database are of approximately equal value, the choice of which to search first may often be a matter of cost, with MEDLINE typically being the less costly option. As noted earlier, PubMed provides free online access to MEDLINE. Other databases, including AIDSLINE, and HealthSTAR are being phased out and their unique journal citations are migrating to PubMed. A new database, called the Gateway (http://gateway.nlm.nih.gov/gw/Cmd) searches PubMED, OLDMEDLINE, LOCATORplus, MEDLINEplus, DIRLINE, Health Services Research Meetings, and Space Life Sciences Meetings.

> **Sources to be searched to identify randomised trials for systematic reviews**
> * The Cochrane Controlled Trials Register (CENTRAL)
> * MEDLINE and EMBASE
> * Other databases as appropriate
> * Journals
> * Conference proceedings
> * Reference lists
> * Sources of ongoing and unpublished studies

Should we continue to handsearch?

Despite the considerable efforts described above to identify reports of controlled trials by searching electronic databases, it is still necessary to "handsearch" journals to identify additional reports. For example, MEDLINE and EMBASE only go back to 1966 and 1974, respectively and despite the efforts to extend MEDLINE back further in time; many earlier reports will never be indexed. Similarly, not all journals published in more recent years are indexed in electronic databases and even for those that are; it is not always possible to tell from the electronic record that the report is a trial.

Personal communication

People who have been working in a particular topic area may know of studies that you have not yet found. Reviewers commonly send a list of the studies they have found to the authors of those studies, asking if they are aware of any other relevant studies. Another approach is to write to the manufacturers of relevant drugs or devices and ask if they are aware of any other studies.

Document your search

It is very important to keep an accurate record of what you have searched, when you searched it and how you searched it. This record will help you avoid having to repeat searches and it will also help people using your review to appraise how well they think you have minimised bias.

Keeping it under control

Keeping track of searches can be a challenge. You may find several reports of the same study, and you will probably find the same report of a study in several databases. So you need some way of keeping track of the references you have looked at, and then some way of grouping together all the reports of a single study. You might like to keep a record of where you found each study, so that you can report how useful different sources were. Some people use reference management software to do all this, such as ProCite, Reference Manager, EndNote or IdeaList. If you like working with databases this is great, and can save time typing in references later on. Other people prefer printing out citations and writing on them. What ever system you choose to use, you will need some system for keeping track of which references you think are relevant, which ones you have ordered from the library, which ones you have received the paper for, etc. It is a good idea to keep a note of which studies you have found and rejected. You may well come across them again later and it can be very frustrating to re-read irrelevant records.

Practice points
- The main advice is simply to get some help from an expert.
- Look at the terms used to index and describe a few studies you already know are relevant to your review, and use these terms in your search strategy.
- Add new terms to your search strategy and then pilot them on part of the database to see whether you get relevant material, before you run it on the whole database.
- Use date limits for your search if appropriate. For example, if drugs, anaesthetic techniques or diseases have only been around since a certain date, there is no point searching before then.
- Other relevant material about search strategies are found in: "Systematic Reviews in Health Care" [21].

Conclusion

It is discussed in this chapter how and where the reviewers should look for studies that may be eligible for inclusion such as *The Cochrane Library*, MEDLINE, EMBASE and other relevant databases that identify appropriate MeSH terms. The inclusion of all relevant studies in projects and systematic reviews is crucial to avoid bias and maximise precision. Furthermore it is discussed which sources there should be searched to identify RCTs for systematic reviews.

REFERENCES

1 Dickersin K, Manheimer E, Wieland S, Robinson KA, Lefebvre C, McDonald S, and CENTRAL Development Group. Development of the Cochrane Collaboration's CENTRAL Register of Controlled Clinical Trials. *Eval Health Prof* 2002; 25: 38–64.

2 Pedersen T, Dyrlund Pedersen B, Møller AM. Pulse oximetry for perioperative monitoring. *The Cochrane Database of Systematic Reviews* 2003; Issue 2. Art. No.: CD002013. DOI: 10.1002/14651858.CD002013.

3 Robinson KA, Dickersin K. Development of a highly sensitive search strategy for the retrieval of controlled trials using PubMed. *Int J Epidemiol* 2002; 31: 150–3.

4 Gregoire G, Derderian F, LeLorier J. Selecting the language of the publications included in a meta-analysis: is there a tower of Babel bias? *J Clin Epidemiol* 1995; 48: 159–63.

5 Moher D, Fortin P, Jadad AR, Juni P, Klassen T, Le Lorier J et al. Completeness of reporting of trials published in languages other than English: implications for conduct and reporting of systematic reviews. *Lancet* 1996; 347: 363–6.

6 Egger M, Zellweger-Zähner T, Schneider M, Junker C, Lengeler C, Antes G. Language bias in randomised controlled trials published in English and German. *Lancet* 1997; 350: 326–9.

7 Juni P, Holenstein F, Sterne J, Bartlett C, Egger M. Direction and impact of language bias in meta-analyses of controlled trials: empirical study. *Int J Epidemiol* 2002; 31: 115–23.

8 Simes RJ. Publication bias: the case for an international registry of clinical trials. *J Clin Oncol* 1986; 4: 1529–41.

9 Dickersin K, Chan S, Chalmers TC, Sacks HS, Smith H. Publication bias and clinical trials. *Control Clin Trial* 1987; 8: 343–53.

10 Simes RJ. Confronting publication bias: a cohort design for meta-analysis. *Stat Med* 1987; 6: 11–29.

11 Begg CB, Berlin JA. Publication bias: a problem in interpreting medical data. *J Roy Stat Soc A* 1988; 151: 445–63.

12 Hetherington J, Dickersin K, Chalmers I, Meinert CL. Retrospective and prospective identification of unpublished controlled trials: lessons from a survey of obstetricians and pediatricians. *Pediatrics* 1989; 84: 374–80.

13 Easterbrook PJ, Berlin JA, Gopalan R, Matthews DR. Publication bias in clinical research. *Lancet* 1991; 337: 867–72.

14 Dickersin K, Min YI. NIH clinical trials and publication bias. *Online J Curr Clin Trial* [serial online] 1993. Doc. No. 50.

15 Song F, Eastwood AJ, Gilbody S, Duley L, Sutton AJ. Publication and related biases. *Health Technol Assess* 2000; 4(10).

16 Smith BJ, Darzins PJ, Quinn M, Heller RF. Modern methods of searching the medical literature. *Med J Aust* 1992; 157: 603–11.

17 Kleijnen J, Knipschild P. The comprehensiveness of Medline and Embase computer searches. Searches for controlled trials of homeopathy, ascorbic acid for common cold and ginkgo biloba for cerebral insufficiency and intermittent claudication. *Pharm Weekblad Sci* 1992; 14: 316–20.

18 Odaka T, Nakayama A, Akazawa K, Sakamoto M, Kinukawa N, Kamakura T et al. The effect of a multiple literature database search – a numerical evaluation in the domain of Japanese life science. *J Med Syst* 1992; 16: 77–81.

19 Rovers JP, Janosik JE, Souney PF. Crossover comparison of drug information online database vendors: Dialog and MEDLARS. *Ann Pharmacother* 1993; 27(5): 634–9.

20 Ramos-Remus C, Suarez-Almazor M, Dorgan M, Gomez-Vargas A, Russell AS. Performance of online biomedical databases in rheumatology. *J Rheumatol* 1994; 21(10): 1912–21.

21 Lefebvre C, Clarke M. Identifying randomised controlled trials. In: Egger M, Davey Smith G, Altman D (eds). *Systematic Reviews in Health Care*. London: BMJ Publishing, 2003.

4

Retrieving the data

John Carlisle

Department of Anaesthetics, NHS Torbay Hospital, Torquay, Devon, UK

In this chapter, I will discuss the methods of data retrieval and storage that help you to subsequently extract and analyse outcomes, bias and confounding factors, with particular reference to the systematic review of experimental studies.

There has been very little empirical research on how different methods of data retrieval and storage affect the results of systematic reviews. Most research has focussed on variables in the early part of the process, such as blinding data extractors to the authors, institute and publishing journal of each trial.

Because of the paucity of evidence I have written a pragmatic chapter based upon my own experience as an author and editor of Cochrane systematic reviews. Therefore you should not accord my conclusions with the same weight you would give to conclusions in other chapters that are based upon more evidence.

Introduction

Your aim is to find out what results your patient can expect from an intervention and how reliable are the effects. To do this you have to retrieve data from studies accurately without introducing bias. You determined the participants, interventions and outcomes for which you want to retrieve data when you planned your protocol (Chapter 2). Your search strategy determined the studies that you found (Chapter 3). In this chapter I will explain how best to retrieve data from those studies.

Stop

You have found studies but you have not yet retrieved data from them. Before proceeding you should review your clinical question and check that the information that you intend to retrieve will answer that question. You should avoid altering your methodology after you have started to retrieve data. The later you make changes, the more likely it is that you will be changing your question to match your results. If you do make changes later on you should make this clear, to yourself and others. One of

Key words: Electronic bibliographies, search strategies, bias, systematic review, outcome.

the tasks of The Cochrane Collaboration's editorial teams (Chapter 9) is to look for differences in the methodologies between a submitted review and the protocol.

Before you "start"

Begin by planning, piloting and redrafting your data extraction form. Read Chapter 8 in the *Cochrane Handbook for Systematic Reviews of Interventions* [1]. More than one person should retrieve data (see section "Getting the data wrong"). You are trying to develop a data extraction form that best promotes precision, accuracy and reliability so that your answer is valid.

Recording retrieved data

Why extract data?

The data you want is already recorded in the studies you have found. However it is difficult to accurately identify, remember and analyse the data you want if you do not unburden them from everything in the study that you do not need. If you do not explicitly extract the data your analyses may be inaccurate, difficult to check and you may fail to identify bias.

Why record extracted data electronically?

You can retrieve the data for each study into a separate paper record and then compare the results and integrate them, usually systematically by transferring the extracted data into a program like RevMan [2]. However if you first retrieve data from each study into software (such as Microsoft's Excel or Access programs) you can make your analyses more complete and easily verified (see below).

What data?

1 *Unique identifiers*

Most electronic bibliographies (such as MEDLINE) assign a unique identifying number to each record in that database. In addition the reference (journal, year, volume, issue, pages) is usually unique. You can take the opportunity to formulate your own unique identifier that reflects the source(s) in which you found the study. If you exclude the study you can modify the identifier to reflect the stage of exclusion. This helps you populate the QUORUM statement algorithm [3].

2 *Search strategies*

The electronic retrieval form is a convenient place to record your search strategies. You can Hyperlink the search strategy to some bibliographic databases that will update your search when you link to them. You can also annotate Figure 4.1 with the search strategy that resulted in the studies you retrieved.

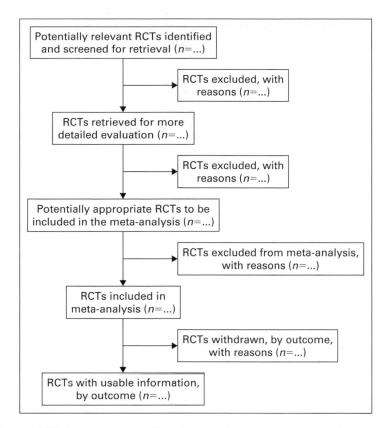

Figure 4.1   QUORUM statement algorithm. RCT: randomised controlled trial

3 *Inclusion and exclusion criteria*

You must verify that you can use the results of a study to answer your question (before you expend time extracting data). For each study you should record the presence of all your inclusion criteria and the absence of any exclusion criteria for: participants, interventions, outcomes, study methodology (e.g. randomly allocated placebo-controlled trials).

4 *Intervention*

Record the number of participants allocated to each intervention, not the number assessed (intention-to-treat analysis). Verify that the controls are adequate enough to be categorised as placebo.

5 *Outcomes*

5.1 Dichotomous outcomes – "it did or did not happen" – are recorded as proportions; the number of participants experiencing an outcome divided by the number allocated to that intervention. Ensure that the unit of analysis corresponds with the unit of allocation: this means that a participant can only be recorded as experiencing an outcome once. If you record each number in different cells you can copy and paste as text into the comparison tables in RevMan.

   5.2 Continuous data – "how much did it happen" – are recorded as the number of participants, the mean and the standard deviation (of the outcome measurement) for each of the allocated groups.

6 *Descriptive variables*

You should record the presence or value of variables even if you do not intend to use subgroup analyses to assess their association with the efficacy of the intervention. Subgroup analyses are difficult to interpret (see other chapters).

7 *Bias within studies*

   7.1 Selection bias depends on two features of a study's methodology: the success of concealing the allocation sequence (for instance telephone allocation) and the unpredictability of the allocation sequence (random sequence).

   7.2 Performance bias depends on both selection bias and blinding of **everyone** who could alter the incidence of the outcomes, including the patient and the anaesthetist.

   7.3 Attrition bias depends on the previous biases and upon unintended consequences of the interventions (thus the preference for intention-to-treat analyses).

   7.4 Detection bias depends on the preceding biases.

Record separately the quality of each study's attempts to reduce each bias. Then you can assess the impact of each independently of the other biases.

Recording retrieved data electronically

Size

- I included 763 randomised controlled trials in my systematic review. The paper pile of single data retrieval sheets would weigh nearly 4 kg and occupy a volume of 5 litres. My flash drive weighs a few grams and fits on a key ring. I extracted data from each study into between 40 and 100 columns in Excel (see below) – my writing would have to be very small to fit this information on one side of A4. I also needed to share the data retrieval forms with colleagues who verified the extracted data: it is expensive to transport 4 kg by post to another country.

Backup

It is both easy to copy and to (accidentally) erase electronic files. A simple solution to keeping track of multiple versions of your file on various media is to name each saved file with the date and place that it is stored.

- My systematic review kept me occupied for over 2 years. I must have spent thousands of hours and nearly £6000 sterling (retrieving studies that were not free).

This sort of investment disciplined me to habitually copy my files. I even e-mailed the latest version to colleagues when I went on holiday in case of drowning or burial in an avalanche!

Program

- I chose to extract data to Microsoft Excel [4] because:
  1.1 I was familiar with it.
  1.2 Most computers I access have it installed (as an anaesthetist I work in many different places – it is time-consuming to arrange installation of novel software on hospital computers).
  1.3 Export of data to other programs is usually easy although occasionally laborious (there are instructions in Excel, RevMan, STATA [5] and other programs).
  1.4 Many programs have been devised to work with data in Excel, including programs that allow you to compare two Excel sheets (see section "Getting the data wrong").

Manipulating retrieved electronic records

If you have found only a few studies you will probably be able to manipulate the data that you have extracted as easily with paper sheets as with an electronic format. But you will find it very difficult to perform the same tasks manually if you have lots of studies to assess.

Counting

Each row is numbered sequentially in Excel, so you know how many studies there are. Excel tells you how many studies you select (or "filter") from the total. If the program does not tell you how many you have selected (it will display the words "filter mode" Figure 4.2).

<u>G</u>o into "<u>T</u>ools" "<u>O</u>ptions" "Calculation" and mark "<u>M</u>anual" (instead of "<u>A</u>utomatic")

Calculations

You can add subgroups (see <u>F</u>ilter and <u>P</u>ivotTable) and you can do other calculations in many software programs. Most of the meta-analytic calculations will be

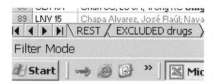

Figure 4.2 Counting: filter mode

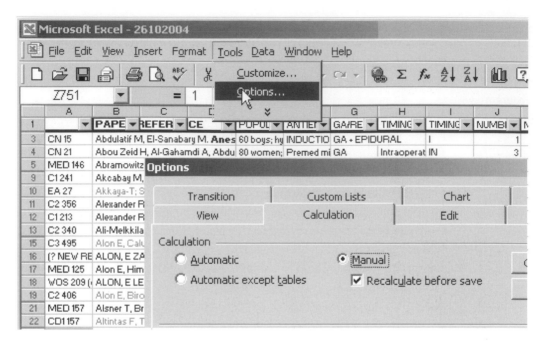

Figure 4.3   Tool option

performed after you have entered your extracted data into RevMan, STATA or another program.

Annotating and linking

You can mark certain records by changing font or by inserting a Comment. You can insert a Hyperlink to another sheet in Excel, to another file (perhaps Word or pdf [6]), or to a web page (perhaps the full text or abstract of the study).

Filter and PivotTable

These two functions allow you to rapidly count how many participants are in a subgroup in one column or in a combination of columns. In this case I had one column "age" with each study categorised as "adult", "child" and "both", and another column "sex" categorised as "male" and "female".

Other factors that affect the validity of your answer

Duplication

Your answer will be skewed if you include the same data more than once. Sometimes duplicate publication is easy to identify because the same authors publish the same

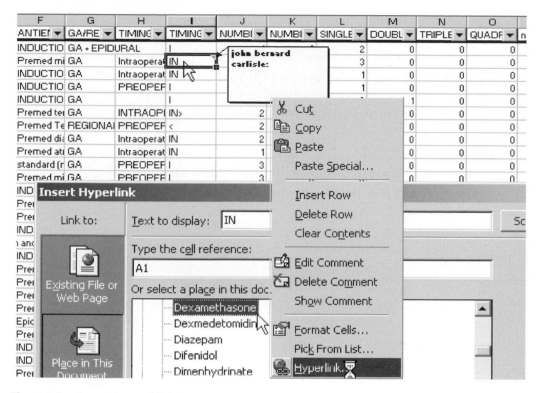

Figure 4.4   Annotating and linking

study (participants, interventions, outcomes) with small variations in the text. Sometimes data are common to multiple studies yet details will be different and the authors will be completely different. This is most likely to occur during or following multicentre studies when authors report results from their own hospitals. It can also occur when results are published during and after completion of a study. You can use Filter, PivotTable and Find to identify authors of more than one paper. If you use 26 columns for surnames beginning with each letter of the alphabet you can use these functions to identify authors who have published together. You can then look for patterns in results.

Author networks and hubs or nodes

You can also start to identify "networks". A network of authors may indirectly connect two other authors who have not published together. Networks analysis allows you to:

- Identify duplicated data when studies have no authors in common.
- Identify possible "hubs" of influence that may affect the methodology and results of studies.

You can measure the degree of "relatedness" between different studies. You can use this measure to order a set of studies and see whether the result (for instance the antiemetic effect of dexamethasone) correlates with the strength of association between studies (in RevMan or in STATA).

If you want to assess network influences on your answer you may need to use social network mapping software. There is freeware available on the web [7].

Getting the data wrong

You will make some errors, both when you retrieve data from studies, and when you transfer it to your record. You can repeat data retrieval on a separate record and then compare the data with the original record. In addition someone else should extract data for two reasons:

1 They are likely to make different errors to you.
2 There is a subjective element to qualitative categorisation of studies.

You can then compare retrieval records manually or if they are electronic, automatically. If you analyse your results, you find extreme (outlying) values, go back to the original papers and check the data retrieval form for extraction errors, such as transposing the placebo results with the intervention results.

Difficult data

Outcome summaries but no details

You are most likely to have problems retrieving outcomes when a study does not present the raw outcome data. For instance there may only be odds ratios, relative risks, differences, standard errors, 95% confidence intervals and so on. Sometimes you can derive the original outcome values or incidences from these data but you are likely to require the assistance of a statistician (see the *Cochrane Handbook for Systematic Reviews of Interventions 4.2*, Chapter 8).

Percentages

A percentage makes the result look more impressive if it exceeds the incidence. It is very easy to make the mistake of retrieving the percentage rather than the incidence. A percentage incidence may be reported that makes no sense, for instance "22% of 34 patients experienced PONV". This equals 7.48 participants! You may only have a graph labelled "%" on the Y-axis from which to estimate the incidences.

Solutions

You should decide before retrieving data what you will do when confronted with such problems to avoid your solution favouring a result towards which you are biased. You should be conservative if you have to estimate the value of a result that you include. This means that you should use the value that reduces any difference between the intervention and control groups.

Summary and practice points

- Logical reasoning, in the absence of contradictory empirical evidence, suggests that you should plan, prepare and pilot your data extraction form. As a minimum this includes all your inclusion and exclusion criteria, methodological variables, outcomes (and their values), subgroup variables and a unique identifier.
- You will makes assumptions. Spend time identifying these assumptions and question whether they are valid (supported by reliable empirical evidence). Your assumptions will bias your results and how you handle issues of dispute.
- Are you sure that electronic data extraction and storage will not help you? Unless you are confident that you will only find a few simple studies you should spend time learning to use an electronic format.
- Consider exporting your electronic data to programs that could help you detect subtle biases and data duplication, perhaps through network analyses.

Research agenda

- The sensitivity of your results and the answer of your clinical question, may depend on how data is extracted and stored.
- There has not been much research into this aspect of systematic reviews.
- Would you like to begin?

RESOURCES

1 http://www.cochrane.dk/cochrane/handbook/hbook.htm
2 http://www.cc-ims.net/RevMan
3 http://www.consort-statement.org/QUOROM.pdf
4 http://office.microsoft.com
5 http://www.stata.com
6 http://www.adobe.com/products/acrobat/readstep2.html
7 http://www.insna.org

REFERENCE

Carlisle J, Stevenson C. Drugs for preventing postoperative nausea and vomiting. *The Cochrane Database of Systematic Reviews* 2006, Issue 3.

Critical appraisal and presentation of study details

Helen Handoll

Teesside Centre for Rehabilitation Sciences, University of Teesside, The James Cook University Hospital, Middlesbrough, UK

The critical appraisal of studies and the succinct presentation of study details are essential aspects of evidence-based anaesthesia. Their primary role is to guide the interpretation of evidence from studies in terms of its validity and applicability. It is necessary to be aware of potential sources of bias that may impact on the reliability of study findings. Similarly, it is important to consider key study characteristics that may affect the relevance of study findings to clinical practice. Formal procedures, such as the use of forms itemising criteria to judge study quality and for the collection of study details, are important to make the process objective and repeatable. There is an underlying need for transparency in methods and reporting.

Introduction

The critical appraisal of studies and the systematic presentation of study details are key components of an evidence-based approach. Both require methodical processes, which should be pre-specified and, where appropriate, piloted. The importance of a written protocol, which includes details of these, cannot be overstated. The preparation and piloting of forms to assess study quality and to gather study details and results are of immense help (see Chapter 4). Similarly of benefit is an outline, which may include draft tables, of what you want to report.

This chapter focuses mainly on the critical appraisal of randomised controlled trials of treatment or preventive interventions and the presentation of study details from these in systematic reviews. Some mention will be made of the similar processes for systematic reviews of tests of diagnostic accuracy.

Critical appraisal

In the context of evidence-based medicine, critical appraisal is the systematic evaluation of the aims, design, conduct, analysis and interpretation of a study in order to assess its value in terms of its relevance (to the question being considered), validity (proximity to the truth) and applicability (usefulness in clinical practice). This evaluation is usually hindered by the inadequate reporting of studies [1]. Given this, reviewers should consider contacting trial investigators for key information missing from trial reports.

Critical appraisal of study reports for systematic reviews is generally a two-stage process. Firstly there is "study selection" where potentially eligible studies are checked to see if they meet the pre-specified inclusion criteria of the review. Then there is "quality assessment" of and data collection from the studies that meet the inclusion criteria.

Study selection

Study selection may involve an initial filtering to exclude those studies that are clearly ineligible, and then a more formal selection process for the remainder. The inclusion criteria for systematic reviews of treatment interventions usually encompass study design, patient population, interventions and outcomes recorded, but may also restrict inclusion to studies reported in full publications or in specific languages. Where practical, the independent assessment by two or more people using forms or some other means of recording their decisions and reasons is recommended. Processes to resolve disagreement should also be stated.

Quality assessment

Upon selecting studies that conform to the review inclusion criteria, the systematic assessment or critical appraisal of study quality is an essential next step. While study "quality" is hard to define absolutely – opinion varies, the essential role of quality assessment is to assist the interpretation of the evidence from a study in terms of its reliability (validity) and, usually, its usefulness (applicability). The results of quality assessment can also be used to decide the inclusion of the results of a study in meta-analyses and as a means to explore heterogeneity, such as in key aspects of study methods, between otherwise similar studies (see Chapters 7 and 8).

Most quality assessment of studies involves an appraisal of aspects of internal and external validity. These are described below.

Internal and external validity

Study validity, also termed "internal validity", is the extent to which the study design and conduct, including analysis, are likely to prevent systematic errors or bias. Four types of systematic bias that could affect the findings of controlled clinical trials are those of selection, performance, detection and attrition (see Box 5.1; also Chapters 7 and 8).

Box 5.1. Sources of systematic bias in controlled clinical trials that can undermine a trial's potential to provide reliable evidence of the effectiveness of anaesthesia interventions under test

Selection bias

Systematic differences between the comparison groups. Random allocation, with prior concealment of allocation, of sufficiently large numbers of trial participants to the trial interventions should prevent this. Where there are sufficient numbers, randomisation should balance both known and unknown confounders (factors other than the interventions under test that influence outcome). The secure concealment of allocation, preventing foreknowledge of trial intervention assignment at randomisation, has been shown to be crucial for preventing selection bias [2].

Performance bias

Systematic differences in care provided apart from the intervention being tested. This can be avoided or diminished by the blinding to trial interventions of those providing and receiving care, and by ensuring comparable care programmes (other than the trial interventions) to all interventions groups. Blinding may not be feasible in trials evaluating some anaesthetic techniques. The standardisation of care protocols is often a challenge: for example, an imbalance in the choice of surgical technique or important differences in postoperative care. Similar training and expertise of health care providers can be an issue here; for example, some allowance needs to be made for the learning curve for new techniques.

Attrition bias (exclusion bias)

Systematic differences between the comparison groups in the loss of participants from the study. These losses could result from protocol deviations (e.g. inappropriate admission into study), participant withdrawals (no longer willing to participate) and exclusions (e.g. because of adverse effects or non-compliance) and dropouts (loss to follow-up). Intention-to-treat analysis where the outcomes of all trial participants are analysed according to the group to which they were allocated at randomisation protects against this bias.

Detection bias (assessment, ascertainment or measurement bias)

Systematic differences in outcome assessment. Blinding of assessors (including trial participants) of outcome is one of the best ways to guard against this. This is not always practical, particularly for trials of physical techniques, but should be possible for at least some outcomes. Nonetheless, independent assessors and the systematic and active follow-up of all trial participants should be possible.

"External validity", also termed applicability or generalisability, is the extent to which the results of a study are applicable outside the study, such as in routine clinical practice.

Various parallel but also different systematic biases pertain to other study designs. For instance, crucial to systematic reviews is "publication bias", where the inclusion of published research only may result in an overestimation or an otherwise incorrect summary of the true effect of an intervention. Indirectly, publication bias and the failure to take into account existing evidence is important also to primary research [3]. An example of bias in diagnostic reviews, where cohort studies are the norm, is "partial verification" where only a selected sample of people evaluated with the "index test" is verified by the "reference standard". A comprehensive summary of the sources of bias and variation in diagnostic studies is provided in Whiting et al. [4].

Quality assessment tools

Many quality checklists and scoring schemes or "tools" have been devised, some of which are quite complex and time consuming to perform. Most "tools" focus on specific types of study design such as controlled trials, diagnostic studies and systematic reviews [5]. Many of the individual items of these tools are in common and reflect generally perceived biases for the different study designs.

There is, however, only limited empirical evidence of a relationship between trial outcomes and a few of the specific criteria generally used to assess the risk of systematic bias in randomised controlled trials. The main finding is that trials with inadequate concealment of allocation tend to result in larger estimates of effect than randomised controlled trials with adequately concealed allocation [2]. Additionally, there is some evidence of an effect from blinding of trial participants, investigators and outcome assessors [6,7]. While there are many aspects in the design and conduct of diagnostic accuracy studies that can lead to bias or variation, there is again only limited evidence about the size and effect of individual aspects [4]. For both types of review, the extent and perhaps direction of bias are likely to be context specific to varying degrees. An underlying difficulty in these investigations and one that applies generally to evidence-based activities is that we do not know the "truth", only that the conforming to good research methods is theoretically more likely to bring us closer to the truth.

Choice of quality assessment tool

When choosing a quality assessment tool, often with a view to adapting it for your own use, it is helpful to consider what aspects of internal and external validity and other features of trial methods are being covered. Given the empirical evidence of a potential effect on study results, essential items of internal validity for randomised controlled trials are concealment of allocation, blinding and, though still unproven but theoretically convincing in terms of an effect, conducting an intention-to-treat analysis.

Some quality assessment and data extraction tools are combined. This can be helpful as various quality criteria may serve as useful prompts to note specific details of study methods rather than to specifically rate these in terms of quality. An easy to use and understand quality assessment tool has obvious advantages. This supports tools with few items and in a checklist (Yes, No, Don't know/Unknown) format. Examples include the Delphi list [8] for randomised controlled trials and QUADAS [9] for diagnostic tests studies. Both of these were devised by consensus methods. Many quality scoring schemes are also practical and can be simple to use. However, summary scores where the scores of individual items are totalled are "problematic" in that they do not reliably distinguish between high and low quality studies [10]. Given this, it is recommended the reporting of quality assessment and any analyses based on the quality assessment should be confined to individual aspects of trial methodology [10,11]. Although the Jadad score [12] is one of the few scores that have been validated for inter-rater and intra-rater consistency, objections to this popular score include its use of a composite score, its over-reliance on reporting accuracy and its restriction to items of internal validity. However, if the assessment of internal validity of a trial indicates it to be seriously flawed, then assessing its external validity may be pointless.

External validity is frequently rated in specific items of other quality tools. This includes the sufficient description of the interventions (for treatment reviews) or diagnostic tests (for diagnostic accuracy reviews), and may also include an appraisal of outcome assessment. Blinded outcome assessment, especially relevant for "soft outcomes", has already been covered in terms of internal validity, but in conjunction with this is the need for active and systematic follow-up. Reliance on retrospective collection from medical records and the failure to assess outcome at set times risks missing important findings, such as adverse events, and hiding or distorting the real effects of interventions or accuracy of diagnostic tests. As well as collecting clinically important outcomes and those that matter to patients, ascertainment of outcome needs to be within an appropriate time frame and thereby sufficient to evaluate longer-term consequences (see Chapter 6).

Performing quality assessment

Consistency in rating or scores can be assisted by explicit formulation of guidelines, such as a list of robust methods that ensure allocation concealment [13]. Where practical, the independent assessment by two or more people using forms or some other means of recording their decisions and reasons is recommended. Masking of authors' names and other identifying information, is costly and time-consuming and may not be worthwhile [14]. Processes to resolve disagreement should also be stated. If necessary, another person could be enlisted to arbitrate.

While the above shows quality assessment to be a scientifically imprecise process, it remains important to undertake a systematic appraisal of study methods and findings. Indeed, it can be viewed as irresponsible to report on trial findings without any consideration or reporting of the biases that might have affected these. And by a formal process, with pre-specified criteria, the assessment of study quality can provide a more rigorous and objective examination of these biases and enable exploration of their potential effects.

Other potentially important sources of bias not usually featuring in a formal appraisal arise from conflicts of interest.

Conflicts of interest and fraud

Readers and reviewers of medical literature need to be aware of the issues of conflicts of interest and of medical fraud.

Important bias may result from conflicts of interest of trial investigators, authors and sponsors. Conflicts of interest arise in clinical trials where decisions and actions of individuals or organisations are or may be taken for personal or corporate benefit or for similarly inappropriate reasons than the interests of patients. While journals are increasingly requiring disclosure of conflicts of interest, it remains difficult to judge whether a conflict of interest, actual or perceived, affected study design, conduct or reporting. There is, however, empirical evidence of the influence of the drug industry on the research agenda (such as choice of inappropriate comparators) and research findings (such as selective publication and reporting of results favourable to company interests) [15,16].

A conflict of interest can lead to medical fraud where there is deliberate misrepresentation of the results of research. Fraud may even entail fabrication of data [17]. Other types of fraud are selective publication, such as multiple publications without cross references or active suppression of reports of unfavourable results, and selective reporting which comprises such activities as the intentional omission of data on adverse outcomes and deliberately ignoring intention-to-treat analysis and presenting the more favourable "per protocol" analyses only [16].

The implementation of reporting standards and the full pre-registration of trials should help not only the critical appraisal of trial methods but also to ensure "fair conduct and reporting" of clinical trials [18].

Reporting standards

Various initiatives have taken place to raise and set the standards of reporting of different types of studies. The CONSORT statement (www.consort-statement.org), endorsed by a growing number of medical journals, provides a detailed breakdown of the essential information required in reports of randomised controlled trials [1,19]. A recent update augmented the guidance for reporting harms-related data [20]. Other statements include those for reporting diagnostic studies [21], non-randomised evaluations [22] and reviews [23].

Clinical trial registration

The requirement to publicly register clinical trials before patient recruitment is gaining momentum [24]. Registration together with the mandatory completion of a "minimal registration data set" should help to avoid selective reporting of trials and trial results [25]. For example, prior identification of primary outcomes may avert outcome reporting bias where other outcomes, more often those attaining statistical significance, are reported [26].

Presentation of study details

The format and content of text and tables presenting the details of studies included in literature reviews and other work depend on the aims, destination and readership of the intended report. A proven format is the presentation of text summaries of the characteristics of the included studies and tabulation of the details of individual studies. Compilation of the table(s) of study characteristics is facilitated by a data extraction form designed with the table in mind. Once complete, the table(s) will help the preparation of the text summaries. Extensive duplication between text and tables should be avoided.

Desirable properties of the table(s) are:
• Consistent and systematic presentation of key information.
• Compatible with review protocol and transparent processes (e.g. mention of key unpublished information received from trial investigators).
• Concise provision of sufficient details, pertinent to the review, that avoids the reader needing, within reason, to consult the original reports or reference books (e.g. abbreviations and acronyms should be defined, preferably in the table footnotes).
• Clear and neat structure and format.

The structure of the "Characteristics of included studies" table of Cochrane (intervention) reviews allows an effective presentation of the key details of individual studies (see Table 5.1). Readers should note that though the location of information is similar in most Cochrane reviews, there is generally acceptable variation in the inclusion and display of study details. Study details tables in systematic reviews in other publications are similar though these often present trial results.

The corresponding table for Cochrane reviews of diagnostic tests is still under development at time of writing. Such a table would probably present concise descriptions of the study design (type of study including whether retrospective or prospective and whether consecutive recruitment, blinding of test interpreters, loss to follow-up or other exclusions, etc.), the study population (sample size and basic characteristics, presenting conditions, eligibility criteria, clinical setting, referral routes, etc.), the index test(s) and comparator or reference test(s), the sequence and

Table 5.1. Structure of and comments on the "Characteristics of included studies" in Cochrane (intervention) reviews

Study identity
This is the unique identifier for the study, often comprising the surname of the first author and the year of publication of the main report.

Methods
Key aspects – typically including the method of randomisation, blinding and intention-to-treat analysis – of study design and conduct are described. Particular aspects of study designs such as for cross-over trials or where the unit of randomisation is not individual patients (such as randomisation of fingers or different limbs, or of groups of people as in "cluster" randomised trials) should also be stated. Quality assessment results or scores may be presented here or in a separate table.

Participants
The overall number of study participants (importantly, the actual number of people randomised) and their basic characteristics (e.g. sex, age, ASA* score, reason for and type of operation, important comorbidities) relevant to the review question. Limited descriptive statistics (e.g. percentage males, mean age and age range) can aid the reader's understanding of the study population.
    Concise account of study inclusion and exclusion criteria.
    The number of participants included in the trial analyses or lost to/available at follow-up may be listed here or, sometimes, in the preceding section.
    Brief details of setting or context (primarily country and trial timing) are recommended.

Interventions
The interventions, and their mode of delivery, should be described sufficiently. Thus for trials of pharmaceutical agents, route of delivery, doses, timing and duration should be recorded. For trials of anaesthetic techniques and strategies, information on who delivered the intervention(s) and setting(s) are often pertinent. Where possible, details of "usual" or "standard" care or what was given to the control group should be provided.
    Details of co-interventions and other aspects of care provided to all treatment groups (e.g. use of antithrombotic agents, sedation) and timing. In a review of "Early extubation for adult cardiac surgical patients", separate tables detailed premedication, induction and maintenance [27].
    Generic drug names (e.g. adrenaline) should be listed instead of or as well as reported drug names.

Outcomes
A list of the reported outcome measures, preferably structured in accordance with the categorisation of outcomes (such as primary and secondary outcomes) given in the protocol and results. Consideration should be given to the explicit documentation of the non-availability of key outcomes, such as adverse effects, and conversely to the minimal reporting of the surrogate or intermediate outcomes (e.g. partial oxygen pressure data, pH values): see Chapter 6.
    A statement of the overall length of follow-up and interim follow-up times, should the main outcome data collection apply to these, is recommended.

(Continued)

Table 5.1. (Continued)

Presentation of further details of the actual measures used should be considered where there is scope for ambiguity: for instance, the scale and direction of VAS[†]-based outcome measures.

Notes
Pertinent information could be whether the study was reported only in a conference abstract; translation obtained of a non-English publication; and important information obtained from trial authors.

Allocation concealment (code)
This specific feature of Cochrane reviews stresses the pivotal role of allocation concealment in the prevention of bias.

---

[*]ASA: American Society of Anesthesiologists' physical status classification; [†]VAS: visual analogue scale.

timing of testing, diagnostic criteria, the methods of test interpretation and any recording of adverse effects. Description of the target condition(s) and reference standard(s) may feature also.

Overall summaries in the text of the studies and study populations will generally draw from the information provided in the study details table(s). Separate sections on "Description" and "Methodological quality" form the preliminary results sections in Cochrane reviews. For multiple comparison reviews, the first section usually presents a breakdown of the trials by comparison as further presented in the main results section. Essentially, the main role of these summaries is to provide information that will inform on the availability, quantity, validity and applicability of the evidence for the review topic.

Summary

The critical appraisal of studies and the succinct presentation of study details are essential components of evidence-based anaesthesia. Both assist the interpretation of the evidence from studies in terms of its validity and, if valid, its applicability.

The formal assessment of study quality should include items that reflect key biases and potential sources of bias, such as the selection bias shown to be associated with failure to conceal allocation before assignment of interventions in randomised controlled trials. Other items may reflect aspects that are likely to have a major impact on the relevance and applicability of study findings.

These considerations also apply to the presentation of study characteristics. A consistent approach using pre-specified methods aiming at objectivity and repeatability is similarly required.

People should not lose sight of the underlying aim of the systematic review process – to identify, assess and summarise the available evidence using systematic, objective and transparent methods in order to inform, where possible, choices in clinical practice.

REFERENCES

1 Moher D, Schulz KF, Altman DG, for the CONSORT group. The CONSORT statement: revised recommendations for improving the quality of reports of parallel-group randomised trials. *Lancet* 2001; 357: 1191–4.

2 Kunz R, Vist G, Oxman AD. Randomisation to protect against selection bias in healthcare trials. *The Cochrane Database of Methodology Reviews* 2002, Issue 4. Art. No.: MR00012. DOI: 10.1002/14651858.

3 Young C, Horton R. Putting clinical trials into context. *Lancet* 2005; 366: 107–8.

4 Whiting P, Rutjes AWS, Reitsma JB, Glas AS, Bossuyt PMM, Kleijnen J. Sources of variation and bias in studies of diagnostic accuracy: a systematic review. *Ann Intern Med* 2004; 140(3): 189–202.

5 Katrak P, Bialocerkowski AE, Massy-Westrop N, Kumar VSS, Grimmer KA. A systematic review of the content of critical appraisal tools. *BMC Med Res Methodol* 2004; 4(22).

6 Schulz KF, Chalmers I, Hayes RJ, Altman DG. Empirical evidence of bias. Dimensions of methodological quality associated with estimates of treatment effects in controlled trials. *JAMA* 1995; 273(5): 408–12.

7 Schultz KF, Grimes DA. Blinding in randomised trials: hiding who got what. *Lancet* 2004; 359: 696–700.

8 Verhagen AP, de Vet HCW, de Bie RA, Kessons AGH, Boers M, Bouter LM et al. The Delphi list: a criteria list for quality assessment of randomised clinical trials for conducting systematic reviews developed by Delphi consensus. *J Clin Epidemiol* 1998; 51(12): 1235–41.

9 Whiting P, Rutjes AWS, Reitsma JB, Bossuyt PMM, Kleijnen J. The development of QUADAS: a tool for the quality assessment of studies of diagnostic accuracy included in systematic reviews. *BMC Med Res Methodol* 2003; 3(25).

10 Juni P, Witschi A, Bloch R, Egger M. The hazards of scoring the quality of clinical trials for meta-analysis. *JAMA* 1999; 282(11): 1054–60.

11 Berlin JA, Rennie D. Measuring the quality of trials. The quality of quality scales. *JAMA* 1999; 282(11): 1083–5.

12 Jadad AR, Moore RA, Carroll D, Jenkinson C, Reynolds DJM, Gavaghan DJ et al. Assessing the quality of reports of randomized clinical trials: is blinding necessary? *Control Clin Trial* 1996; 17(1): 1–12.

13 Schultz KF, Grimes DA. Allocation concealment in randomised trials: defending against deciphering. *Lancet* 2004; 359: 614–8.

14 Berlin JA. Does blinding of readers affect the results of meta-analyses? *Lancet* 1997; 350: 185–6.

15 Lexchin J, Bero LA, Djulbegovic B, Clark O. Pharmaceutical industry sponsorship and research outcome and quality: systematic review. *BMJ* 2005; 326: 1167–70.

16 Melander H, Ahlqvist-Rastad J, Meijer G, Beermann B. Evidence b(i)ased medicine – selective reporting from studies sponsored by pharmaceutical industry: review of studies in new applications. *BMJ* 2003; 326: 1171–3.

17 Miller RD. The place of research and the role of academic anaesthetists in anaesthetic departments. *Best Prac Res Clin Anaesthesiol* 2005; 16(3): 353–70.

18 Rennie D. Fair conduct and fair reporting of clinical trials. *JAMA* 1999; 282(18): 1766–8.

19 Altman DG, Schulz KF, Moher D, Egger M, Davidoff F, Elborne D et al. The revised CONSORT statement for reporting randomized trials: explanation and elaboration. *Ann Intern Med* 2001; 134(8): 663–94.

20 Ioannidis JPA, Evans SJW, Gotzsche PC, O'Neill RT, Altman DG, Schulz K et al. Better reporting of harms in randomized trials: an extension of the CONSORT statement. *Ann Intern Med* 2004; 141(10): 781–8.

21 Bossuyt PM, Reitsma JB, Bruns DE, Gatsonis CA, Glasziou P, Irwig L et al. The STARD statement for reporting studies of diagnostic accuracy: explanation and elaboration. *Ann Intern Med* 2003; 138(1): W1–W12.

22 Des Jarlais DC, Lyles C, Crepaz N, and the TREND Group. Improving the reporting quality of nonrandomized evaluations of behavioral and public health interventions: The TREND statement. *Am J Public Health* 2004; 94(3): 361–6.

23 Moher D, Cook DJ, Eastwood S, Olkin I, Rennie D, Stroup DF et al. Improving the quality of reports of meta-analyses of randomised controlled trials: the QUOROM statement. *Lancet* 1999; 354: 1896–1900.

24 De Angelis C, Drazen JM, Frizelle FA, Haug C, Hoey J, Horton R et al. Clinical trial registration: a statement from the International Committee of Medical Journal Editors. *Lancet* 2004; 364: 911–2.

25 De Angelis CD, Drazen JM, Frizelle FA, Haug C, Hoey J, Horton R et al. Is this clinical trial fully registered? A statement from the Internal Committee of Medical Journal Editors. *Lancet* 2005; 365: 1829.

26 Chan A-W, Hrobjartsson A, Haabr MT, Gotzsche PC, Altman DG. Empirical evidence for selective reporting of outcomes in randomized trials. Comparison of protocols to published articles. *JAMA* 2004; 291(20): 2457–65.

27 Hawkes CA, Dhileepan S, Foxcroft D. Early extubation for adult cardiac surgical patients. *The Cochrane Database of Systematic Reviews* 2003, Issue 4. Art. No.: CD0003587. DOI: 10.1002/14651858.

6

Outcomes

Ann Møller

The Cochrane Anaesthesia Review Group, Department of Anaesthesiology, Herlev University Hospital, Herlev, Denmark

When making decisions in health care all relevant outcomes should be considered. Clinically relevant outcomes are patient orientated, and measure directly how a patient feels, functions or survives. Examples of clinically relevant outcomes in anaesthesia could be mortality, postoperative morbidity, postoperative nausea and vomiting (PONV) and postoperative pain. Other relevant outcomes relate to length of stay in hospital, intensive care admittance, quality of life measures, and costs.

Different types of trials measure different types of outcomes, and trial quality is an equally important factor in estimating treatment effectivity. Surrogate outcomes are sometimes used instead of the real outcome in question, because they save time, money and number of patients. Surrogate outcomes are, however, not very reliable and extreme care should be taken if a surrogate outcome measure is used as the base of clinical decisions.

Introduction

When we consider the implementation of an intervention in health care practice, we want to know how this affects our patients. The randomised controlled trial measures the effects of the intervention in question on the outcomes decided by the investigators. The optimal clinical trial explores the effects of a well-described, well-defined, clinically relevant intervention on all relevant outcomes, including benefits and harms, costs and ease of practice. However, this ideal situation is rarely the case. When a systematic review is being prepared, it is often revealed that very few studies have patient relevant outcomes, often outcomes are poorly defined and studies evaluating costs and ease of practice are very rare.

This chapter will describe types of outcome data, deal with evaluation of outcome data, and explain the difficulties with the use of surrogate outcomes.

Key words: Outcome measure, endpoint, surrogate outcome measures, randomised controlled trial, clinical relevance, POEMs.

Clinically relevant outcomes

A clinically relevant outcome measures directly how a patient feels, functions or survives [1]. Clinically relevant outcomes are generally subject to direct patient interest; those are endpoints that patients will often ask about. (Will I survive this operation, doctor?) Typical clinically relevant outcomes in the field of anaesthesia could be perioperative mortality, major postoperative complications such as respiratory failure, myocardial infarction, infections and surgical complications needing secondary surgery. Postoperative pain and PONV would also be considered clinically relevant outcomes.

Some other outcomes may be of relevance to patients as well as the health care staff. Length of stay in postoperative care unit (PACU), intensive care unit (ICU) or in hospital may be very relevant for patients, staff and hospital administrators.

Another relevant outcome could be "ease of practice". When different interventions are compared, one can be much easier to perform than the other. This could be exemplified in trials comparing different types of nerve blocks, catheter insertion, etc., but it could also be of direct relevance to patients (as one drug administration per day compared to four). Whenever relevant, this outcome should be included in trials.

Whether costs should be considered a relevant outcome has been discussed a lot. In countries, where patients have to pay for their treatments, this is definitely a patient relevant outcome. In countries, where health care is free, this may not be of direct relevance for patients, but it certainly is relevant for hospital administrators, and should be included when weighing the pros and cons at specific treatment.

Patient satisfaction

Patient satisfaction can be measured in multiple ways and results can be surprising. Nevertheless, the success of an intervention is dependent upon how the patients feel and think about it. So patient satisfaction measures will always be relevant in clinical trials [2,3].

Other considerations

Outcomes can be positive or negative. Mortality is negative and survival is positive. A postoperative complication is a negative outcome and a patient case with no complication is positive. Tradition tells us to count the "bad happenings" – but it could be argued, that the number of successful patient cases could be just as good a measure.

Rare outcomes, such as death during anaesthesia or other rare complications are difficult, or even impossible to deal with in randomised controlled trial – even in non-randomised clinically controlled trials it might be difficult to get enough of the rare outcomes to show a difference or relationship. These types of outcomes are best described in large cohort studies:

At its most extreme, the intervention might improve one aspect of the disease – level of symptoms or patient satisfaction – while other aspects deteriorate – leading to serious complications or even death.

Outcomes exemplified

Mortality

As a dichotomous outcome and the most final endpoint of all, mortality is often considered the hard outcome of all. This is true indeed. Fortunately, however, mortality is rare in anaesthesia trials, and trials will have to be extensive to show a difference in mortality. Nevertheless, mortality should most often be included as an outcome of trials and systematic reviews.

Morbidity

Examples of morbidity related outcomes in anaesthesia will be the common post-operative complications, such as respiratory failure, myocardial infarction, infections, wound complications, etc. In some cases more rare outcomes may be relevant, most often such that are directly related to the surgical procedure in question or the type of anaesthesia (as the incidence of post-spinal headache after spinal anaesthesia). All of these examples are also dichotomous – meaning that they are either there or they are not.

Other anaesthesia related clinical outcomes

Examples of continuous outcomes related to anaesthesia are PONV, postoperative pain, postoperative cognitive dysfunction and quality of life measures. These can all be measured on a continuous scale and require specific statistical handling (see Chapter 7).

Other relevant outcomes

Other relevant outcomes that are not directly clinically relevant are related to duration of stay in hospital or in ICU, re-admissions to hospital, emergency visits and related to costs; cost per patient per day or cost per episode of care.

Of relevance to the clinician are outcomes like ease of practice, time consumption, etc.

POEMs

POEMs is short for Patient Oriented Evidence that Matters, and was first described by Shaughnessy et al. in 1994 in *The Journal of Family Practice* [4]. The concept of POEMs has mostly been used in journals and articles about general practice, but the idea can be transformed to other specialities as well. The major idea is that articles about primary care topics that measure patient oriented outcomes (morbidity, mortality and quality of life) should change practice, if the reported results are valid.

Types of trials

The randomised controlled trial

The randomised controlled trial focuses on the intervention, and the effect of the intervention on the chosen outcomes. The process of randomisation has the purpose of keeping all other factors than the intervention equally distributed between the groups, trying to isolate the effect of the intervention. In other words, the baseline risk is the same in the two groups. The intervention, however, may affect more than one outcome. For example brain surgery for epilepsy may improve the symptoms of epilepsy in some patients, but cause loss of vision in some patients as well. Mortality may be different between the groups. The costs are definitely not the same and quality of life may be affected. When deciding to perform an operation, the clinician will have to consider all the relevant outcomes. It can be a good idea to produce a list of benefits and harms, or pros and cons.

This is true for most clinical interventions. The randomised trial is about effect of intervention and does not explain why or how an intervention is working, or why it is not.

The cohort study (epidemiological research/regression analysis)

The regression analysis or multivariate analysis is about relations. The typical analysis starts with the outcome, mortality for example. A number of factors the investigators think may be of importance are chosen, and the relations analysed. The results will show whether there is a statistic correlation between the outcome and the factor in question. The multivariate analysis "cleans" away the influence the factor may have on each other. It is very important to stress that though this type of research is about relations it does not show cause relationship. The major use of these studies is in the generation of hypotheses. A cohort study may show that patients with 80% oxygen during surgery have fewer infections than those with a lower oxygen percent. However, a randomised trial will be needed to see if raising the oxygen content to 80% will change the infection risk.

Qualitative research

Qualitative research is very different from the traditional quantitative research in more than one way. In qualitative research there is no numbers or calculation. The methodology is, however, a very useful supplement to the quantitative trials. The qualitative research is very much about "how" and "why", and gives us information on why patients prefer one intervention to the other, how they feel about what is being done to them, and eventually what they would like to change. In this type of research the individuals being researched give us their ideas of what they consider relative outcomes to be.

Outcome related bias

Different types of bias are related to outcomes in clinical trials:

1 *Outcome bias*: Outcome bias occurs when there is a selective reporting of positive outcomes in a trial. The example is that a multitude of outcomes has been measured, and at the end of the trial, the investigators choose to report only the outcomes that showed significance. This is extremely common, especially in trials with many physiological measurements (surrogates). This type of bias is overcome by strict adherence to the protocol, and favourably publishing the protocol prior to the trial performance.

2 *Detection bias*: This type of bias occurs when the outcome assessors hope for a specific result of the trial or have strong beliefs that the intervention either works or does not work. This type of bias is best overcome by having blinded outcome assessors with no relation to the trial performance.

Surrogate outcome

A surrogate endpoint can be defined as a laboratory or physiologic measurement used as a substitute for an endpoint that measures directly how a patient feels, functions, or survives. Surrogate endpoints have several drawbacks. Firstly, a change in the surrogate endpoints does not itself answer the essential questions: What is the objective of treatment in this patient? Secondly, the surrogate endpoint may not closely reflect the treatment target. Thirdly, the use of a surrogate endpoint has the same limitations as the use of any other single measure of the success or failure of treatment – it ignores all the other measures. Reliance on a single surrogate endpoint as a measure of therapeutic success or intervention success usually reflects a narrow or naïve clinical perspective [5]. When flipping through a variety of anaesthesia journals one will find surprisingly many articles, which measures only surrogates [6].

So why would investigators continue to perform trials that measure only surrogates, such as blood pressure, cardiac output, central venous pressure or a variety of laboratory findings?

The reasons are many. These trials are much easier to perform. Patients can be included, anaesthetised, outcome measured within one day and at a minimal cost and effort – even during the performance of daily clinical work. Being an anaesthetist makes you familiar with the registration and interpretation of various clinical signs. But beware. What is a great help in keeping the anaesthetised patient stable and safe may well mislead you, if new interventions should rely on trials with just one, or a few clinical signs as outcomes.

In order to rely on a surrogate outcome as a substitute for the true outcome in question, there has to be a very strong correlation between the surrogate and the real outcomes. And this correlation has to go both ways. That is the surrogate should be present in all patients with the true outcome, and all the patients in whom the surrogate is present should suffer (or obtain) the true outcome. This is only very rarely the case – and in many instances, the relation between the surrogate and the true outcome has not been investigated [7].

Trials with surrogate outcomes should be considered preliminary or hypothesis generating and should never be the basis of a clinical decision, let alone the

Examples of former trials with surrogate outcomes
- Bone density was used as a measure of bone strength and fracture rate in osteoporotic women in trials investigating the effect of fluoride on the fracture rate. In 1990 Riggs demonstrated that even fluoride increased bone density, the fracture rate and increased skeletal fragility [8].
- Ventricular ectopy is associated with sudden cardiac death. Encainide and flecainide effectively reduce ventricular ectopy and were used for years in order to prevent cardiac death in patients with ventricular ectopy. In 1991 Echt et al. demonstrated that there was an excess of deaths due to arrhythmia and deaths due to shock after acute recurrent myocardial infarction in patients treated with encainide or flecainide [9].

Practice points
1 A clinically relevant outcome measures directly how a patient feels, functions or survives. A trial or systematic review should try to include all clinical relevant outcomes.
2 Trial design depends on the type of outcome in question. Typical trial types are randomised controlled trial, cohort study and qualitative trials.
3 A surrogate endpoint can be defined as a laboratory or physiologic measurement used as a substitute for an endpoint that measures directly how a patient feels, functions or survives. Trials with surrogate outcomes must be considered preliminary and results taken with extreme care.
4 Large, definitive trials with clinically relevant outcomes should always be performed before new interventions are accepted.

implementation of new interventions. Large, definitive trials with clinically relevant outcomes should always be performed before new interventions are accepted.

Conclusions

In conclusion, the major purpose of clinical trials is to support decision-makers in health care with reliable documentation of high scientific and methodological quality. In order to do so the trial must be large enough, well performed and address all clinical relevant outcomes as well as other relevant outcomes.

REFERENCES

1 Temple RJ. *Clinical Measurement in Drug Evaluation*. New York: J Wiley, 1995.

2 Heidegger T, Nuebling M, Husemann Y. Consistency in anaesthetic care – Patients' attitudes matter. *BMJ* 2003; 327(7420): 931.

3 Heidegger T, Nuebling MI, Germann R, Borg H, Fluckiger K, Coi T et al. Patient satisfaction with anesthesia care: information alone does not lead to improvement. *Can J Anaesth* 2004; 51(8): 801–5.

4 Ebell MH, Barry HC, Slawson DC, Shaughnessy AF. Finding POEMs in the medical literature. *J Fam Pract* 1999; 48(5): 350–5.

5 Greenhalgh T. *How to Read a Paper. The Basics of Evidence Based Medicine*, London: *BMJ Books*. 2nd edition. 2003.

6 Lauritsen J, Moller AM. Publications in anesthesia journals: Quality and clinical relevance. *Anesth Analg* 2004; 99(5): 1486–91.

7 Gotzsche PC, Liberati A, Torri V, Rossetti L. Beware of surrogate outcome measures. *Int J Technol Assess Health Care* 1996; 12(2): 238–46.

8 Riggs BL, Hodgson SF, Ofallon WM, Chao EYS, Wahner HW, Muhs JM et al. Effect of Fluoride Treatment on the Fracture Rate in Postmenopausal Women with Osteoporosis. *New England Journal of Medicine* 1990; 322(12): 802–9.

9 Echt DS, Liebson PR, Mitchell LB, Peters RW, Obiasmanno D, Barker AH et al. Mortality and Morbidity in Patients Receiving Encainide, Flecainide, Or Placebo – Cardiac-Arrhythmia Supression Trial. *New England Journal of Medicine* 1991; 324(12): 781–8.

7

The meta-analysis of a systematic review

Nathan Pace

Department of Anesthesiology, University of Utah, Salt Lake City, Utah, USA

Meta-analysis (MA) uses numerical tools to synthesise effect measures from the data discovered in the literature search of randomised controlled trials (RCTs) for a systematic review (SR). An effect measure is a single number that contrasts the results of two different treatments. Commonly used effect measures for binary data are the risk ratio (RR) or the odds ratio (OR); the one or the other is calculated for each included study. Statistical methods for an MA are straightforward. A summary effect measure for data from all included studies is the desired output of the MA and is displayed in a forest plot. It is critically important to minimise bias in estimating this value. Techniques in MA to identify and/or minimise bias include the funnel plot, the exploration of clinical and statistical heterogeneity and the use of sensitivity analysis.

Introduction

Suppose that an anaesthesiologist reads an SR of most improbable research studies comparing cyclopropane versus diethyl ether general anaesthesia for aortic valve surgery. The conclusion offered is that the cyclopropane is favoured because the summary RR for mortality is 0.6 (95% confidence interval (CI) 0.45 to 0.8) with an I^2 statistic of 80%. From whence did these numbers appear? What do they mean?

A fundamental distinction must be drawn between an SR and an MA. Most commonly an SR is the result of a predetermined and orderly process for retrieving previously published RCTs comparing outcomes from two treatments for a specific disease or clinical problem. After the retrieval of these publications, the characteristics and results of each study are extracted and entered into a database. What has been done and reported – the discovered clinical trials – might vary considerably from the best methods of clinical trial methodology for studying an intervention under all relevant circumstances. While each study used in an SR is an RCT, an SR is observational research; the literature search of an SR can only discover what has been done and reported. Methods for a mathematical synthesis of the observed

Key words: Bias, clinical heterogeneity, effect measures, forest plot, quality assessment, RR, OR, sensitivity analysis, statistical heterogeneity.

results have been developed; these methods are known as MA. It is possible, but not mandatory, that an MA be performed to calculate from the results of all studies a single summary estimate of treatment effect.

SR data: study characteristics

The characteristics to be extracted from the report of a study include the nature of the participants, the specifics of the interventions, the types of outcomes reported, and the details of experimental design and study methods. These characteristics are the determinants of including or excluding a study in an SR. The nature of the participants include demographics and diseases; for example, if an SR is oriented to anaesthesia for children, then the maximum age of patients in each study should exclude adults. In a study of postoperative pain management, an example of the specifics of the interventions might be the pharmaceutical agents (fentanyl versus morphine), the routes of administration (oral versus intravenous), the protocol for administration (time contingent versus on-demand), the doses, etc. The outcomes could be mortality, morbidity (myocardial infarction, postoperative vomiting, neurological complications, etc.), and variables reflecting the process of anaesthetic care (time to awakening postoperatively, hospital charges, pain scores, etc.). For each SR, outcomes are specified as primary or secondary; if a study meets all other inclusion criteria, but does not report any designated primary or secondary outcomes, it will be excluded from the SR. Besides using the nature of the participants, the specifics of the interventions, and the types of outcomes reported to include or exclude studies within an SR, these characteristics may prove useful later in the MA for performing sub-group analyses.

The MA of an SR should be conducted to minimise bias – bias being any deviation of the results from the true state of nature. The history and development of clinical trials in medicine has prompted statisticians to discover multiple flaws in study design that allow or promote bias. The sources of bias in clinical trials have been labelled:

1 *Selection bias*: systematic differences between the patients receiving each treatment.
2 *Performance bias*: systematic differences in care being given to study patients other than the preplanned treatments being evaluated.
3 *Attrition bias*: systematic differences in the withdrawal of patients from each of the two treatment groups.
4 *Detection bias*: systematic differences in the ascertainment and recording of the outcomes.

There are extensive lists of various specific examples of bias within these four broad categories. At present the main focus of bias detection in an SR is to grade studies by: (1) the randomisation process for allocation of patients to treatment groups; (2) the concealment of the allocation process from the patients and the study recruiters; (3) the blinding (masking) of patients, physicians, nurses, and outcome assessors concerning the assigned treatment; and (4) the analysis of results from patients dropped from the study. A part of MA is to test the sensitivity of the summary estimate of treatment effect according to the biases present in the studies included in the SR by asking the question: "Do the results differ between studies with and without evidence of bias"? [1] This is known as sensitivity analysis.

Sub-group analyses are another aspect of an MA. Suppose that a substantial literature exists comparing two antiemetics for prevention of postoperative emesis. In some studies the investigators included only teenagers while in other studies all patients were octogenarians. If all studies used good experimental methods, then there is no bias in their results. However, it may be more meaningful to combine separately studies of teenagers and studies of octogenarians. This is sub-group analysis [2].

SR data: observed study outcomes

Anaesthesia research studies report the data of things that vary – the variables, for example blood pressure, age, sex, ASA physical status score, etc. Readers of medical research have become familiar with the importance of properly categorising the types of data before undertaking an analysis. Broadly speaking, data is either categorical or quantitative. Categorical data types include binary variables (yes/no, sometimes denoted dichotomous; e.g. mortality), ordinal variables (an ordered outcome; e.g. maximal dermatomal level of spinal anaesthesia), and nominal variables (categories not allowing ranking: e.g. ethnicity, eye colour, etc.). Quantitative data is most commonly called a continuous variable, such as height, heart rate, plasma propofol concentration, etc. Quantitative data also includes counts (the number of episodes of nausea) and time-to-event (days of life following surgery). While there appears to be a similarity between an ordinal variable such as Mallampati score and a continuous variable such as mean pulmonary artery pressure, strictly speaking an ordinal variable is only defined at previously specified levels (Mallampati score: 1, 2, 3, or 4) while mean pulmonary artery pressure can be measured to an arbitrarily chosen precision.

Because an SR is always focused on comparing two treatments, the study outcomes are stored in specialised tables such as Table 7.1 that shows binary outcomes from an SR published in *The Cochrane Library* [3]. Binary outcomes are usually of greater interest than are continuous variables in an SR.

The table headers precisely identify the comparison treatments and the exact outcome being collected; the outcome for binary data can be either an adverse or a beneficial event. The first column indicates the last name of the lead author and the year of publication of the included study. It is also possible to include sub-categories; in Table 7.1, there are 14 studies of a new treatment versus 1 of 4 different other treatments – here denoted A (7 studies), B (3 studies), C (4 studies), and

Table 7.1. Typical SR data. The data in this table are taken from Ref. [3]. The first column indicates the last name of the lead author and the year of publication of the included study as cited by Zaric et al.

Comparison: Lidocaine versus other local anaesthetics

Outcome: Transient neurologic symptoms (adverse event)

Study	Lidocaine		Other local anaesthetic	
	Events (rate %)	Sample size	Events (rate %)	Sample size
Sub-category A (lidocaine versus bupivacaine)				
Hampl (1995)	9 (32)	28 *	0 (0)	16
Pollock (1996)	16 (15)	107 *	0 (0)	52
Hampl (1998)	4 (27)	15 *	0 (0)	30
Salmela (1998)	3 (20)	15 *	0 (0)	30
Keld (2000)	9 (26)	35 *	1 (3)	35
Aouad (2001)	0 (0)	100	0 (0)	100
Philip (2001)	1 (3)	30	2 (7)	28 *
Sub-category B (lidocaine versus mepivacaine)				
Salmela (1998)	3 (20)	15	11 (37)	30 *
Liguori (1998)	6 (22)	27 *	0 (0)	30
Salazar (2001)	1 (3)	40	3 (8)	40 *
Sub-category C (lidocaine versus prilocaine)				
Hampl (1998)	5 (33)	15 *	1 (3)	30
Martinez-Bourio (1998)	4 (4)	98 *	1 (1)	102
de Weert (2000)	7 (20)	35 *	0 (0)	35
Østgaard (2000)	7 (14)	49 *	2 (4)	50
Sub-category D (lidocaine versus procaine)				
Hodgson (2000)	11 (31)	35 *	2 (6)	35
Le Truong (2001)	8 (27)	30 *	0 (0)	30

* Treatment with higher event rate.

D (2 studies). Some studies have more than two treatments relevant to the SR. In such cases it may be appropriate to subdivide data of a study into two or more sub-categories (Salmela, 1998: sub-category A and B; Hampl, 1998: sub-category A and C). The table displays the number of events, the number of patients (sample size) and the event rate. It is easy to identify the studies showing higher rate of adverse events for the new treatment (e.g. Hampl, 1995: 32% versus 0%) and the other treatment (e.g. Philip, 2001: 3% versus 7%). Similar tables are used for quantitative data. The "Other Treatments" group might well be those receiving a placebo or standard active treatment.

Effect measures

Two contrasting statistical approaches to reporting outcomes must be appreciated to understand an MA. Most journal articles comparing two treatments perform hypothesis testing. A null hypothesis of no difference is created and the observed sample values are used to calculate a test statistic; if the value of the test statistic is sufficiently improbable, the null hypothesis is rejected and the alternative hypothesis is accepted. For example, Keld, 2000 (Table 7.1) has event rates of 26% (9 events in 35 patients) versus 3% (1 event in 35 patients) for the lidocaine versus bupivacaine. Typically, a Pearson chi squaned test would be calculated to test the null hypothesis that the two treatments and the adverse event rates are independent. For Keld, 2000, the test statistic (Pearson chi squared) has a value of 7.5 with one degree of freedom; the associated probability value being less than 0.01, the null hypothesis of independence would be rejected. The alternative hypothesis that there is a relationship between treatment and adverse events would be accepted; this would conform to an intuitive appreciation that a rate of 26% is much more than a rate of 3%.

In an MA, the statistical approach is known as parameter estimation. A parameter is an unknown number that characterises a population; parameters cannot be measured, but are estimated from sample values. In an MA, the sample values of outcomes from the two treatment groups are combined to create an effect size for each study. This is done whether or not the original publication included a calculation of effect size. The effect size is a single numerical estimate that contrasts the effects of the two treatments. Four types of effect sizes are in common use for binary outcomes; all express the outcome in one group relative to the outcome in the other group (Box 7.1).

Risk is a frequently used term in medicine; it is the probability of an outcome – a number between 0 and 1. If the risk is 0.1, then for every 100 patients the event occurs in 10 patients. Odds is a concept from gambling, but is used also in medicine. If there are 10 patients with an event and 90 without an event, the odds are 1 to 9 (written as the ratio 1:9 or as the decimal fraction 0.111…). Risk and odds are mathematically convertible:

$$\text{risk} = \frac{\text{odds}}{1 + \text{odds}} \; ; \; \text{odds} = \frac{\text{risk}}{1 - \text{risk}}.$$

Risk and odds for the two treatment groups may be combined in four ways.

The RR describes the multiplication of risk that occurs with the use of the new treatment whereas the OR describes the multiplication of odds that occurs with the use of the new treatment. The RR is more easily understood than the OR. In Keld, 2000, patients in the new treatment group were nine times more likely to experience an adverse event (Box 7.2; RR = 9.00 (1.20, 67.31)); this was statistically significant since the 95% CI did not span 1.00. It is apparent that the RR must be interpreted in light of the event rate in the group receiving the standard or placebo treatment. An RR of 2 is possible with a risk pair of 0.30 and 0.15 and a risk pair of 0.04 and 0.02.

Box 7.1. Methods for calculation of binary effect measures

These formulas are used by the software RevMan version 4.2.8.

The data from a study can be redisplayed as a 2 by 2 table:

	Count of events	Count of non-events	Total counts
New treatment	a	b	$a + b$
Other treatment	c	d	$c + d$

where a, b, c, and d are the count of patients with each outcome.

Four treatment effects can be calculated:

$$RR = \frac{a/(a + b)}{c/(c + d)};$$

$$OR = \frac{ad}{bc};$$

$$RD = \frac{a}{a + b} - \frac{c}{c + d}; \text{ and}$$

$$NNT = \frac{(a + b)(c + d)}{a(c + d) - c(a + b)}$$

The RR is the risk of an event in the new treatment group ($a/(a + b)$) divided by the risk of an event in the other treatment group ($c/(c + d)$).

The OR is the odds of an event in the new treatment group (a/b) divided by the odds of an event in the other treatment group (c/d).

The RD is the difference of risks for the two treatment groups.

The NNT is the number of patients receiving the new treatment necessary to produce one more event; it is the inverse of the RD.

The precision of the estimates is given by a 95% CI which is derived from the standard error; the standard error is calculated by common statistical formulas. For example, the

standard error of the log RR is $\sqrt{\dfrac{1}{a} + \dfrac{1}{c} - \dfrac{1}{(a + b)} - \dfrac{1}{(c + d)}}.$

If no events are reported for the treatment groups, then the RR and OR are declared not estimable. Essentially there is no information for creating ratios of outcomes; this is also the case for the calculation of the OR if all patients have an event. For Aouad, 2001 (Table 7.1), 200 patients had no adverse events; the RR and OR cannot be calculated. If there are no events in the control group but events occurred in the new treatment group or vice versa, the calculation of an RR and OR is still possible. By statistical convention, a small value (0.5) is added to all cells of the 2 by 2 table. Thus for Hampl, 1995 (Table 7.1), the RR is 11.14 (0.69, 179.55) and the OR is 16.08 (0.87, 297.61); neither is statistically significant.

An MA should list or display the calculated effect measure for each study. In Table 7.2 the treatment effects and weights have been added. The lack of precision

---

Box 7.2. Calculation of binary effect measures

The data in this box is taken from Ref. [3]. The data from Keld (2000) (Table 7.1) is listed in a 2 by 2 table.

	Count of events	Count of non-events	Total counts
Lidocaine	$a = 9$	$b = 26$	$a + b = 35$
Bupivacaine	$c = 1$	$d = 34$	$c + d = 35$

$$\text{RR} = \frac{a/(a + b)}{c/(c + d)} = \frac{9/35}{1/35} = 9.00.$$

$$\text{OR} = \frac{ad}{bc} = \frac{9 \times 34}{26 \times 1} = 11.77.$$

$$\text{RD} = \frac{a}{a + b} - \frac{c}{c + d} = \frac{9}{35} - \frac{1}{35} = \frac{8}{35} = 0.23.$$

$$\text{NNT} = \frac{(a + b)(c + d)}{a(c + d) - c(a + b)} = \frac{35 \times 35}{9 \times 35 - 1 \times 35} = 4.35.$$

For Keld (2000), RR = 9.00 (1.20, 67.31); OR = 11.77 (1.40, 98.85); RD = 0.23 (0.07, 0.38); NNT = 4.35 (2.63, 14.29). For RR and OR, if the 95% CI does not span 1, the RR and OR are declared to demonstrate a statistically significant treatment effect. For RD, if the 95% CI does not span 0, the RD is declared to demonstrate a statistically significant treatment effect. For Keld (2000), the RR, OR, and RD all show a treatment effect. The interpretation of the NNT is more complicated.

for estimates of RR in small studies is readily apparent. The RR of Hampl, 1995 (Table 7.2) is slightly over 11, but the 95% CI is very broad: from 0.69 to 179.55; this treatment effect would be declared not statistically significant. The overall impression of the 16 RRs (3 studies with RR < 1, 12 studies with RR ≥ 1, 1 study with RR not estimable) in Table 7.2 is for values considerably above 1; however, only 4 studies have RRs with a 95% CI not spanning 1 (sub-category A: Keld, 2000; sub-category C: Hampl, 1998; sub-category D: Hodgson, 2000, Le Truong, 2001).

The risk difference (RD) is always calculable even if no events occur. It is an absolute measure of treatment effect. For Aouad, 2001 (Table 7.2) the RD is 0.00 (−0.02, 0.02). The RD must also be interpreted in light of the typical number of events in the standard treatment group. An RD of 0.02 could be from a study with risks of 0.60 and 0.58, or it could be from a study with risks of 0.03 and 0.01.

Arguments among statisticians persist about the most meaningful effect measure for binary variables. The RR is usually favoured for ease of interpretation, consistency, and mathematical properties [4,5]. The number needed to treat (NNT) may have some utility for summarising the results, but does not have statistical properties necessary for summary and is very vulnerable to misinterpretation

Table 7.2. Typical SR data: individual study effect sizes. The data, weights, and RRs in this table are taken from Ref. [3]. Weights are calculated by a fixed effect model for all studies. RRs and weights are estimated by the software RevMan version 4.2.8

Comparison: Lidocaine versus other local anaesthetics				
Outcome: Transient neurologic symptoms (adverse event)				
Study	Lidocaine	Other	Weight (%)	RR (95% CI)
Sub-category A (lidocaine versus bupivacaine)				
Hampl (1995)	9/28	0/16	2.8	11.14 (0.69, 179.55)
Pollock (1996)	16/107	0/52	3.0	16.19 (0.99, 264.78)
Hampl (1998)	4/15	0/30	1.5	17.44 (1.00, 304.11)
Salmela (1998)	3/15	0/30	1.5	13.56 (0.75, 246.76)
Keld (2000)	9/35	1/35	4.4	9.00 (1.20, 67.31)
Aouad (2001)	0/100	0/100	No weight	Not estimable
Philip (2001)	1/30	2/28	9.2	0.47 (0.04, 4.87)
Sub-category B (lidocaine versus mepivacaine)				
Salmela (1998)	3/15	11/30	32.6	0.55 (0.18, 1.67)
Liguori (1998)	6/27	0/30	2.1	14.39 (0.85, 244.06)
Salazar (2001)	1/40	3/40	13.3	0.33 (0.04, 3.07)
Sub-category C (lidocaine versus prilocaine)				
Hampl (1998)	5/15	1/30	3.0	10.00 (1.28, 78.12)
Martinez-Bourio (1998)	4/98	1/102	4.4	4.16 (0.47, 36.60)
de Weert (2000)	7/35	0/35	2.2	15.00 (0.89, 252.96)
Østgaard (2000)	7/49	2/50	8.8	3.57 (0.78, 16.35)
Sub category D (lidocaine versus procaine)				
Hodgson (2000)	11/35	2/35	8.9	5.50 (1.31, 23.03)
Le Truong (2001)	8/30	0/30	2.2	17.00 (1.03, 281.91)
All (lidocaine versus bupivacaine, mepivacaine, prilocaine, and procaine)				
	94/674	23/673	100.0	

CI: Confidence interval.

because of varying baseline risk [6]. For continuous data such as blood pressure, the effect size is the mean difference – also known as the weighted mean difference (WMD). This is calculated from the mean and standard deviation of each treatment group in a study; a 95% CI of the WMD is also calculated.

Summary effect measures and heterogeneity

MA is a two-stage process. After the estimation of the individual study treatment effects, a summary treatment effect estimate is calculated as a weighted average of the treatment effects of each individual study. Compared to the difficulty of choosing which studies to include in an SR, the statistical methods for the summary treatment effect estimate are well established [7]. In a general form, the equation of the weighted average is:

$$\text{weighted average} = \frac{\text{sum of (estimate} \times \text{weight)}}{\text{sum of weights}} = \frac{\sum T_i W_i}{\sum W_i}.$$

The weights are chosen to reflect the amount of information contained in each study. It must be emphasised that the summary treatment effect estimate is not calculated by simply summing the events and patient counts for all studies (Table 7.2; 94/674 versus 23/673). As a simple example, the weighted average of the integers 4, 7, and 7 is 6, not 5.5. The WMD, RR, OR, and RD all may be used for the calculation of a summary treatment effect estimate. The exact forms of the T_i and W_i depend on the type of treatment effect variable and on the details of the statistical model used to create the summary effect. For example, the W_i may be a function of the number of patients in a study or may be the standard error of the individual study treatment effect. In the presentation of the results of MA, the weights of the individual studies are normalised to a percentage so that the total weight sums to 100%. In Table 7.2, the weights range from a lowest value of 1.5% to a highest value of 32.6%; since Aouad, 2001 does not have an estimable RR, it has no weight at all. With the calculation of the summary treatment effect, a standard error is also calculated. The standard error is then used to compute a z statistic as a statistical test of overall effect and to calculate a 95% CI on the summary treatment effect.

Clinician readers of the medical literature recognise that every study comparing treatments has unique features. Thus, in assembling a pool of studies comparing the same treatments, inevitably there is variability. Any kind of variability among studies in an SR may be termed heterogeneity. There is the clinical diversity of the participants (age, gender, associated illnesses, etc.), the implementation of the interventions (dose, route, associated therapies, etc.) and the measurement of outcomes (hospital mortality, 30 day mortality, etc.); this is described as clinical heterogeneity. There is also variability in trial design and quality (sometimes called methodological heterogeneity).

Concerning the role of heterogeneity, two points of view may be adopted in the statistical calculation of the summary effect; these are called a fixed effect model (FEM) and a random effects model (REM). In the FEM it is believed or assumed that every study has the same true effect of treatment in both magnitude and direction; any observed differences are due solely to chance variation. If the observed variation of treatment effect among studies becomes large, then a different assumption may be chosen. In an REM it is assumed that the various studies are not measuring an identical treatment effect, but rather these are similar, related treatment effects that have a distribution of values (usually assumed to be Gaussian). Heterogeneity (clinical or

Table 7.3. Typical SR Data: summary treatment effect sizes. The weights, RRs, and heterogeneity statistics in this table are taken from Ref. [3]. RRs, weights and heterogeneity statistics are estimated by the software RevMan version 4.2.8

Comparison: Lidocaine versus other local anaesthetics

Outcome: transient neurologic symptoms (adverse event)

	FEM		REM	
	Weight (%)	RR 95% CI	Weight (%)	RR 95% CI
Lidocaine versus bupivacaine ($n = 6$)	22.5	7.60 (3.00, 19.30)	33.8	6.65 (2.05, 21.56)
	Heterogeneity chi squared $= 6.30, df = 5, P = 0.28; I^2 = 20.6\%$.			
Lidocaine versus mepivacaine ($n = 3$)	48.1	1.09 (0.50, 2.38)	22.9	1.05 (0.15, 7.45)
	Heterogeneity chi squared $= 5.78, df = 2, P = 0.06; I^2 = 65.4\%$.			
Lidocaine versus prilocaine ($n = 4$)	18.3	6.14 (2.31, 16.32)	28.5	5.62 (2.07, 15.23)
	Heterogeneity chi squared $= 1.21, df = 3, P = 0.75; I^2 = 0.0\%$.			
Lidocaine versus procaine ($n = 2$)	11.1	7.80 (2.19, 27.77)	14.8	6.94 (1.94, 24.86)
	Heterogeneity chi squared $= 0.52, df = 1, P = 0.47; I^2 = 0.0\%$.			
Lidocaine versus all other local anaesthetics ($n = 15$)	100.0	4.23 (2.71, 6.60)	100.0	4.36 (1.99, 9.56)
	Heterogeneity chi squared $= 28.10, df = 14, P = 0.01; I^2 = 50.2\%$.			

CI: Confidence interval.

methodological) that cannot be explained may be incorporated into the summary effect size by using the REM.

A chi squared test for statistical heterogeneity exists and is usually reported within an MA. In the typical SR this chi squared test lacks power to detect heterogeneity. There is a variation of the chi squared statistic (known as the I^2 statistic) that allows quantification of heterogeneity; this describes the percentage of variability that is due to heterogeneity rather than sampling error [8]. I^2 ranges from 0% to 100%; a value of I^2 greater than 50% is often considered to indicate substantial heterogeneity.

Table 7.3 displays the summary RRs and weights for the four sub-categories of Table 7.1. The summary RRs are different for the two models; for example, in the sub-category lidocaine versus bupivacaine the RR for an FEM is 7.60 and the RR for an REM is 6.65. The difference of the summary RRs between the models is solely due to the difference in weighting; the RR for each study is identical for both models. A main consequence of the REM is to widen the 95% CI. For the sub-category lidocaine versus mepivacaine, the 95% CI has grown from (0.50, 2.38) to (0.15, 7.45) for REM. The I^2 statistic shows that there is substantial statistical heterogeneity for the sub-category lidocaine versus mepivacaine (65.4%) and for the overall summary RR (50.2%).

Managing heterogeneity

What should be done if there is substantial statistical, clinical and/or methodological heterogeneity? Of course simple errors in data extraction and data entry must be excluded. A change to a different effect measure may reduce the heterogeneity, for example using RR in place of RD. In the extreme case, the authors of an SR may decide that the studies have extremely disparate results in both the magnitude and the direction of treatment effect; they may forsake the inclusion of an MA. With such a disproportion of study results, an averaged value for the treatment effect could be very misleading. Heterogeneity may also ensue from bias in the included studies. It has been empirically demonstrated that if studies with a lower methodological quality such as failure to conceal random allocation are included in an MA, the treatment effect will be overestimated by about 30% [9].

Heterogeneity of an MA may be explored by seeking factors in some studies that systematically modify the treatment effect. This is called sub-group analysis. For example, are there certain types of patients, variations in the interventions, differences in concomitant care, or the timing of outcome assessment that produce true variation? [2]. If such factors can be identified, then studies with these characteristics might be removed from an overall summary treatment effect with a resulting reduction or elimination of statistical heterogeneity. There are statistical tests of interaction for comparing summary treatment effects [10]; this test can be used to compare the RRs of two sub-categories. In the sub-categories of Table 7.3, the RR for the lidocaine versus mepivacaine comparison is significantly different from the RRs for the other three comparisons (mepivacaine: 1.09; and bupivacaine: 7.60, prilocaine: 6.14, procaine: 7.80). With such large differences in the magnitude of the RRs (Table 7.3), it is reasonable to eliminate the three studies comparing lidocaine versus mepivacaine from the MA; the overall summary RR increases from 4.23 to 7.13 and the heterogeneity I^2 statistic shrinks from 50.2% to 0%.

If statistical heterogeneity cannot be explained, one analytical approach is to report the results using an REM. As previously noted, the CI of summary treatment effect under an REM will be wider as it incorporates both statistical error and statistical heterogeneity. There is a difference in interpretation between an FEM and an REM. For an FEM the fixed effect estimate and its CI addresses the question "what is the best estimate of the treatment effect"? The random effects estimate and its CI address the question "what is the average treatment effect"? The CIs for both an FEM and an REM treatment effect estimate give precision bounds on the weighted average. The CI for REM does not describe the variability of treatment effect among the studies.

Graphical tools

An MA produces a large quantity of description and analysis. As seen in Tables 7.1–7.3 these elements include: (1) the treatments being compared, (2) the outcome (event) of interest, (3) an abbreviated citation for each included study including the year of publication, (4) the counts of events and sample size for the two treatment groups, (5) the identity of the chosen effect estimate and the calculated value for each study with CI, (6) the model (FEM versus REM) and weight for each study, (7) the summary treatment effect estimate – both for sub-categories and all included studies, (8) the heterogeneity statistics – both for sub-categories and all included studies, and (9) the statistical test for overall effect – both for sub-categories and all included studies. The "forest plot" – a CI plot – is a highly developed graphical method for displaying simultaneously a table and a figure as shown in Figure 7.1.

This has been particularly well implemented in the freely available software (RevMan) used by The Cochrane Collaboration [11]. Each study is represented by a square (sized by the study weight) with a horizontal line extending to either side of this block representing the CI. There is a vertical line at the value of identical effect. The eye can easily discern which studies are statistically significant in that the CI line does not cross the line of identical effect. Diamonds represent the summary effects for sub-categories and for all studies; the width of diamonds represents the CI. Figure 7.1 omits the lidocaine versus mepivacaine studies. In the bottom part of the graph the tally of events (84 in 592 lidocaine patients and 9 in 573 other local anaesthetic patients), the summary RR value (7.13), the graphical display of the diamond of the summary RR being well away from the value of identical effect (RR = 1), and the high value of the z statistic ($z = 6.44$, $P < 0.00001$) mutually reinforce the conclusion that the adverse event transient neurologic symptoms is much more likely after lidocaine spinal anaesthesia. The I^2 statistic ($I^2 = 0.0\%$) shows an FEM without statistical heterogeneity.

Since many SRs have several primary outcomes, multiple secondary outcomes, and safety data of adverse events, an SR may have multiple forest plots. Other plots may also appear in an SR. For example, a funnel plot is a commonly used graphical display for appraising the possibility of bias in the retrieval of studies [12,13].

Resources, problems, and promises

Of the hundreds of publications concerning SRs, a smaller number specifically focus on techniques for MA. These include monographs by statisticians and handbooks

Review: Transient neurologic symptoms following spinal anaesthesia with lidocaine versus
          other local anaesthetics
Comparison: Lidocaine versus other local anaesthetic (excluding mepivacaine)
Outcome: 01 Transient Neurologic Symptoms

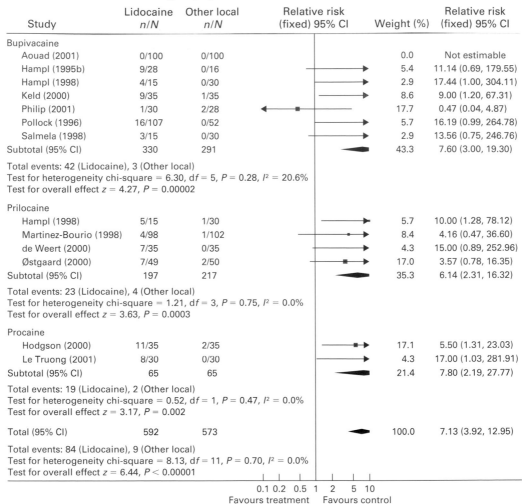

Study	Lidocaine n/N	Other local n/N	Relative risk (fixed) 95% CI	Weight (%)	Relative risk (fixed) 95% CI
Bupivacaine					
Aouad (2001)	0/100	0/100		0.0	Not estimable
Hampl (1995b)	9/28	0/16		5.4	11.14 (0.69, 179.55)
Hampl (1998)	4/15	0/30		2.9	17.44 (1.00, 304.11)
Keld (2000)	9/35	1/35		8.6	9.00 (1.20, 67.31)
Philip (2001)	1/30	2/28		17.7	0.47 (0.04, 4.87)
Pollock (1996)	16/107	0/52		5.7	16.19 (0.99, 264.78)
Salmela (1998)	3/15	0/30		2.9	13.56 (0.75, 246.76)
Subtotal (95% CI)	330	291		43.3	7.60 (3.00, 19.30)

Total events: 42 (Lidocaine), 3 (Other local)
Test for heterogeneity chi-square = 6.30, df = 5, $P = 0.28$, $I^2 = 20.6\%$
Test for overall effect $z = 4.27$, $P = 0.00002$

Prilocaine					
Hampl (1998)	5/15	1/30		5.7	10.00 (1.28, 78.12)
Martinez-Bourio (1998)	4/98	1/102		8.4	4.16 (0.47, 36.60)
de Weert (2000)	7/35	0/35		4.3	15.00 (0.89, 252.96)
Østgaard (2000)	7/49	2/50		17.0	3.57 (0.78, 16.35)
Subtotal (95% CI)	197	217		35.3	6.14 (2.31, 16.32)

Total events: 23 (Lidocaine), 4 (Other local)
Test for heterogeneity chi-square = 1.21, df = 3, $P = 0.75$, $I^2 = 0.0\%$
Test for overall effect $z = 3.63$, $P = 0.0003$

Procaine					
Hodgson (2000)	11/35	2/35		17.1	5.50 (1.31, 23.03)
Le Truong (2001)	8/30	0/30		4.3	17.00 (1.03, 281.91)
Subtotal (95% CI)	65	65		21.4	7.80 (2.19, 27.77)

Total events: 19 (Lidocaine), 2 (Other local)
Test for heterogeneity chi-square = 0.52, df = 1, $P = 0.47$, $I^2 = 0.0\%$
Test for overall effect $z = 3.17$, $P = 0.002$

Total (95% CI)	592	573		100.0	7.13 (3.92, 12.95)

Total events: 84 (Lidocaine), 9 (Other local)
Test for heterogeneity chi-square = 8.13, df = 11, $P = 0.70$, $I^2 = 0.0\%$
Test for overall effect $z = 6.44$, $P < 0.00001$

0.1 0.2 0.5 1   2   5 10
Favours treatment   Favours control

Figure 7.1   Typical SR data: the forest plot. This is figure 2 from Ref. [3]. Copyright Cochrane Library,
             reproduced with permission.

by The Cochrane Collaboration [14–16]. Several journals regularly publish papers
on MA methods including the *British Medical Journal* and *Statistics in Medicine*.

In the past MA has been criticised as a silly synthesis of disparate data. This criticism continues. Specific examples of discrepancies between meta-analytic summary
statistics and subsequent large RCTs have been noted; in one report about one-third
of the outcomes in the latter trials were discordant with the previous MA [17]. This

has led some prominent statisticians to still favour the narrative review [18]. Other statisticians have emphasised the need for a careful exploration of heterogeneity by sub-category and sensitivity analyses in every MA [9]. It may be necessary in some SRs to use advanced statistical methods to avoid bias [19].

There are statistical issues that remain unresolved. Since the methodological quality of research articles vary and since articles of poorer quality tend to exaggerate treatment benefit, should a research quality score be used to weight the summary statistic? If so, how? [1] Meta-analytic methods are being extended to SRs of observational studies, studies of prognosis, and studies of diagnostic tests; these methods are still under development.

To recapitulate, MA is a set of techniques to calculate summary treatment effect statistics from the data of two or more RCTs comparing two treatments. While the performance of an SR with MA is original research, this is observational research. The data elements come from what has been done – which may differ from what should have been done. The MA results are tentative and provisional. Each updating of an SR may require revision of the MA if additional relevant studies are found. MA can provide relevant evidence for policy decisions in medicine [20].

Summary

MA of RCTs has been criticised as an incautious synthesis of disparate data. Also, there are specific examples of discrepancies between meta-analytic summary statistics and the results of subsequent large RCTs evaluating the same therapies. The MA of an SR is a research tool; it is transparent and available. It can be used correctly or incorrectly. There must be a careful exploration of clinical heterogeneity in every MA which can provide relevant evidence for policy decisions in medicine by estimating summary effect measures contrasting treatment choices. While the performance of an SR with analysis is original research, this is observational research. The data elements come from what has been done – which may differ from what should have been done. The results of MA are tentative and provisional. Each updating of an SR may require revision of the MA if additional relevant studies are found.

REFERENCES

1 Moher D, Pham B, Jones A, Cook D, Jadad A, Moher M, Tugwell P, Klassen T. Does quality of reports of randomised trials affect estimates of intervention efficacy reported in meta-analyses? *Lancet* 1998; 352: 609–13.

2 Glasziou P, Sanders S. Investigating causes of heterogeneity in systematic reviews. *Stat Med* 2002; 21: 1503–11.

3 Zaric D, Christiansen C, Pace NL, Punjasawadwong Y. Transient neurologic symptoms (TNS) following spinal anaesthesia with lidocaine versus other local anaesthetics. *The Cochrane Database of Syst Rev* 2005, Issue 4. Art No.: CD003006. DOI: 10.1002/14651858. pub2.

4 Deeks J. Issues in the selection of a summary statistic for meta-analysis of clinical trials with binary outcomes. *Stat Med* 2002; 21: 1575–1600.

5 Furukawa T, Guyatt G, Griffith L. Can we individualize the "number needed to treat"? An empirical study of summary effect measures in meta-analyses. *Int J Epidemiol* 2002; 31: 72–6.

6 Smeeth L, Haines A, Ebrahim S. Numbers needed to treat derived from meta-analyses – sometimes informative, usually misleading. *BMJ* 1999; 318: 1548–51.

7 Whitehead A, Whitehead J. A general parametric approach to the meta-analysis of randomised clinical trials. *Stat Med* 1991; 10: 1665–77.

8 Higgins J, Thompson S, Deeks J, Altman D. Measuring inconsistency in meta-analyses. *BMJ* 2003; 327: 557–60.

9 Egger M, Ebrahim S, Smith D. Where now for meta-analysis? *Int J Epidemiol* 2002; 31: 1–5.

10 Altman D, Bland J. Interaction revisited: the difference between two estimates. *BMJ* 2003; 326: 219.

11 *Review Manager (RevMan), 4.2 for Windows Edition*. Copenhagen: The Nordic Cochrane Centre, The Cochrane Collaboration, 2003.

12 Egger M, Smith D, Schneider M, Minder C. Bias in meta-analysis detected by a simple, graphical test. *BMJ* 1997; 315: 629–34.

13 Chan A-W, Altman D. Identifying outcome reporting bias in randomised trials in PubMed: review of publications and survey of authors. *BMJ* 2005; 330: 753–6.

14 Egger M, Smith D, Altman D. *Systematic Reviews In Health Care: Meta-Analysis In Context*, 2nd Edition. London: BMJ Publishing Group, 2001.

15 Higgins J, Green S (eds). *Cochrane Handbook for Systematic Reviews of Interventions 4.2.5*, The Cochrane Library. Chichester, UK: John Wiley & Sons Ltd, 2005.

16 Cooper H, Hedges L. *The Handbook of Research Synthesis*, 1st edition. New York: Russell Sage Foundation, 1994.

17 LeLorier J, Gregoire G, Benhaddad A, Lapierre J, Derderian F. Discrepancies between meta-analyses and subsequent large randomised, controlled trials. *New Eng J Med* 1997; 337: 536–42.

18 Bailar III J. The promise and problems of meta-analysis. *New Eng J Med* 1997; 337: 559–61.

19 Higgins J, Spiegelhalter D. Being sceptical about meta-analyses: a Bayesian perspective on magnesium trials in myocardial infarction. *Int J Epidemiol* 2002; 31: 96–104.

20 Lee A, Gin T. Applying the results of quantitative systematic reviews to clinical practice. *Anesth Analg* 2002; 94: 372–7.

8

Bias in systematic reviews: considerations when updating your knowledge

Harald Herkner

Editor Cochrane Anaesthesia Review Group, Specialist Internal Medicine, Intensive Care Medicine, Cochrane Anaesthesia Group, Department of Emergency Medicine, Vienna General Hospital/Medical University of Vienna, Währinger Gürtel, Vienna, Austria

This chapter is divided into two sections: (1) Bias within single studies and (2) bias between studies in systematic reviews. The general concept of bias is discussed in the beginning. Particular forms of bias like selection, attrition or detection bias are presented together with potential answers to the problem. The association between potential bias and trial quality is illustrated, as well as the impact of realisation versus reporting and the assessment of trial quality. The first part ends with special considerations regarding bias and quality assessment in diagnostic studies. The main part related to bias at the between-study level contains a description of publication bias and related biases, how it happens, how it may be prevented, and how to deal with it. Further biases like those resulting from choice of databases, biased inclusion criteria, differentially delayed publication, publication language and analysis are also discussed.

Introduction

Traditional narrative reviews were frequently criticised for giving a potentially biased view of a topic [1]. Systematic reviews aim at avoiding many of the biases contained in traditional narrative reviews, but nevertheless there is still potential for numerous biases even in elaborate systematic reviews.

Dealing with biases and compiling systematic reviews belong together. A well-known definition of systematic reviews says [2]: *the application of scientific strategies that limit bias by the systematic assembly, critical appraisal and synthesis of all relevant studies on a specific topic.* Noteworthy this definition already contains the term bias.

Key words: Selection bias, information bias, CONSORT, trial quality, STARD, publication bias, language bias, delayed publication.

A general definition of bias, "bias stands for any systematic error in the design, conduct, analysis or interpretation of a study that result in conclusions that are different from the truth". The two basic forms of bias are:

1 Selection bias (differential exclusion or absence of participants),

2 Information bias (differential accuracy of measurements).

Bias can appear in many situations and was hence characterised with numerous different terms. Many of these terms are explained in detail below. Nonetheless, all these distinct forms can be finally ascribed to the two basic forms of selection and information bias.

Component parts used for systematic reviews are studies of individual patients or participants. Unit of analysis of the primary studies are individual persons, and a number of biases may occur at this level. Systematic reviews itself can be described as clustered studies. The respective unit of analysis is at the level of the published studies, representing clusters of individual persons. A number of potential biases may operate at this level, too. Systematic reviews may contain all usual forms of biases within the clusters, but in addition, there is also potential for bias between the clusters.

Within-study biases/trial quality

If biased studies are summarised, the bias may remain unchanged. Therefore a systematic review is not a good means to remove bias from the studies itself. The lower trial quality, the higher is the chance for potential bias. Unfortunately almost all studies bear a potential for bias to some extent. More perturbing is the empirical evidence that the quality of many clinical trials is generally weak, and that this affects its conclusions [3]. Therefore trial quality is crucial. If the findings are flawed the conclusions of systematic reviews may be invalid. Formal assessment of trial quality is a major part of systematic reviews to estimate the potential for bias.

Moreover, study quality is not a simple concept. Quality may relate to internal validity as well as to external validity [4]. Internal validity is determined by design, conduct and analysis of the study and is a matter of bias. On the other hand, external validity is related to the generalisability of the study results to the actual clinical situation. It depends on the population studied, the kind and details of the intervention, the setting of the study as well as the outcome modalities, like definition of the outcomes or timing of follow-up, and must always be judged in context. However, with regard to this chapter trial quality is primarily related to internal validity and hence potential for bias.

Bias and quality assessment in randomised controlled trials

Randomised controlled trials (RCTs) are considered the potentially most unbiased form of clinical epidemiological study designs if conducted appropriately. Furthermore randomisation may avoid measurable and non-measurable confounding.

The process of randomisation should enable us to ascribe an effect directly to the examined intervention, because ideally the intervention group and control group are equal in all aspects except the intervention.

Nevertheless, there is always potential for bias in RCTs. Typical and specific forms of bias found in RCTs includes the following.

Selection bias: biased allocation to intervention or control group

The major aim of randomisation is to make the comparison groups similar in all aspects apart from the intervention. Therefore confounding and selection can be averted, and changes in the outcome can with some restrictions be attributed to the intervention. To facilitate random allocation of the intervention, the *allocation sequence must be unpredictable* (*random*) and this sequence must be concealed to the participant and the enrolling investigator. Knowledge about the sequence may lead to selection of patients according to other prognostic factors. Hence an observed effect cannot be attributed to the intervention alone any more.

Allocation concealment is known to be a major quality item in the appraisal of RCTs.

Performance bias: unequal care for the intervention and control group

A good means to avoid performance bias is the introduction of blinding investigators and participants to the intervention. A number of additional advantages can be achieved: participants comply better (attrition bias less likely), and also measures to blind the outcome assessor are much easier (reduce information bias). However *blinding of the intervention* is not always possible, and ethical concerns were raised when sham operations were performed to blind the control arm of an arthroscopy study [5].

Information (Detection) bias: different outcome assessment in the comparison groups

Knowledge of the intervention may influence the assessment of the outcome, in particular if it includes judgement of the assessor. The more subjective an outcome measure is, the more it is prone to detection bias. Results may be biased, if the quality or extent of outcome assessment differs between the intervention and control group. *Blinding the outcome assessor* to the intervention is important to reduce this form of bias. Unlike blinding of the intervention, it is theoretically possible to blind the outcome assessor in any situation. Lack of blinding may be associated with an inflation of the effect, therefore this is regarded as another important quality criterion.

Attrition bias: differential loss to follow-up or handling of protocol deviations

This flaw is a form of selection bias and happens if participants from the intervention or control group are differentially selected or lost at the stage of outcome assessment.

Protocol deviations that may lead to exclusions of participants may include protocol deviations or non-adherence to treatment. Loss to follow-up may arise due to unrecognised deaths of patients, non-compliance, moving away, etc. Many of the factors associated with protocol deviations and loss to follow-up are also associated with prognostic factors like socioeconomic status, educational status and health consciousness. A useful rule of thumb is that if *loss to follow-up is less than 20%* then attrition bias is not very likely. If loss to follow-up or exclusion of participants exceeds these 20%, results must be judged with caution.

Further, if protocol deviations occur it is important that the analysis is performed according to the *intention-to-treat* principle to maintain the advantages of random allocation. The effect demonstrated by an intention-to-treat analysis is usually more conservative (closer towards the null) than per protocol analyses, but it is less biased.

The empirical evidence

There is empirical evidence underlining the influence of such biases on the reported effects of interventions. They are, however, not entirely consistent and they may depend on the underlying condition, the interventions and the nature of the outcome. For example information bias will not be a major problem if the outcome is all cause mortality. On the other hand there is potential for information bias if assessment depends highly on the judgement of an investigator who has already an idea of the studied effect [3,6].

Realisation versus reporting

Design, conduct and analysis are not necessarily identical with reporting of the methods. A well-performed study can be badly reported and vice versa. In fact badly reported studies usually contain a number of flaws, and well-reported studies tend to have a better quality. Bad reporting was empirically shown to be associated with bad methods [3]. Therefore the principle of "guilty until proven innocent" [7] is generally applied.

As a consequence to the implications of low quality of reporting the CONSORT statement was published [8], which aims to standardise reporting of RCTs. This statement contains a number of items related to the methods of RCTs, and can be used to systematically present the quality of trials included in a systematic review, for example, in the form of a table. This statement should improve the quality of reporting, reduce bias, and make it easier to judge which biases are to be expected. This is important, because when dealing with a systematic review we must always be aware, that our raw material is the reports of studies and usually not the raw data of the studies itself.

Assessing trial quality of RCTs

There are currently two methods to assess study quality: (1) composite scales and
(2) the component approach.

Composite scales yield to produce a summary value describing the quality of a study.
Numerous composite scores are published, where different weights are given to the
core items: Randomisation, Blinding, Follow-up. Jüni et al. [9] examined the relative
effect of 25 different quality scores and found that the different scores yielded very
contradictory results. Therefore the composite approach seems to be of limited value.

Accordingly it is current practice to *assess each component* of study quality separately. Proposed components are allocation concealment, blinding of the outcome
assessor and intention-to-treat analysis [7]. These items may be classified as (a) adequate; (b) unclear or (c) inadequate.

The information collected on study quality should then be used to perform sensitivity analyses. The procedure is explained in detail in Chapter 7. These analyses aim
to examine whether the summary effect is robust to varying study quality, that is, see
whether a summary effect changes if only studies with, for example adequate blinding of the outcome assessor are included. Incorporating study quality scores to
weight studies in a meta-analyses is not recommended.

Omission of low-quality studies

As study quality may affect conclusions of systematic reviews, it might be tempting
to assemble only studies of satisfactory quality and omit weak studies to avoid bias in
systematic reviews. However, this strategy is prone to introduce selection bias at the
between-study level itself and is therefore discouraged. Additionally, too rigorous
standards of quality bear the potential to obscure adverse events and harmful effects
of interventions [10]. It is necessary to carefully balance the benefits of a wider spectrum of studies when including also unpublished reports and data from observational studies to the disadvantages of potential biases.

Quality assessment of abstracts

Usually papers are presented as abstracts first. However, only half of these abstracts
are followed by a full publication [11]. To obtain the full picture it is preferable to
include such abstracts. However, it is usually not possible to sufficiently judge the
quality of such abstracts, unless study authors can provide more details.

In summary assessment of trial quality should be a routine procedure in systematic reviews.

Bias and quality assessment in diagnostic studies

RCTs are appropriate to evaluate diagnostic tests, but they are employed infre-
quently in this context. If randomised controlled studies of diagnostic tests are to be

quality assessed, the above criteria should be considered. Most studies evaluating diagnostic tests are cohort, case–control and cross sectional studies. These studies are subject to numerous forms of bias additionally to those found in RCTs. The potential for bias is much larger, and for each study type there are some crucial points where bias may arise.

Specifically signified biases are as follows.

Spectrum bias

A form of selection bias which arises if the sample is not representative of the population of interest leading to a distortion of the diagnostic value of a test. Stratified analysis can abate this problem. However it is related to the spectrum effect, which is a varying performance of a diagnostic test in subgroups of patients according to their clinical presentation and severity of the disease. There are methods to determine in which situations this spectrum effect may lead to a spectrum bias [12].

Selection bias in case–control studies

If the cases are not representative of all cases in the population (e.g. very sick patients from teaching hospitals) there may be selection bias.

A similar situation arises if controls are not representative of the population that produced the cases.

Ascertainment bias

Ascertainment bias represents a form of information bias and arises if the reference standard is not applied with the same rigour in test positive and test negative participants.

Incorporation bias

Incorporation bias may appear if the test of interest and the reference standard are not independent, for example when the test of interest is part of the diagnostic criteria that are used to confirm the disease status.

Verification bias

Verification bias is a form of selection bias which happens if not all participants undergo reference testing. A well-known example is the use of prostate biopsy as reference standard in a study of prostate specific antigen (PSA) to diagnose prostate cancer. Biopsy was not performed in all men PSA negative, hence it is not clear how many of the PSA negative men indeed had prostate cancer. There are however statistical methods to deal with this problem [13].

A *treatment paradox* may be introduced if participants may receive treatment between the first test and the reference test.

The empirical evidence

There is empirical evidence for the effect of these design-related biases on the diagnostic test characteristics [14]. The relevant design items associated with a distortion of diagnostic test characteristics are:

• Using a case–control design (versus cohort study).
• Different reference standards depending on test result.
• Unblinded assessment of the test and reference standard.

Further Lijmer described that the quality of reporting influenced the diagnostic characteristics; lack of describing the test of interest, the reference standard or the study population resulted in distortions of the diagnostic test characteristics.

In general, there are more diagnostic studies per topic in systematic reviews of diagnostic tests as compared with systematic reviews of interventions. However, the quality of diagnostic trials is frequently low. Following the study of Lijmer and the successful development of the CONSORT statement it was aimed to develop a standard for reporting as a first step to improve trial quality. The Standards for Reporting of Diagnostic Accuracy (STARD) initiative was established. Complete and accurate reporting should allow the reader to detect the potential for bias in the study. Current versions of this statement can be downloaded from http://www.consort-statement.org/Statement/revisedstatement.htm. Bias at the between-study level: Publication bias and related biases, "Between-study bias" can be considered to have three stages [15]:

1 Prepublication bias occurs in the performance of research.
2 Publication bias refers acceptance or rejection of a manuscript.
3 Postpublication bias occurs in publishing interpretations, reviews, and meta-analyses of published clinical trials.

Between-study bias can be categorised as selection bias and information bias. Selection bias may arise if the studies included in a systematic review do not represent all studies performed on this topic or if they are selected according to the outcome. Information bias may occur for example if the quality of extraction of study results depends on the risk factor. Post hoc definitions of outcome variables to be extracted may suffer from information bias, because frequently more than one result is presented for an outcome in the original studies.

Publication bias

Publication bias is defined as the publication or non-publication of research findings, depending on the nature and direction of the results [16].

In a survey Dickersin et al. found that up to 20% of all RCTs and 14% of completed trials remain unpublished. Significantly less unpublished trials favoured a new therapy than published trials did [17].

Sutton et al. found publication bias in about half of 48 meta-analyses examined from *The Cochrane Database of Systematic Reviews* [18]. Inferences changed in around 10% of reviews after the bias was adjusted for.

Studies with significant results are more likely to get published than studies without significant results, leading to publication bias [17,19–26].

Publication bias does appear in the classical field of clinical medicine, but also in reports of complementary medicine [27]. Since trials that show positive effects are more likely to be published, systematic reviews based on published studies can give misleading conclusions about treatment effectiveness, and patients may thus be exposed to useless or even harmful therapies [28].

Publication bias may have several sources: Investigators, authors, peer reviewers, editors, sponsors and funding bodies may all be responsible for the existence of publication bias, but some evidence suggests that authors and investigators are the main source [26]. A study of manuscripts for a highly cited medical journal indicated, that there was no major impact of the editorial process on the selection of significant studies for publication [29].

There are several methods to detect publication bias, including simple graphical (funnel plot) and more complex statistical methods. Both are described in detail in Chapter 7.

Prevention of publication bias

Registries of clinical trials

Soon after publication bias was recognised by the medical scientific community, a priori registration of clinical trials was considered a way to enhance publication regardless of the results [19]. This strategy was considered the most effective measure to reduce publication bias. Many trial registers are set up now [30], but there are still many unsolved issues. In member states of the European Union there is now a compulsory registration of clinical trials of interventions to a database (EudraCT) since 2004 EudraCT has been established in accordance with the EU-Directive 2001/20/EC [31]. Additionally major medical journals require how a trial registry number at submission of manuscripts.

Medical editors' trial amnesty

To encourage authors to publish controlled clinical trials the editors of nearly 100 international medical journals called for the "Medical editors' trial amnesty". This initiative against publication bias was to increase the number of published trials with non-significant results [32], but was not as successful as expected [33].

Peer-reviewed electronic journals

Another aspect of publication bias is the space limitation and need to be newsworthy of conventional paper journals. Peer-reviewed electronic journals without limitation of space might provide a solution to this paradox. To maintain the integrity of medical publication, editorial policy needs to be changed to accept clinical trials for publication, based only on the methodological criteria and not on the impact of their findings [34].

Yielding at peer reviewers and editors Newcombe suggested that biasing decisions on a posteriori power does not eliminate the publication bias, but *a priori power* should be the criterion of choice [35].

In summary prevention may be due to electronic journals without space restrictions, changed editorial policies stressing quality more than impact of the findings, and prospective registries for trials [26].

Retrieval bias

Choice of databases

Nieminen and Isohanni have noted and empirically defined coverage bias against European journals in the MEDLINE database. This bias can lead to lower citation counts of European research [36]. Articles published in non-indexed journals are rarely located, and hence may be missing in systematic reviews if they are based on MEDLINE only. EMBASE on the other hand is incomplete, too. The actual degree of reference overlap between MEDLINE and EMBASE depends on the topic, with reported overlap values in particular areas ranging from 10% to 75%, although they have been found to return similar numbers of relevant references [37]. This is discussed in more detail in the Cochrane Handbook for Systematic Reviews of Interventions [37]. Retrieval bias may be introduced when omitting one of these large databases if some studies are covered by a database selectively more frequent according to the outcome.

There may also be variations between disciplines, like an under-representation of specialities in high-impact journals. On average only 1 in 15 of the main research reports published in some leading non-specialist medical journals were surgical. A potential for a speciality based publication bias was postulated, as such papers are more difficult to locate [38]. Searching the major databases (MEDLINE and EMBASE) alone may therefore not be sufficient. In some fields an extended searching of specialised databases and trial registries identified an important number of additional RCTs [39].

Grey literature

Many trials are published at conferences as abstracts or elsewhere. However, these results can differ significantly from those presented later in paper publications [11]. The grey literature is therefore an important source of information for systematic reviews. Results from systematic reviews of full paper publications tended to give more favourable results than those that also included the grey literature [40]. In contrast the quality of data usually cannot be assessed in reports from the grey literature unlike for fully published papers. Again the reduction of between-study biases is at the cost of potentially uncontrolled introduction of within-study biases. In summary it is recommend that all systematic reviews should at least attempt to identify trials reported in the grey literature.

Unpublished studies

Location of unpublished studies is an important issue in systematic reviews (see Publication bias). It may be performed by contacting leading authors, experts in the field or specialist medical associations, or searching trial registries. A failure to locate such studies would lead to a bias summary effect. On the other hand there is an association between publication status and trial quality [41]. Inclusion of unpublished studies may therefore introduce bias itself. To date, however, inclusion of unpublished studies is encouraged rather than discouraged.

Biased inclusion criteria

Selective inclusion of studies depending on the nature and direction of the results due to manipulation of inclusion criteria may lead to a flawed systematic review [16]. Predefined inclusion criteria are a means to reduce this bias. Moreover, there is evidence that using at least two reviewers has an important effect on reducing the possibility that relevant reports will be discarded [42].

Time lag bias

Another aspect of between-study bias was the notion of differential delay in the publication of studies according to the results. In a survey Stern and Simes found that median time to publication in studies yielding a $P < 0.05$ was 4.7 years as compared to 8.0 years in studies with non-significant results [25]. Comparable results were found for multicentre studies [43]. Delay in publication does appear to involve active withholding of results, which are not at random [44] and therefore underline the potential for bias. Evolvement over time including contradiction of original findings can be found also in highly cited high-impact research [45]. This has important implications for systematic reviews, because for new areas of research positive studies may dominate the literature and the full picture will be visible with a delay of several years. Regular updates of systematic reviews are therefore necessary, as is done in Cochrane reviews.

Multiple publication bias

The problem of multiple publications of the same data has been an issue for a long time [46]. Publication of several reports from one study happens frequently and may lead to an overestimation of treatment effects [47]. Duplicate publication appears to be more than simple copying. Different patterns of duplicate publication could be identified according to the presented sample and the chosen outcome [48]. One-third of duplicates were sponsored by the pharmaceutical industry. The number of authors, the impact factor of the publishing journal and the citation rate were virtually the same for original and duplicate publications, whereas the names of the authors were different between publications in two-thirds of the studies. In contrast to the above time lag bias, duplicates were published with a median delay of only 1 year [48]. Accordingly, duplicate publication may be difficult to detect, but as studies with significant results are more likely to be duplicated this may inflate treatment effects in systematic reviews.

Citation bias and reference bias

This bias may arise if a search is based only on contacting experts in the field and checking the reference lists of other studies and reviews [49]. It has been a major problem for narrative non-systematic reviews. Analysing narrative review articles that discuss interventions against house dust mites for people with asthma Schmidt and Gøtzsche found evidence for severe reference bias. In 90% of the narrative articles interventions were recommended, which were shown to have no effect in a systematic Cochrane review [1]. As described above it is not unusual for highly cited publications to be challenged and refuted over time [45]. A review based on reference lists alone can therefore not be called systematic, and will have a high potential for bias.

Language bias

Publishing research reports in non-English language dramatically limits the international readership. Therefore for significant results English language publication is preferably sought. Consequently there are more reports of significant results found in English language journals as compared with non-English language journals [50,51]. The quality of non-English articles was found to be comparable to English language articles [52]. Restriction of studies according to publication language was frequently observed in the 1990s [53], because translations can be tedious and costly. As the potential effects of language bias are understood now, the general advice of The Cochrane Collaboration is to avoid any language restrictions [37].

"Place of publication" bias

In the field of tropical medicine authors from countries with a low development index are under-represented. An imbalance of international representation exists among editorial and advisory boards of the ISI referenced journals on tropical medicine. Only 1.7–7.7% of the articles published in the six leading tropical medicine journals in 2000–2002 were generated exclusively by scientists from countries with a low human development index [54].

Outcome reporting bias

This bias is sometimes referred to as "publication bias in situ". More than one outcome is frequently reported in original studies, and sometimes more than one method is used to describe effects or differences. This term describes the selective reporting of results and selective use of favourable types of statistical methods according to the nature or direction of the expected effect [55]. Predefined data extraction rules and analysis protocols for systematic reviews may help to avoid this form of bias.

Practice points

What we know

There is empirical evidence that biases can significantly distort reported effects of interventions and diagnosis in single studies. Bad reporting is associated with bad methods.

Publication bias can be found frequently. Many trials remain unpublished or are delayed depending on significance of results. Inferences of reviews can change after the bias was adjusted for. MEDLINE and EMBASE overlap and cover many studies, but both are incomplete. Unrestricted search strategies using as many sources of studies, independent duplicate searching and inclusion of studies, predefining data to be extracted, employing extraction forms and independent duplicate data extraction are means to reduce between-study biases.

What we think we know

For trial quality assessment compound methods appear better than composite scales. Authors and investigators may be the main source of publication bias. There is some empirical evidence for the importance of citation bias. Limited evidence exists for the impact of outcome reporting bias, duplicate publication bias, language bias and database bias.

What we do not know
Direction of some biases may be unpredictable depending on the actual situation. Details of publication and related bias remain open, hence standards to identify unpublished work are lacking. Inclusion of unpublished studies may introduce bias because they may be of poor quality, but incompleteness of reviews produces bias, too.

Summary

There is empirical evidence that studies with significant results are published or cited earlier and more frequently than those with non-significant or unfavourable results. There is some empirical evidence for the existence of citation bias. Limited evidence exists for outcome reporting bias, duplicate publication bias, language bias and database bias. Investigators, peer reviewers, editors and funding bodies may all be responsible for the existence of publication bias, but some evidence suggests that authors and investigators are the main source [26]. Unrestricted search strategies using as many sources of studies, independent duplicate searching and inclusion of studies, predefining data to be extracted, employing extraction forms and independent duplicate data extraction are means to reduce between-study biases when producing a systematic review. As for primary studies, the quality of a systematic review can only be judged if reporting is appropriate. Readers of systematic reviews have to consider the possibility of inherent biases; therefore it is reasonable to use standards for reporting. Well-recognised resources are the Cochrane Handbook for Systematic Reviews of Interventions [37], the QUOROM statement for systematic reviews of RCTs, and the MOOSE statement for systematic reviews of observational studies (http://www.consort-statement.org/Initiatives/complements.htm).

REFERENCES

1 Schmidt LM, Gøtzsche PC. Of mites and men: reference bias in narrative review articles: a systematic review. *J Fam Pract* 2005; 54(4): 334–8.
2 Cook DJ, Sackett DL, Spitzer WO. Methodologic guidelines for systematic reviews of randomized control trials in health care from the Potsdam Consultation on Meta-Analysis. *J Clin Epidemiol* 1995; 48(1): 167–71.
3 Schulz KF, Chalmers I, Hayes RJ, Altman D. Empirical evidence of bias. Dimensions of methodological quality associated with estimates of treatment effects in controlled trials. *JAMA* 1995; 273: 408–12.
4 Campbell DT, Stanley JC. Experimental and quasi-experimental designs for research on teaching. In: Gage NL (ed.). *Handbook of Research on Teaching*. Chicago: Rand McNally, 1963.

5 Moseley JB, O'Malley K, Petersen NJ, Menke TJ, Brody BA, Kuykendall DH, Hollingsworth JC, Ashton CM, Wray NP. A controlled trial of arthroscopic surgery for osteoarthritis of the knee. *New Engl J Med* 2002; 347(2): 81–8.

6 Moher D, Pham B, Jones A, Cook DJ, Jadad AR, Moher M, Tugwell P, Klassen TP. Does quality of reports of randomised trials affect estimates of intervention efficacy reported in meta-analyses? *Lancet* 1998; 352: 609–13.

7 Jüni P, Altman DG, Egger M. In: Egger M, Smith GD, Altman DG (eds). *Systematic Reviews in Health Care: Meta-analysis in Context*, London: BMJ Books, 2001, p. 100.

8 Moher D, Schulz KF, Altman DG. (2001) The CONSORT statement: revised recommendations for improving tühe quality of reports of parallel-group randomised trials. Retrieved November 2 2005 from WWW. http://www.consort-statement.org

9 Jüni P, Witschi A, Bloch R, Egger M. The hazards of scoring the quality of clinical trials for meta-analysis. *JAMA* 1999; 282(11): 1054–60.

10 Chou R, Helfand M. Challenges in systematic reviews that assess treatment harms. *Ann Intern Med.* 2005; 142(12): 1090–9.

11 Scherer RW, Dickersin K, Langenberg P. Full publication of results initially presented in abstracts. A meta-analysis. *JAMA* 1994; 272: 158–62.

12 Goehring C, Perrier A, Morabia A. Spectrum bias: a quantitative and graphical analysis of the variability of medical diagnostic test performance. *Stat Med.* 2004; 23(1): 125–35.

13 Punglia RS, D'Amico AV, Catalona WJ, Roehl KA, Kuntz KM. Effect of verification bias on screening for prostate cancer by measurement of prostate-specific antigen. *New Engl J Med* 2003; 349(4): 335–42.

14 Lijmer JG, Mol BW, Heisterkamp S, Bonsel GJ, Prins MH, van der Meulen JH, Bossuyt PM. Empirical evidence of design-related bias in studies of diagnostic tests. *JAMA* 1999; 282: 1061–6.

15 Chalmers TC, Frank CS, Reitman D. Minimizing the three stages of publication bias. *JAMA* 1990; 263(10): 1392–5.

16 Egger M, Dickersin K, Davey Smith G. In: Egger M, Smith GD, Altman DG (eds). *Systematic Reviews in Health Care: Meta-analysis in Context*, London: BMJ Books, 2001.

17 Dickersin K, Chan S, Chalmers TC, Sacks HS, Smith Jr H. Publication bias and clinical trials. *Control Clin Trials* 1987; 8(4): 343–53.

18 Sutton AJ, Duval SJ, Tweedie RL, Abrams KR, Jones DR. Empirical assessment of effect of publication bias on meta-analyses. *BMJ* 2000; 320(7249): 1574–7.

19 Simes RJ. Publication bias: the case for an international registry of clinical trials. *J Clin Oncol* 1986; 4: 1529–41.

20 Simes RJ. Confronting publication bias: a cohort design for meta-analysis. *Stat Med* 1987; 6: 11–29.

21 Begg CB, Berlin JA. Publication bias: a problem in interpreting medical data. *J Roy Statist Soc A* 1988; 151: 445–63.

22 Easterbrook PJ, Berlin JA, Gopalan R, Matthews DR. Publication bias in clinical research. *Lancet* 1991; 337: 867–72.

23 Dickersin K, Min Y, Meinert C. Factors influencing publication of research results. *JAMA* 1992; 267: 374–8.

24 Dickersin K, Min YI. NIH clinical trials and publication bias. *On-line J Curr Clin Trials* 1993; 28 April: Doc No. 50.

25 Stern JM, Simes RJ. Publication bias: evidence of delayed publication in a cohort study of clinical research projects. *BMJ* 1997; 315(7109): 640–5.

26 Song F, Eastwood AJ, Gilbody S, Duley L, Sutton AJ. Publication and related biases. *Health Technol Assess* 2000; 4(10): 1–115.

27 Zimpel T, Windeler J. Publications of dissertations on unconventional medical therapy and diagnosis procedures – a contribution to "publication bias". *Forsch Komplementarmed Klass Naturheilkd* 2000; 7(2): 71–4.

28 Egger M, Davey Smith G. Misleading meta-analysis. *BMJ* 1995; 310: 752–4.

29 Olson CM, Rennie D, Cook D, Dickersin K, Flanagin A, Hogan JW, Zhu Q, Reiling J, Pace B. Publication bias in editorial decision making. *JAMA* 2002; 287(21): 2825–8.

30 Tonks A. Registering clinical trials. *BMJ* 1999; 319(7224): 1565–8.

31 EudraCT European Clinical Trials Database [WWW Document]. 2001, April 1. Retrieved November 2 2005 from WWW. https://eudract.emea.eu.int/eudract/index.do

32 Smith R, Roberts I. An amnesty for unpublished trials. *BMJ* 1997; 315: 622.

33 Roberts I. An amnesty for unpublished trials. *BMJ* 1998; 317: 763–4.

34 Song F, Eastwood A, Gilbody S, Duley L. The role of electronic journals in reducing publication bias. *Med Inform Internet Med* 1999; 24(3): 223–9.

35 Newcombe RG. Towards a reduction in publication bias. *BMJ (Clin Res Ed)* 1987; 295(6599): 656–9.

36 Nieminen P, Isohanni M. Bias against European journals in medical publication Databases. *Lancet* 1999; 353(9164): 1592.

37 Higgins JPT, Green S (eds). [updated May 2005]. Cochrane handbook for systematic reviews of interventions 4.2.5. Retrieved November 2 2005 from WWW. http://www.cochrane.org/resources/handbook/hbook.htm

38 Magos A, Cumbis A, Katsetos C. Bias against publication of surgical papers. *Lancet.* 2000; 355(9201): 413.

39 Savoie I, Helmer D, Green CJ, Kazanjian A. Beyond Medline: reducing bias through extended systematic review search. *Int J Technol Assess Health Care* 2003; 19(1): 168–78.

40 Burdett S, Stewart LA, Tierney JF. Publication bias and meta-analyses: a practical example. *Int J Technol Assess Health Care* 2003; 19(1): 129–34.

41 Sterne JA, Juni P, Schulz KF, Altman DG, Bartlett C, Egger M. Statistical methods for assessing the influence of study characteristics on treatment effects in "meta-epidemiological" research. *Stat Med* 2000; 21(11): 1513–24.

42 Edwards P, Clarke M, DiGuiseppi C, Pratap S, Roberts I, Wentz R. Identification of randomized controlled trials in systematic reviews: accuracy and reliability of screening records. *Stats Med* 2002; 21: 1635–40.

43 Ioannidis JP. Effect of the statistical significance of results on the time to completion and publication of randomized efficacy trials. *JAMA* 1998; 279(4): 281–6.

44 Blumenthal D, Campbell EG, Anderson MS, Causino N, Louis KS. Withholding research results in academic life science: evidence from a national survey of faculty. *JAMA* 1997; 277: 1224.

45 Ioannidis JP. Contradicted and initially stronger effects in highly cited clinical research. *JAMA* 2005; 294(2): 218–28.

46 Gøtzsche PC. Multiple publication of reports of drug trials. *Eur J Clin Pharmacol* 1989; 36(5): 429–32.

47 Tramer MR, Reynolds DJ, Moore RA, McQuay HJ. Impact of covert duplicate publication on meta-analysis: a case study. *BMJ* 1997; 315(7109): 635–40.

48 von Elm E, Poglia G, Walder B, Tramer MR. Different patterns of duplicate publication: an analysis of articles used in systematic reviews. *JAMA* 2004; 291(8): 974–80.

49 Gøtzsche PC. Reference bias in reports of drug trials. *BMJ* (*Clin Res Ed*) 1987; 295(6599): 654–6.

50 Egger M, Zellweger-Zähner T, Schneider M, Junker C, Lengeler C, Antes G. Language bias in randomised controlled trials published in English and German. *Lancet* 1997; 350: 326–9.

51 Juni P, Holenstein F, Sterne J, Bartlett C, Egger M. Direction and impact of language bias in meta-analyses of controlled trials: empirical study. *Int J Epidemiol* 2002; 31: 115–23.

52 Moher D, Fortin P, Jadad AR, Juni P, Klassen T, Le Lorier J, Liberati A, Linde K, Penna A. Completeness of reporting of trials published in languages other than English: implications for conduct and reporting of systematic reviews. *Lancet* 1996; 347: 363–6.

53 Gregoire G, Derderian F, Le Lorier J. Selecting the language of the publications included in a meta-analysis: is there a tower of Babel bias? *J Clin Epidemiol* 1995; 48: 159–63.

54 Keiser J, Utzinger J, Tanner M, Singer BH. Representation of authors and editors from countries with different human development indexes in the leading literature on tropical medicine: survey of current evidence. *BMJ* 2004; 328: 1229–32.

55 Phillips CV. Publication bias in situ. *BMC Med Res Methodol* 2004; 4: 20.

9

The Cochrane Collaboration and the Cochrane Anaesthesia Review Group

Tom Pedersen[1] and Ann Møller[2]

[1]The Cochrane Anaesthesia Review Group, Centre of Head-Orthopaedics, University of Copenhagen, Rigshospitalet, Copenhagen, Denmark
[2]The Cochrane Anaesthesia Review Group, Department of Anaesthesiology, Herlev University Hospital, Herlev, Denmark

The Cochrane Collaboration is an international non-profit and independent organisation, dedicated to making up-to-date, accurate information about the effects of health care readily available worldwide. It produces and disseminates systematic reviews of health care interventions and promotes the search for evidence in the form of clinical trials and other studies of interventions. The major product of the Collaboration is *The Cochrane Database of Systematic Reviews*, which is published quarterly as part of *The Cochrane Library.* Those who prepare the reviews are mostly health care professionals who volunteer to work in one of the many Collaborative Review Groups (CRGs), with editorial teams overseeing the preparation and maintenance of the reviews, as well as application of the rigorous quality standards for which Cochrane reviews have become known. In 2000 the Cochrane Anaesthesia Review Group (CARG) was established and is situated in Copenhagen. The scope covers anaesthesia, perioperative medicine, intensive care medicine, resuscitation and emergency medicine. CARG published 24 reviews in *The Cochrane Library*, Issue 4, 2005.

What is The Cochrane Collaboration?

The Cochrane Collaboration is an international non-profit and independent organisation, dedicated to making up-to-date, accurate information about the effects of health care readily available worldwide. The Cochrane Collaboration is the largest organisation in the world engaged in the preparation and maintenance of systematic reviews. The Collaboration aims to help people make well-informed decisions by preparing, maintaining and promoting the accessibility of systematic reviews of the effects of interventions in all areas of health care. The Cochrane Collaboration was founded in 1993 and named after the British epidemiologist, Archie Cochrane. It is

Key words: The Cochrane Collaboration, systematic reviews, evidence-based medicine (EBM).

comprised of 50 CRGs; 11 Field Groups; 11 Methods Groups; 12 Cochrane Centres and The Cochrane Collaboration Steering Group.

The Cochrane Collaboration is supported by hundreds of organisations from around the world, including health service providers, research funding agencies, departments of health, international organisations and universities. There are currently 13 000 people contributing to the work of The Cochrane Collaboration in almost 100 countries. This involvement continues to grow at a rapid rate. The number of people involved in the Collaboration has more than doubled since 2000.

Although there is a great deal of work that remains to be done, much has already been accomplished. *The Cochrane Database of Systematic Reviews*, the main product of The Cochrane Collaboration, now contains the full text of 2435 completed Cochrane reviews, each of which will be kept up-to-date as new evidence accumulates and other ways of improving them are identified. There are also 1606 published protocols for reviews in progress, and hundreds more at a pre-protocol stage. Several hundred newly completed reviews and protocols are added each year to *The Cochrane Library*; and several hundred reviews are updated.

It has been estimated that approximately 10 000 Cochrane reviews are needed to cover all health care interventions that have already been investigated in controlled trials, and these reviews will need to be assessed for updating and updated, if necessary, at the rate of 5000 per year. If the growth in The Cochrane Collaboration continues at the pace of the last few years, there will be 10 000 Cochrane reviews during the next 10 years. However, this will require continuing and evolving partnership and collaboration. The Cochrane Collaboration will need to continue to attract, and support, the wide variety of people who contribute to its work, and make it easier for these people to contribute.

The Cochrane Collaboration is a major focus of activity, and a rich source of information within the evidence-based medicine (EBM) movement. The term EBM originated at McMaster University in Canada. EBM has been defined as "the conscientious, explicit and judicious use of the best evidence in making decisions about the care of individual patients" [1–3]. Thus, to practise EBM is to integrate clinical expertise with the best available external evidence from systematic research. The practice of EBM is described by David Sackett [3]. The use of EBM in anaesthesia and perioperative medicine was recently overviewed [4–6].

In 1972, the British epidemiologist Archie Cochrane published his view of the principles on which the delivery of health care should be based [7]. He wrote: "It is surely a great criticism of our profession that we have not organised a critical summary, by specialty or subspecialty, adapted periodically, of all relevant randomised controlled trials". Cochrane's criticism is still relevant, in that people wanting to make well-informed decisions about health care are often confronted with hundreds of thousands of potentially relevant research reports. No one can be expected to sift through these mountains of evidence to discover which forms of health care are more likely to do good than harm. Put simply, Cochrane stated that limited resources should be used equitably to provide care of proven benefit. Cochrane promoted randomised controlled trials as the most reliable source of evidence on which to base decisions about the effectiveness of health care interventions. He advocated the compilation of a comprehensive catalogue of definitive reviews of scientifically valid clinical trials for each speciality. These regularly updated reviews could be consulted to assist with clinical decision-making. Medical interventions would thus be scientifically based on properly planned and executed clinical trials (distilled where possible into equally scientifically valid reviews) rather than on anecdote, habit, selective experience, faulty memory or a skewed sample of the relevant clinical trials as is often the case. The impact of Cochrane's book [7] Effectiveness and Efficiency was not fully recognised at the time, but it captured the essence of today's EBM movement. Cochrane's vision of a reliable, comprehensive and accurate medical database, *The Cochrane Library*, is approaching reality.

Structure of the Collaboration

CRGs

The main work of The Cochrane Collaboration is carried out by 50 CRGs, within which the Cochrane reviews are prepared and maintained. The members of these groups: researchers, health care professionals, people using the health services (consumers) and others, have come together because they share an interest in generating reliable, up-to-date evidence relevant to the prevention, treatment and rehabilitation of particular health problems or groups of problems.

To become part of The Cochrane Collaboration, each CRG is required to prepare a plan outlining how it will contribute to the Collaboration's objectives. This plan describes who will have responsibility for planning, co-ordinating and monitoring the Group's work (a co-ordinating editor, supported by an editorial team). It also describes how the Group will identify and assemble in a specialised register as high a proportion as possible of all the studies relevant to its declared scope; and who, drawing on the studies in this register, will take responsibility for preparing and maintaining which reviews. Every Group appoints an individual to organise and manage the day-to-day activities of the Group: a Review Group Co-ordinator. The primary task of a CRG is to conduct and regularly update systematic reviews of prevention and health care issues within the scope of its group. Each CRG creates a specialised register of methodologically sound controlled studies, relevant to their group, of both published and unpublished studies in all languages to avoid publication bias, which means that journal appears to favour trials with positive results [8].

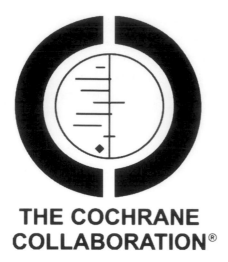

THE COCHRANE COLLABORATION®

Figure 9.1   *The Cochrane Collaboration Logo*: Illustrates a systematic review of data from 7 randomised controlled trials (RCT) comparing one health care treatment with a placebo. Each horizontal line represents results of one trial. The shorter the line means the more certain the result. The diamond is the combined result, if it is to the left then treatment is beneficial. If a horizontal line touches the vertical one then the trial found no clear difference between the treatments. If the horizontal line is to the right, or the diamond is to the right of the vertical line then the treatment is not good, and may do more harm than good

The work of CRGs is supported by people working in Methods Groups, Fields, the Consumer Network and Centres (Figure 9.1).

Methods Groups

The science of research synthesis is still relatively young and evolving rapidly. Methods Groups have been established to develop methodology and advise the Collaboration on how the validity and precision of systematic reviews can be improved. For example, the Statistical Methods Group is assessing ways of handling different kinds of data for statistical synthesis. The Applicability and Recommendations Methods Group is exploring important questions about drawing conclusions regarding implications for practise, based on the results of reviews.

Fields

Fields focus on dimensions of health care other than health problems, such as the setting of care (e.g. primary care), the type of consumer (e.g. older people) or the type of intervention (e.g. vaccines). People associated with Fields search specialist sources for relevant studies, help to ensure that priorities and perspectives in their sphere of interest are reflected in the work of CRGs, compile specialised databases, co-ordinate activities with relevant agencies outside the Collaboration, and comment on systematic reviews relating to their particular area.

Consumer Network

The Cochrane Consumer Network provides information and a forum for networking among consumers involved in the Collaboration, and a liaison point for consumer groups around the world.

Centres

The work of CRGs, Methods Groups, Fields and the Consumer Network is facilitated in a variety of ways by the work of a dozen Cochrane Centres around the world. They share responsibility for helping to co-ordinate and support members of the Collaboration in areas such as training, and they promote the objectives of the Collaboration at national level. The work of CRGs, Methods Groups, Fields/ Networks and the Consumer Network is facilitated in a variety of ways by the work of more than a dozen Cochrane Centres around the world. They share responsibility for helping to co-ordinate and support members of the Collaboration in areas such as training, and they promote the objectives of the Collaboration at national level.

Steering Group

All registered CRGs, Methods Groups, Fields, the Consumer Network and Centres are eligible to vote in the election of members to the Collaboration's Steering Group, and at its annual general meeting. The Steering Group meets twice a year, once during the annual Cochrane Colloquia and on one other occasion. In between its two main meetings, the Steering Group's various working groups hold regular meetings by teleconference. Steering Group decisions are guided by goals and objectives set out in the Collaboration's Strategic Plan. The Cochrane Collaboration's work is based on 10 key principles (Table 9.1).

The Cochrane Database of Systematic Reviews

An important contribution of The Cochrane Collaboration is the identification of controlled studies and creation of a specialised register. This register houses the identified trials that can be accessed to conduct systematic reviews. The reviews

Table 9.1. The 10 key principles of The Cochrane Collaboration

---

1 *Collaboration* by internally and externally fostering good communications, open decision-making and team work.

2 *Building on the enthusiasm of individuals* by involving and supporting people of different skills and background.

3 *Avoiding duplication* by good management and co-ordination to maximise economy of effort.

4 *Minimising bias* through a variety of approaches such as scientific rigour, ensuring broad participation and avoiding conflicts of interest.

5 *Keeping up-to-date* by a commitment to ensure that Cochrane reviews are maintained through identification and incorporation of new evidence.

6 *Striving for relevance* by promoting the assessment of health care interventions using outcomes that matter to people making choices in health care.

7 *Promoting access* by wide dissemination of the outputs of the Collaboration, taking advantage of strategic alliances, and by promoting appropriate prices, content and media to meet the needs of users worldwide.

8 *Ensuring quality* by being open and responsive to criticism, applying advances in methodology, developing systems for quality improvement.

9 *Continuity* by ensuring that responsibility for reviews, editorial processes and key functions is maintained and renewed.

10 *Enabling wide participation* in the work of the Collaboration by reducing barriers to contributing and by encouraging diversity.

---

prepared within the Collaboration are published in *The Cochrane Database of Systematic Reviews*, and can be revised and updated every 3 months if necessary. All outcomes from The Cochrane Collaboration are published electronically on CD-ROM and via the Internet. For a more detailed introduction to the Cochrane Collaboration: http://www.cochrane.org/docs/newcomersguide.htm

The Cochrane Library

The Cochrane Library is a unique source of reliable and up-to-date information on the effects of interventions in health care. Published on a quarterly basis, the Cochrane Library is designed to provide information and evidence to support decisions taken in health care and to inform those receiving care. It provides a database of other identified completed reviews; a register of bibliographic information on over 250 000 controlled trials and information about the CRGs (Table 9.2). *The Cochrane Library* is widely acknowledged as the best single source of evidence about the effects of health care interventions. It contains *the Cochrane Controlled Trials Register*, which is now recognised as the most comprehensive bibliography of published reports of controlled trials available.

Table 9.2. *The Cochrane Library* EBM databases

The Cochrane Library consists of a regularly updated collection of EBM databases. The databases and the current numbers of records in 2005 are:

Database	Total records
The Cochrane Database of Systematic Reviews (Cochrane reviews)*	4041
Database of Abstracts of Reviews of Effects (DARE)**	5340
The Cochrane Central Register of Controlled Trials (CENTRAL)	454 449
The Cochrane Database of Methodology Reviews (Methodology Reviews)***	20
The Cochrane Methodology Register (Methodology Register)	7059
Health Technology Assessment Database (HTA)	4620
NHS Economic Evaluation Database (NHS EED)	15 884
About The Cochrane Collaboration and the Cochrane CRGs (About)§	90

*Comprises 2435 Complete Reviews and 1606 Protocols. **Comprises 4540 Abstracts and 800 other reviews. ***Comprises 11 Reviews and 9 Protocols. §The Cochrane Collaboration, 1; CRGs, 50; Fields, 11; Methods Groups, 11; Networks, 1; Centres, 12; Possible Cochrane entities, 4.

CARG

The idea of forming the CARG first arose in 1997. CARG was established in February 2000 in Copenhagen. The main goal of CARG is to conduct systematic reviews of randomised controlled trials and other controlled clinical trials of interventions [5,6]. CARG's scope covers anaesthesia, perioperative medicine, intensive care medicine, resuscitation and emergency medicine. The individual tasks of the editorial office are described in Table 9.3.

The editorial process

A review is initially registered by a CRG in the Cochrane Title base as a *title*. That *title* will **then** become a *protocol*, which prospectively sets out what is being tested, why, and how it will be done. The complete *systematic review* adheres to the protocol in order to maintain uniformity and minimise bias. Systematic reviews performed by CARG are reviews of studies in which evidence has been systematically searched for, studied, assessed and summarised according to predetermined criteria.

Titles

To register a title with CARG, a potential author needs to submit a registration form (available from either the CARG's web site: http://www.carg.dk or on request from the Review Group Co-ordinator: jane_cracknell@yahoo.com). The completed registration form should include: authors' contact details, a preliminary title and a synopsis describing the background, participants, interventions, outcomes and

Table 9.3. The tasks of the Cochrane Anaesthesia Review Group (CARG)

The Co-ordinating Editors have overall responsibility for CARG. They assure the quality of all publications and make the final decision on whether a title is registered; a protocol or review is published. The other responsibilities includes:

- Manage the development and growth of the Group.
- Disseminate *The Cochrane Library* through the Group.
- Provide information on group activities and performance.
- Ensure the effectiveness and efficiency of the Group.
- Represent the Group and The Cochrane Collaboration.
- Help the Steering Group attain its objectives.

The Review Group Co-ordinator (RGC) is responsible for the smooth daily running and effectiveness of CARG. The other responsibilities includes:

- Liaises with, and supports authors, editors and peer reviewers.
- Co-ordinates the production of a review from title registration, through the editorial process, to publication in *The Cochrane Library.*
- Submits approved module (all approved reviews) to the publisher.
- Communicates with publishers.
- Recruits new members.

The Trials Search Co-ordinator is a full-time paid member of staff. He is responsible for trial identification and manages the CRG's specialised register (database of trials). The other responsibilities includes:

- Submits the register for inclusion in *The Cochrane Library's* Controlled Trials Register.
- Helps authors with searching.
- Co-ordinates the hand-searching process.
- Maintains the members' directory.
- Provides secretarial support to the editorial base.

The Consumer Co-ordinator

- Recruits consumers to comment on all CARG protocols and reviews;
- Collects and collates the consumer comments.
- Liaises with and supports CARG's consumers and the RGC.
- Liaises with the Cochrane Consumer Network.

The Handsearch & Communication Co-ordinator

- Hand-searching process.
- Fundraising.
- The CARG web site and the newsletter.

key words. After the title has been approved by all CARG's editors, and the Review Group Co-ordinator has excluded any potential duplication of work or conflicts of interest with other Cochrane Groups, the title is registered. The author is then sent guidelines for writing a systematic review "Tips for authors" [9] advised to download (http://www.cochrane.org/cochrane/hbook.htm) and read the Cochrane Handbook for Systematic Reviews of Interventions [10] and glossary and sent details of Cochrane training workshops.

Protocols and reviews

Protocols and reviews are prepared using The Cochrane Collaboration's Review Manager, Software Review Manager (Revman 4.2) [11] (which can be downloaded from http://www.cochrane.org/cochrane/revman.htm). Authors who do not have the computer capability to access RevMan 4.2 should contact the editorial office. The Review Group Co-ordinator acknowledges receipt of the protocol in the editorial office, and forwards the protocol, along with guidelines for editing (see http://www.carg.dk: "Tips for editors and peer referees") to the assigned CARG content and statistical editors, two peer referees and a consumer panel. The editor and peer referees evaluate and comment on the review title, background, objectives, selection criteria, search strategy, methodology and the language of the protocol. The protocol and later the systematic review (the principal output of the Collaboration) will be published electronically in successive issues of *The Cochrane Library's Database of Systematic Reviews*. The CARG published, in Issue 4, 2005 of *The Cochrane Library* Issue 4, 2005, 24 reviews and 48 protocols in *The Cochrane Library*.

Updating

Authors are expected to include new trials and update their reviews every 2 years, or in response to criticism from readers. Those updates will then be published electronically in *The Cochrane Library*. The editorial office will provide each author with additional annual references within the scope of the review from the specialised register. The updated review will be edited by the same editorial team. If the author does not update the review, it may be re-allocated or withdrawn.

Specialised register

The CARG maintains a register of more than 25 000 randomised controlled trials and clinical controlled trials related to anaesthesia, perioperative medicine, intensive care medicine, pre-hospital medicine, resuscitation and emergency medicine. The register is maintained on ProCite software, and searches for trials are executed quarterly. Trials included in the register are tagged SR-ANAESTH, and the tag term may be searched in *The Cochrane Library*. Access to the register is available to authors and other members of the CARG.

Consumer representation

One of the goals of The Cochrane Collaboration is to make Cochrane evidence accessible to consumers through *The Cochrane Library*. CARG is liaising with other Review Consumer Groups in order to set up good communications and learn how to successfully involve the public within our group. At present, the CARG has only a few consumers but we are in the process of collaborating with other consumer groups. More information is given in *the Cochrane Consumers Network's* web site (www.cochraneconsumers.com).

> **Practice points**
>
> The Cochrane Collaboration is an international organisation that aims to help people make well-informed decisions about health care by preparing, maintaining and promoting the accessibility of systematic reviews of the effects of health care interventions.
>
> - The major product of the Collaboration is the Cochrane Database of Systematic Reviews, which is published quarterly as part of *The Cochrane Library*.
> - One of the aims of the CARG is to conduct systematic reviews of randomised controlled trials and other controlled clinical trials of interventions in anaesthesiology.

Conclusion

The necessity of The Cochrane Collaboration and EBM has become widely recognised by health professionals and lay people alike. This is for several reasons. Firstly, hard evidence to support many treatments is simply not available because properly designed studies have not been performed. Secondly, the evidence may exist, but may not be easily accessible to those making the decisions. Thirdly, even when available, the evidence may not be accepted by those delivering care, particularly if it seems to be in conflict with perceived wisdom or personal experience or if it threatens a vested interest. The vision statement of The Cochrane Collaboration for the future is:

Health care decision-making throughout the world will be informed by high quality, timely research evidence, and The Cochrane Collaboration will play a pivotal role in the production and dissemination of this evidence across all areas of health care.

REFERENCES

1 Sackett DL, Rosenberg WM, Gray JA et al. Evidence-based medicine: what it is and what it isn't [Editorial]. *BMJ* 1996; 312(7023): 71–2.
2 Sackett DL, Richardson WS, Rosenberg WM et al. *Evidence-Based Medicine. How to Practice and Teach Evidence-Based Medicine.* Edinburgh: Churchhill Livingstone, 1997.

3 Evidence-based medicine. A new approach to teaching the practice of medicine. Evidence-Based Medicine Working Group [See comments]. *JAMA* 1992; 268(17): 2420–5.

4 Pronovost PJ, Berenholtz SM, Dorman T et al. Evidence-based medicine in anesthesiology. *Anesth Analg* 2001; 92: 787–94.

5 Pedersen T, Møller AM. How to use evidence-based medicine in anaesthesiology. *Acta Anaesth Scand* 2001; 45: 267–74.

6 Pedersen T, Møller AM, Cracknell J. The mission of the Cochrane Anaesthesia Review Group: preparing and disseminating systematic reviews of the effect of health care in anesthesiology. *Anesth Analg* 2002; 95: 1012–18.

7 Cochrane A. *Effectiveness and Efficiency. Random Reflections on Health Services.* London: Nuffield Provicial Hospitals Trust, 1972.

8 Crombie IK. *Critical Appraisal.* London: BMJ Publishing Group, 1999.

9 Cracknell J, Pedersen T, Møller A, Bismuth L. (2005). Tips for authors [WWW Document], from World WideWeb: http://www.cochrane-anaesthesia.suite.dk/tips_reviewers.html

10 Higgins JPT, Green S (eds). Cochrane Handbook for Systematic Reviews of Interventions 4.2.5 [Updated May 2005]. In: *The Cochrane Library*, Issue 3. Chichester, UK: John Wiley & Sons, Ltd, 2005.

11 Review Manager (RevMan) [Computer program]. Version 4.2 for Windows. Copenhagen: The Nordic Cochrane Centre, The Cochrane Collaboration, 2003.

10

Integrating clinical practice and evidence: how to learn and teach evidence-based medicine

Steven Knight[1] and Andrew Smith[2]

[1]Department of Anaesthetics, Wythenshawe Hospital, Manchester, UK
[2]Department of Anaesthetics, Royal Lancaster Infirmary, Lancaster, UK

Integrating the principles of evidence-based medicine (EBM) into daily practice is an important but often difficult task. Despite the obstacles due to lack of knowledge, skills and resources, many tools exist to help learn and teach EBM. Educational programmes in EBM have been shown to change the behaviour of clinicians, improving critical appraisal skills and improving the implementation of EBM in the clinical workplace. Established educational activities, such as the journal club, can be modified to place EBM at their core. Access to sources of evidence at the point of delivering care to patients can assist evidence-based decision-making. Sources of pre-appraised evidence, including evidence-based guidelines, can speed up the process of applying evidence to practice. Strategies to disseminate evidence, such as educational programmes, clinical decision support systems and audit, can be useful tools to help change the practice of colleagues.

Introduction

The principles of evidence-based medicine (EBM) are well described [1] and the integration of these principles into practice is an important part of the daily work of clinicians [2]. However, three conditions need to be satisfied before EBM will work in practice. First, practitioners need the *motivation* to look for the evidence base for their work. The benefits of EBM have been outlined previously in this book, but for us, keeping up to date with relevant research is primarily a matter of professional pride. Second, people also need the *opportunity* to practise EBM. While clinical medicine and nursing are full of such opportunities, we do not always take them. Some of the reasons for this are explored in the next section. Lastly, we need to be equipped with the *tools and skills* to enable evidence-based practice. This chapter

Key words: Critical appraisal, journal club, implemenation of evidence.

will explore some of the obstacles to these conditions, and offer some strategies and practical suggestions to help learn and teach evidence-based anaesthesia.

The process of practising EBM can be summarised in five steps [3]:

1 formulate the clinical problem into an answerable question,
2 efficiently locate the best evidence with which to answer the question,
3 appraise the evidence to assess its validity and usefulness,
4 implement the results of the appraisal process in our clinical practice,
5 evaluate our performance.

Although this summary of the process is succinct, practising clinical medicine in this way presents challenges. Problems may arise at each step, and can vary with the type of question being asked, the environment in which we are working, the extent of our knowledge of the subject and the patient we are applying the answer to. It can be helpful to have some idea of the obstacles that lie between our desire to practise EBM and our ability to do so.

We will examine:

- difficulties in applying research evidence to practice,
- approaches to teaching evidence-based practice,
- strategies for implementing evidence-based anaesthesia (and EBM in general) and the evidence to support such strategies.

What prevents clinicians from using evidence more often?

The following is a consideration of some important obstacles to evidence based practice [4,5].

Lack of awareness of a gap in personal knowledge

Practitioners need to be aware of gaps in their knowledge in order to be able to formulate clinical questions. Without this insight, the process of seeking the best available evidence to support a given course of action cannot begin.

Lack of ability to formulate a clinical question

A clinical question needs to be properly formulated to allow a structured search for evidence to be undertaken. If the question is vague, or does not adequately relate to the clinical problem, the resulting search for information to answer the question will be more difficult. For example, the question "How can I relieve shoulder pain after an arthroscopy"? would be harder to answer with a literature search than the question "Are opioids as effective as an interscalene block for the relief of pain following shoulder arthroscopy"? Not only does formulating a precise question help focus the literature search, the discipline of having to specify it carefully helps us to think more clearly about the clinical problem.

Lack of access to information resources

The search for information with which to answer a clinical question depends on access to appropriate resources. These exist in a variety of formats, both printed and electronic, including textbooks, journals and bibliographic indices of the medical literature. The internet has revolutionised the availability of information, but problems with information retrieval still occur.

Lack of computers with internet access in the workplace is a major barrier to evidence-based practice. Slow or unreliable computers, organisational blocks on access to appropriate web sites, or lack of institutional subscriptions to the required resource also hinder the search for the best available evidence.

If the scope of the available resources is limited, then other problems arise. The resources may be out of date, may contain incorrect information or may be incomplete. Most of us will have endured the frustration of discovering that the required journal volume is the only one missing from the library shelf!

Lack of skills in retrieving and interpreting information from available resources

A well-formulated clinical question and access to high-quality resources are only of value if an appropriate search strategy is employed to find the necessary information. The amount of information available and the multiple ways in which it is presented can be bewildering, and an inadequate search may lead to information being missed and subsequent failure to answer the clinical question correctly.

A lack of skills to interpret and synthesise many pieces of evidence, some of which may have contradictory conclusions, can be another barrier to evidence-based practice. When faced with a complex collection of information, it may be easier to abandon the attempt to answer a clinical question, rather than process the information and draw a conclusion based upon the best evidence.

Difficulty in changing clinical practice in the light of evidence

Finding an answer to a clinical question does not automatically lead to a change in practice by an individual or within an organisation. It may be that the resources, financial or otherwise, are not available to implement the desired change. Key personnel may object to the changes, for many reasons. Current practice may be too entrenched to allow change to occur. The practitioner who wishes to instigate change may occupy a relatively junior position in the hierarchy of the organisation and therefore may not be in a position to influence policy. This is especially true of nurses.

Lack of time

Studies describing the barriers to evidence-based practice have reported lack of time as a major concern to many clinicians [4,5]. The demands of modern medical practice, particularly the "production pressure" on the part of managers, limit the amount of time available for educational activities, and many clinicians feel that the time spent in systematic pursuit of the answers to their clinical questions is a luxury they cannot afford. However, we feel that this is a rather blinkered view and suggest that it is time that clinicians exert conflicting pressure on management to emphasise that promoting effective, high-quality care by using the best available evidence may take time in the short term but that this time is well spent in the longer term.

The above issues represent some of the barriers to evidence-based practice. However, these difficulties can be successfully overcome, and the process of implementing EBM can be very rewarding.

Strategies for learning and teaching evidence-based practice

The objective of teaching programmes in EBM is to improve the skills and knowledge of participants in the programme, thereby helping them to improve their clinical decision-making abilities, and so, improve patient outcomes. Such teaching is effective. A systematic review [6] and a study using a validated questionnaire [7] have demonstrated significant increases in knowledge and skills of participants in EBM courses. Furthermore, educational approaches that integrate EBM skills teaching with daily clinical work have been found to be more effective at changing behaviour than classroom-based courses [6].

However, providing good quality educational opportunities can be difficult. Some problems that may arise include:
• lack of adequately trained faculty,
• lack of resources for educational materials,
• lack of time in the educational programmes of the target group.
Additionally, support for evidence-based skills teaching may be lacking at an organisational level because it is difficult to demonstrate an improvement in patient outcomes following educational interventions to improve skills in EBM [8,9].

How then should we go about creating opportunities for learning and teaching EBM? Many resources are available, for instance:
• dedicated courses run in specialist centres,
• distance learning courses delivered via the internet,
• integrating teaching sessions within existing educational programmes,
• delivering teaching in the clinical workplace.
Dedicated courses in specialist centres are likely to be expensive and will only have the capacity to teach a minority of practitioners, but can provide a core group of

individuals with knowledge that they can disseminate. Distance learning courses may be more cost effective, and be available to more people. Participants may lack the self-discipline to complete the course, but can work at their own pace, in their own time. Integrating critical appraisal skills teaching with existing educational programmes may be time and cost effective, but the lack of suitably qualified faculty to provide the teaching may be a problem. Delivering teaching in the clinical workplace may be an effective technique for changing behaviour [6], but may present time management challenges within the demands of a large clinical workload. The approach taken will depend on many factors, including financial resources available, the presence of skilled tutors locally, the number of people that need to be taught and the time available for such teaching.

However, the ideas of EBM are simple, and a little knowledge together with a lot of enthusiasm for using available opportunities will go a long way.

Practical techniques for learning and teaching EBM

General

It is important to regard the process of EBM as an integral part of clinical practice and education, rather than it being an "optional extra". There are numerous existing structures, which can be easily adapted to incorporate EBM techniques. Perhaps the most powerful influence is the experience of seeing a colleague whom one respects trying to "live out" EBM in practice. Further, if they are not yet expert at it, but are clearly still learning for themselves, this is even more impressive, as it demonstrates both humility (in that they recognise the limits to their knowledge and skills) but also the commitment to lifelong learning which characterises the most highly-regarded anaesthesia teachers [10].

Another vital behaviour we encourage is that of asking for help. This sometimes requires courage as it shows up an individual's ignorance. However, if we can overcome this, it allows us to gain from the knowledge and skills of others.

Generating and formulating questions

The heart of EBM is asking questions inspired by problems in clinical practice. These occur frequently, but often remain unanswered as they are not followed up. One strategy for making sure that these learning opportunities are not missed is to set up a "clinical question bank". Anyone can submit a question to the bank, and selected questions can be used to initiate the search for "Critically Appraised Topics (CATs)", described in more detail below, or to provide the topic and material for deeper appraisal in the journal club (see below). The bank of questions can be maintained by the departmental administrator and, to provide an incentive, individuals can be ranked at the end of each year on how many questions they have posed!

A more immediate technique is for teachers to issue an "educational prescription" [11] when the question first arises. These specify the clinical problem that gave rise to the question, the question to be answered, who is to answer it, and when it is to be done by. The learner is then given the task of "filling" the prescription. Another variant allows learners to issue prescriptions for their seniors. As well as reinforcing the impression that everyone is learning together, this helps prepare trainees for *their* future role as teachers too.

Searching

Information access in the workplace

Teaching critical appraisal skills in the clinical workplace has been shown to improve knowledge and change behaviour of participants [6].

The provision of high-quality sources of information (the "evidence cart") in the workplace to facilitate critical appraisal skills teaching has been described [12]. This resource consisted of printed and electronic materials available on a trolley, on the ward, for immediate access by the medical team. The presence of the "evidence cart" was found to increase the extent to which clinicians sought evidence to answer their clinical questions. Therefore, access to information sources in the clinical workplace is useful for the teaching and implementation of evidence-based practice. The provision of internet linked computers in the operating theatre suite can be very useful. Clinical questions that have been raised during preoperative assessment rounds can be investigated before, or between, cases. Similarly, access to electronic information sources on intensive care units can help anaesthetists to search for evidence in their daily practice.

Appraisal

Critical reading of research articles is nothing new. It has been a central skill in academic life and journal editing for many years. What is new is the idea that practising clinicians should learn to make sense of the evidence themselves, instead of relying on expert opinion. The aim now is to use research evidence to make us better clinicians rather than better researchers (though reading the reports of others' work often brings a good understanding of the research process too). While this sounds democratic, it means that we all need at least some understanding of critical appraisal techniques.

Critically appraised topics

CATs are summaries of evidence-based answers to clinical questions, and can be a useful tool to help teach EBM skills [11]. A CAT consists of the following components:
- a brief summary of the question,
- the steps taken to find the evidence (the search strategy),
- a brief synthesis of the evidence,
- the conclusion, or clinical "bottom line".

The questions for CATs can be made relevant by basing them on problems encountered in daily practice. For example, during a preoperative assessment of a patient for an elective abdominal aneurysm repair, the use of perioperative beta-blockade may be considered. However, it may be that neither the consultant nor the trainee anaesthetist is sure about the evidence for the risks and benefits of this intervention. This problem can form the basis of a CAT:

- The problem is formulated into an answerable clinical question: Does the use of perioperative beta-blockade reduce the postoperative morbidity and/or mortality for abdominal aneurysm repair?
- An appropriate search strategy is devised (see Chapter 3), possibly with the assistance of the medical librarian.
- Once identified and retrieved, the relevant studies are subjected to critical appraisal. This process can be undertaken as a group exercise as part of the journal club (see below).
- The evidence is synthesised into an answer to the clinical question, and presented as the clinical "bottom line".
- A short summary of the process is written, given a date for review, and added to the collection of CATs previously written. This process can also be done as part of an educational meeting.

By using commonly encountered problems as the basis for CAT writing, the practical benefits of EBM readily become apparent. Requiring participants in an educational programme to prepare CATs based on questions generated by their clinical experiences can be a valuable way to disseminate critical appraisal skills. Also, a collection of up-to-date CATs can form a bespoke evidence-based resource, tailored for local use, for future reference.

Teaching critical appraisal skills using the journal club format

The journal club is a familiar event in most postgraduate medical education programmes. Traditionally, it consists of a group of doctors and other practitioners who listen to a colleague present a summary of a paper from a recent journal. The presentation is followed by a discussion of the paper and its strengths and weaknesses. The extent to which the paper is subject to critical appraisal and consideration of its likely impact on clinical practice depends on the skills of those present.

The traditional journal club provides a forum for appraisal of published research and has the advantage of being a timetabled and established educational activity. The format of the journal club can be modified to allow skills of critical appraisal and EBM to be taught [13].

A programme of critical appraisal skills teaching using the journal club format is undertaken by one of the authors of this chapter in a busy anaesthesia department. The weekly timetabling of the journal club provides a relatively protected time when members of staff, both consultant and trainee, are able to attend. The course consists of ten 1 h sessions, with a curriculum based around four modules.

Level 1: Basic principles of critical appraisal

This introductory module aims to give trainees (and any experienced clinicians who also want to take part) an understanding of the basic principles of critical appraisal. A good place to start is with randomised controlled trials (RCTs) as these are familiar to most anaesthetists and it is possible to compare them against well-known standards for trial reporting (see for instance the CONSORT guidelines at www.consort-statement.org).

Level 2: Increasing relevance to practice

Once participants understand how to deal with published evidence, it is rewarding to put it to use in answering clinical questions, using the techniques described above.

Level 3: The anatomy of the anaesthesia journal

Whilst the RCT tends to predominate in clinical anaesthetic research, and this is a good starting point, journals contain other types of writing too. The focus of this module, then, is to understand the functions and structures of these different pieces. Exploration of the different types of paper, such as systematic reviews, traditional reviews, case-control and cohort studies, can be made, as well as consideration of the role of editorial pieces and correspondence.

Level 4: The nature and limits of evidence

This advanced level module can also be tied into clinically relevant material. A useful starting point is a sharing of ideas on the clinical topic of the paper, which introduces the notion that the same anaesthetic problem can be successfully managed in a number of ways, and there is often no single "textbook" technique. This leads on to a discussion of the evidence base and theoretical justification for each option, which in turn paves the way for exploring the relationship between knowledge and practice more generally. It is often instructive to choose an older, "classic" paper as it can be surprising how poorly conducted such studies can be by modern standards.

The programme was evaluated [14]. Participants felt more confident about critically appraising the literature after the course and self-reported understanding of terms relating to EBM also improved. The course also demonstrated that, with the availability of a suitably experienced tutor, critical appraisal skills teaching could be integrated into the existing programme of medical education of trainee doctors without additional financial resources.

Practical suggestions for running a journal club are given in the Box.

Practice points: Running a journal club session
- Organisation is important. It is best if a timetable is prepared for a few months in advance and the topics to be addressed are publicised beforehand.
- Journal clubs are social occasions as well as educational ones and drinks and possibly also food should be provided. This will encourage attendance, especially if you are planning to hold the session early in the morning or at lunchtime.
- A supportive senior clinician should lead the session. Setting the right tone is important – participants should not be afraid to contribute, even if this means showing their lack of knowledge. Enthusiastic trainees may lead the session but this should be in the presence of, and under the supervision of, their senior.
- Clinically relevant papers should be chosen wherever possible. The choice of topics will depend on the interests and needs of those present, but less specialised clinical material allows very junior anaesthetists to contribute and may therefore influence clinical practice more widely in the department of anaesthesia.
- We suggest that each person should have his or her own copy of the paper. These should be made available at least a few days before the meeting so that everyone can read the article through carefully before the meeting starts. Whilst some journal clubs encourage presenters to summarise articles, this can introduce a bias and we think it is better to read the authors' original words. In addition, each participant then has a reminder of what has been discussed to take away and keep.
- Sometimes, games may be used to enliven the session. For instance, splitting the participants into two teams, who take turns to debate the pros and cons of the article, referring to the text as they do so, can be fun, especially if a "referee" is appointed, complete with football shirt, whistle and stopwatch!

Integrating evidence into practice

Using pre-appraised evidence

The process of implementing evidence-based practice can be made easier by using sources of pre-appraised evidence that present summaries of critically appraised evidence, systematic reviews and other collations of information. Examples include *The Cochrane Database of Systematic Reviews* (www.thecochranelibrary.com), Clinical Evidence (www.clinicalevidence.com) and the UK National Institute for Health and Clinical Excellence (NICE) (www.nice.org.uk). Readers need to be aware, however, if such publications represent pure "evidence" or, in the case of some NICE guidance, the evidence "interpreted" by consensus groups. Whilst this is quite acceptable, it should always be made clear. The use of such sources can make the work of implementing evidence-based practice easier because they provide extensive critical appraisal of the medical literature. Other advantages include:

- they are easy to access,
- they are updated frequently,
- their contents are peer reviewed.

Disadvantages include:

- they are not comprehensive; not all clinical questions will have been addressed by all, or indeed any, of the sources,
- the clinical questions addressed may not be applicable to individual practice or patients,
- internet access is required for the latest versions.

Pre-appraised evidence sources do not remove the need for clinicians to have critical appraisal skills. The conclusions of some systematic reviews are controversial, and not universally accepted. Systematic reviews may have methodological flaws and may draw the wrong conclusions. Clinicians need to have critical appraisal skills and be able to make their own judgements about the validity of evidence, and about its applicability to individual patients in their own practice.

Clinical guidelines

Clinical guidelines can be another useful tool for implementing evidence-based practice. Guidelines are defined by the World Health Organisation [15] as:

"systematically developed evidence-based statements which assist providers, recipients and other stakeholders to make informed decisions about appropriate health interventions."

As well as guideline documents, this definition also encompasses protocols, consensus statements, expert committee recommendations and integrated care pathways.

From a public health and policymakers' perspective, guidelines offer various benefits [16]. They can:

- reduce variations in practice,
- discourage outdated and inefficient practice,
- highlight areas where gaps in evidence exist and so guide the research agenda,
- be used as standards against which clinical performance can be measured,
- improve the efficiency of health care delivery, freeing valuable resources.

By these means, the goals of improving practice and patient outcomes can be realised [17].

There are also disadvantages associated with guideline use:

- they may not be evidence based,
- harm can be done if a guideline makes the wrong recommendation,
- they may be difficult to apply to individual patients,

- local circumstances may not allow implementation of the guideline due to lack of resources among other factors,
- they may limit professional judgement by being too prescriptive.

Guidelines with a sound and explicit evidence base, compatibility of recommendations with existing values and no requirement for extra resources, skills or knowledge are more likely to be implemented [18]. Evidence based, robust guidelines that are transparent to critical appraisal are more likely to be used and are a valuable tool for evidence-based practice.

> **Practice points: the key principles of guideline writing**
> - systematic review and synthesis of the evidence,
> - explain the methodology of the guideline clearly to allow the guideline to be critically appraised,
> - make recommendations in a clear, accessible way that allows flexibility and application of the guideline to individual circumstances,
> - periodically review and update the guideline.

Organisations exist which produce evidence-based guidelines, such as the Scottish Intercollegiate Guidelines Network (www.sign.ac.uk) and the National Institute for Health and Clinical Excellence (www.nice.org.uk). An appraisal tool from the Appraisal of Guidelines for Research and Evaluation collaboration (www.agreecollaboration.org) can be used to assess the quality of guidelines.

Strategies to change behaviour

Applying the process of EBM to our clinical practice often leads to the conclusion that our practice must change, and consequently we need to consider ways in which we can influence the practice of others. The provision of high quality, well presented, robust evidence is the first step in this process. Once we have the evidence, there are many ways in which changes in behaviour can be encouraged in others [19].

Educational interventions

Various educational methods can be used to influence clinical practice:
- distribution of educational materials,
- conferences, courses and small group teaching,
- educational outreach,
- use of local opinion leaders.

Distributing educational materials such as booklets, posters or audiovisual media is relatively inexpensive, and may be useful as one part of a wider process. Courses and conferences, although useful, are generally less effective at changing behaviour than workshops [20]. Educational outreach, defined as a personal visit by a trained person to a health care provider in his or her own setting, can also be an effective method of changing behaviour [21]. The use of local opinion leaders, defined as health professionals nominated by their colleagues as being educationally influential, to disseminate advice, is less well supported by evidence [22], possibly because it is not always clear how to identify local opinion leaders. However, as we noted above, it is quite possible that a respected colleague who tries to practice EBM will be, or will become, a local opinion leader.

Clinical decision support systems

Clinical decision support systems are electronic or non-electronic systems designed to aid in clinical decision-making. Examples include electronic prescribing systems that issue reminders about drugs, including interactions, toxicity profiles and the need to monitor levels. Other systems may suggest certain investigations for a particular set of circumstances, or attach reminder notes to an anaesthetic chart. The purpose of these systems is to allow evidence-based recommendations to be delivered at the point of patient care, tailored to individual patients. They can be effective instruments for improving the quality of care that we deliver [23].

Other interventions

Other techniques can be employed to help to implement change. Audit and feedback, financial interventions and mass media campaigns have all been used with generally positive effects [19].

Some of the techniques outlined will be beyond the reach of most clinicians, but some are relatively simple tools to aid in the implementation of evidence-based practice. For example, small group teaching, printed educational materials and audit and feedback processes are low-cost and low-technology interventions that can yield improvements to practice. In general, combinations of different techniques to change behaviour are more likely to be successful than techniques used singly.

Practice points: changing behaviour

- Persuading others to change their practice relies on the provision of robust evidence that is clinically relevant: pre-appraised evidence sources can make finding the evidence a more manageable task.
- Implementation strategies are more likely to succeed if a combination of techniques is used.
- Low-cost, low-technology strategies can work well!
- Clinical decision support systems can be a useful way of bringing evidence directly into the clinical workplace.
- Audit processes can give encouragement to the change process by demonstrating the benefits of the implemented changes.

Summary

This chapter has explored some of the obstacles to the teaching and practice of evidence-based anaesthesia and suggested some solutions. The difficulties encountered are far from insurmountable, and the environment in which anaesthetists work can be favourable for both teaching and implementing evidence-based practice:

- The diversity of clinical conditions that anaesthetists manage provides an excellent opportunity for asking clinical questions.
- Operating theatre work offers many opportunities for high-quality teaching and exploration of clinical questions.
- Critical care medicine provides a more traditional ward environment for clinical workplace teaching.
- Anaesthetists' working environments are increasingly provided with internet linked computers.
- Teaching programmes are usually well organised and can incorporate critical appraisal skills teaching.
- Protected time for journal clubs can allow this educational activity to become an important part of EBM skills teaching.
- Anaesthesia is a large speciality, and can therefore exert influence within organisations to bring about evidence-based practice.

The integration of pre-appraised evidence, clinical guidelines and clinicians' own appraisal of the literature can be implemented into a rational practice by using a variety of techniques to change our own behaviour and that of our colleagues.

Acknowledgments

We thank the European Society of Anaesthesiology for permission to reproduce material from a refresher course lecture "Getting evidence into practice: how to read a paper and run a journal club", delivered at the 2005 meeting in Vienna.

FURTHER READING

1 The UK Centre for Evidence-Based Medicine, based in Oxford, has an excellent web site that provides a large number of EBM resources. (www.cebm.net)
2 David Sackett's book "Evidence Based Medicine – how to practice and teach EBM" [11] is a very readable general introduction to EBM.

REFERENCES

1 Sackett DL, Rosenberg WM, Gray JA, Haynes RB, Richardson WS. Evidence based medicine: what it is and what it isn't. *BMJ* 1996; 312(7023): 71–2.

2 Whitcomb ME. Why we must teach evidence-based medicine. *Acad Med* 2005; 80: 1–2.

3 Greenhalgh T. How to read a paper. The basics of evidence based medicine, 2nd edition. London: BMJ Publishing Group, 2001.

4 Ely JW, Osheroff JA, Ebell MH, Chambliss ML, Vinson DC, Stevermer JJ, Pifer EA. Obstacles to answering doctors' questions about patient care with evidence: qualitative study. *BMJ* 2002; 324(7339): 710.

5 Green ML, Ruff TR. Why do residents fail to answer their clinical questions? A qualitative study of barriers to practicing evidence-based medicine. *Acad Med* 2005; 80(2): 176–82.

6 Coomarasamy A, Khan KS. What is the evidence that postgraduate teaching in evidence based medicine changes anything? A systematic review. *BMJ* 2004; 329(7473): 1017.

7 Fritsche L, Greenhalgh T, Falck-Ytter Y, Neumayer HH, Kunz R. Do short courses in evidence based medicine improve knowledge and skills? Validation of Berlin questionnaire and before and after study of courses in evidence based medicine. *BMJ* 2002; 325(7376): 1338–41.

8 Dobbie AE, Schneider FD, Anderson AD, Littlefield J. What evidence supports teaching evidence-based medicine? *Acad Med* 2000; 75(12): 1184–5.

9 Parkes J, Hyde C, Deeks J, Milne R. Teaching critical appraisal skills in health care settings. *The Cochrane Database of Syst Rev* 2001, Issue 3. Art. No.: CD001270. DOI. 10.1002/1465185.

10 Cleave-Hogg D, Benedict C. Characteristics of good anaesthesia teachers. *Can J Anaesth* 1997; 44: 587–91.

11 Sackett DL, Straus SE, Richardson WS, Rosenberg W, Haynes RB. *Evidence-based Medicine: How to Practice and Teach EBM*, 2nd edition. Edinburgh: Churchill Livingstone, 2000.

12 Sackett DL, Straus SE. Finding and applying evidence during clinical rounds: the "evidence cart". *JAMA* 1998; 280(15): 1336–8.

13 Milbrandt EB, Vincent JL. Evidence-based medicine journal club. *Crit Care* 2004; 8(6): 401–2.

14 Knight S, Smith AF. Using the journal club format to foster critical appraisal skills in anaesthetic trainees. *Eur J Anaesthesiol* 2003; 20(Suppl 30): 7.

15 World Health Organisation. *Guideline for WHO guidelines*. EIP/GPE/EQC/2003.1 2003.

16 Woolf SH, Grol R, Hutchinson A, Eccles M, Grimshaw J. Clinical guidelines: potential benefits, limitations, and harms of clinical guidelines. *BMJ* 1999; 318(7182): 527–30.

17 Grimshaw JM, Russell IT. Effect of clinical guidelines on medical practice: a systematic review of rigorous evaluations. *Lancet* 1993; 342(8883): 1317–22.

18 Grol R, Dalhuijsen J, Thomas S, Veld C, Rutten G, Mokkink H. Attributes of clinical guidelines that influence use of guidelines in general practice: observational study. *BMJ* 1998; 317(7162): 858–61.

19 Grol R, Grimshaw J. From best evidence to best practice: effective implementation of change in patients' care. *Lancet* 2003; 362(9391): 1225–30.

20 O'Brien MA, Freemantle N, Oxman AD, Wolf F, Davis DA, Herrin J. Continuing education meetings and workshops: effects on professional practice and health care outcomes. *The Cochrane Database of Syst Rev* 2001, Issue 1. Art. No.: CD 003030. DOI: 10.1002/14651858.

21 O'Brien MA, Oxman AD, Davis DA, Haynes RB, Freemantle N, Harvey EL. Educational outreach visits: effects on professional practice and health care outcomes. *The Cochrane Database of Syst Rev* 1997, Issue 4. Art. No.: CD000409. DOI: 10.1002/14651858.

22 O'Brien MA, Oxman AD, Haynes RB, Davis DA, Freemantle N, Harvey EL. Local opinion leaders: effects on professional practice and health care outcomes. *The Cochrane Database of Syst Rev* 1999, Issue 1. Art. No.: CD000125. DOI: 10.1002/14651858.

23 Kawamoto K, Houlihan CA, Balas EA, Lobach DF. Improving clinical practice using clinical decision support systems: a systematic review of trials to identify features critical to success. *BMJ* 2005; 330(7494): 765.

11

Involving patients and consumers in health care and decision-making processes: nothing about us without us

Nete Villebro[1] and Janet Wale[2]

[1]Department of Anaesthesiology, H:S Bispebjerg University Hospital, Copenhagen, Denmark
[2]Cochrane Consumer Network, Perth, Australia

This chapter sets out to emphasise the place for patient-centred care with provision of the relevant information and effective communication that forms the basis of informed consent to, and preparation for, an occasion of anaesthesia. Patient-relevant outcomes are important to consider in clinical research that sets out to inform best practice and health care management in the anaesthetic environment. Many patients do want to be informed in a way that allows them to prepare for an episode of anaesthesia and to work toward improving outcomes.

Introduction

Receivers of health care, also termed consumers or patients, are involved in the systematic review process within The Cochrane Collaboration. This is in line with thinking that the best systematic reviews of health care interventions are those produced by teams comprising users, practitioners and researchers [1].

The Cochrane Collaboration defines a consumer as an individual who has unique personal experiences that allow him or her to provide an effective health care user or receiver perspective to a systematic review question. The term is used more broadly than for patients actively under treatment and the role of consumers in Cochrane Review Groups (Pregnancy and Childbirth, Breast Cancer, Haematological Malignancies) is the subject of a number of publications [2–4]. Consumers are also actively involved in the editorial process of the Cochrane Anaesthesia Review Group (CARG).

People have a right to be involved in decisions that involve their own bodies and their own value systems as well as financial commitments to health care, both

Key words: Patient-centred care in anaesthesia, shared decision-making, well-informed decision, patient-relevant anaesthesia outcome measures.

individually and by health systems. Large amounts of health care information, of varying quality, are available through the media, the internet, corporate organisations and health care providers. Yet in many ways consumers are increasingly on their own in the quest to make the right health decisions for themselves and their family and to identify sources of information knowing the role of vested interests around profiting from illness. To make a well-informed decision requires awareness (obtained from evidence-based, relevant and up-to-date information) of the potential benefits, uncertainties, physical risks, and psychological, moral, social and financial costs involved.

This chapter sets out to highlight the concept of the informed patient who takes an active role in shared decision-making with their health care providers, in the context of anaesthesia. Patient-centred care is considered in the sense that an individual has the right for information about their health care in the context of their own medical history, physical and psychological characteristics, personal and social values. These personal inputs have an important role in informed consent, reducing anxiety and optimising health outcomes and increasing patient and provider satisfaction.

The informed patient and shared decision-making

If a patient wishes to be actively involved in their health care and to understand the options open to them then shared decision-making is an important process. A well-informed patient is able to discuss openly with their physician the benefits and possible harms of treatment together with any alternatives. The end decision is passed through a filter of the patient's knowledge, personal characteristics, beliefs and values [5]. A consultation between a patient and physician is often seen as part of a ritual that involves a large degree of trust on the part of the patient. Many patients believe they have to be "good" for the doctor. This is interpreted as not questioning the physician's judgements in any way, which prevents them asking questions, no matter how important to them. They may feel obliged to accept the physician, his manner, and the treatment he proposes and delivers without querying options or stating any discomfort and concerns [6].

A physician generally has, limited time for consultation. Prior to an anaesthetic occasion of service, this may take place in an environment that is lacking in terms of space, convenience, privacy free of interruption and availability of necessary equipment. Under these circumstances a patient is often ill or under stress so that they may not be clear headed, rational nor ready to hear about risks, costs and the relative benefits and harms of one procedure or treatment compared with another, especially if the consultation takes place the day before, the morning of, or immediately before a required procedure. These factors can introduce a high degree of tension into the interaction.

Patients differ in how involved they want to be in decision-making about their health care. The same patient may also feel differently under different circumstances. Nevertheless, it is important that accessible information is made available, with the time to discuss it or for an individual to peruse that information on their own in private. A better understanding of a person's health care and the decisions about treatment and care may be particularly important for procedures such as joint replacement or coronary angioplasty. For example, a study of a group of patients requiring angioplasty showed that an education and counselling programme, as well as the conventional ward care and education provided to the control group, helped those patients with anxiety about the procedure. This benefit passed on to their caregivers so that everyone coped better in the longer term [7].

Trust

Entwistle in an editorial [8] explained that a patient is likely to feel safer and more able to engage in an open discussion about treatment options when he or she is confident that the health professional will listen to their concerns. They want their questions to be answered honestly and in a way that respects their views. Studies report a clear relationship between patients' trust in their physicians and their preference for involvement in treatment decision-making. Those who preferred an active role were likely to have moderate to high levels of trust in the patient–physician relationship. Patients with high levels of trust played a passive role [9–11].

A physician's motivation and orientation towards patients is important ethically, socially and psychologically for the patient. This is no more so than with interventions requiring an anaesthetist, where a person is indeed vulnerable.

Patient-centred care

When we talk about patient-centred health care we are referring to a relationship in which the values of the patient, their family and carers are incorporated into the decision-making process about which intervention(s) are to be used and the development of an agreed care-management plan. The required principles and concepts are: communication, balanced information and consideration of patient-centred values and outcomes [12]. Most studies on patient-centred care are based in primary care and outpatient clinics; and patient-centred care is an important issue in the treatment of chronic conditions [13].

Communication and information

Information and effective communication are crucial to informed patient consent and shared decision-making that incorporates a sense of feeling respected and able to make a meaningful contribution to the decision-making process [14–16]. It is important that the process of obtaining consent is adapted to match a person's ability to comprehend information [17]. Many patients do not know what information might be relevant to their clinical situation – so it is the physician's responsibility to provide the appropriate information. In this way physicians are able to guide patients to decisions as well as making recommendations. Similarly, patients do not always want detailed information when giving informed consent, particularly for decisions that are inevitable, involve life or death or when only one medically reasonable option exists [18].

Decision aids (http://decisionaid.ohri.ca/AZinvent.php) have been developed to inform choices in health care and to improve the process of informed consent [19]. It may be that patients reach the same decision as their physician but they are more comfortable with it [20,21].

Systems of care

Medical intervention is aimed at increasing the length and quality of life. Yet our culture today is often driven by technological imperative – bigger and better equipment, more measurements, faster and more efficiency. Unfortunately treatment may result in little benefit or even adverse events and hospitalisation in itself can cause harm. In this environment a place remains to encourage patients to have realistic expectations of health care and of their personal role in it. Within clinical governance, administrators and staff take responsibility to ensure that appropriate structures, processes and monitoring systems are in place to ensure clinical safety and quality, on a collective and individual level. Population health, health equality and the responsiveness of the health system to the legitimate expectations of the population are considered as human rights. We expect respect for personal dignity, autonomy of the individual to make choices about health, confidentiality of personal health information, prompt attention to health needs with basic amenities (clean waiting rooms, adequate beds and food in hospitals) as well as access to social support networks, choice of institution and individual providing care (World Health Organisation Framework for Health System Performance Assessment 2000).

Anaesthesia and surgical procedures have improved dramatically over the years in terms of drugs, materials, equipment, training and standards of care. Anaesthesia is relatively safe and methods of anaesthesia used largely depends on physician preferences and hospital practice. In an environment of escalating health care costs, systems of care are also changing with reduced lengths of stay in hospital following procedures under anaesthesia, increasing use of endoscopy and laser surgical techniques and wide use of day surgeries. When presenting at a health care facility on the morning of a procedure under anaesthetic or sedation in order to return home on the same day (or to an aftercare facility for social, administrative or clinical reasons) the turnaround time, recovery and comfort in the immediate postoperative period, and patient discharge become very important.

Evidence-based practice

Evidence-based health care is dependent on an effective transfer of information (evidence) and its incorporation into practice. The values of patients, their families and carers and service providers form an inherent part of evidence-based practice. Clinical practice guidelines are developed to improve health outcomes for patients as well as to improve the quality and consistency of health care.

Outcomes

Providing information to patients is aimed at improving health outcomes. For a patient before surgery this may result in a reduction in the number of complications, length of stay in hospital, reduced need for pain relief (where they are less stressed because they know what to expect), and increased confidence and sense of satisfaction about their health care [22]. Yet "bottom line" clinical variables are often used as the measures of effectiveness of clinical care. These include: death, especially if untimely; incidence of disease (strokes and cardiac episodes); use of health care systems and cost effectiveness. Clinical controlled trials often use surrogate measures that are easy to follow over a short period of time (e.g., blood pressure, bone mineral density, blood and biochemical markers) but their relationship to the bottom line variables or patient well-being is not well defined. Subjective experience of illness; discomfort, which includes pain, nausea, breathlessness, fatigue; disability, loss of function in activities of daily living, work or recreation and independent living; dissatisfaction and emotional reaction to disease or its care and destitution; loss of financial or social status as a result of illness are other commonly used outcome measures in clinical studies [23].

A mismatch of the concerns and needs of consumers and what is determined in health care research [24–26] has led to consumer input into health care decision-making, policy and funding of research proposals [27]. Outcomes of importance to consumers and patient groups are vital for health research as a measure of quality of life and well-being [16]. In the systematic review process the study outcomes are integral to the relevance and quality of Cochrane reviews. These are limited by the design and process of included studies and are measured in a way that enables statistical analysis and meta-analysis, that is, a consistent way of measuring outcomes across studies. Kelson [28] concluded that Review Groups varied considerably in the extent to which they involved consumers in developing reviews and that there was no apparent consensus on the importance attached to patient-defined outcomes.

The individual patient: health care provider role in anaesthesia

Many people want to know more about what is happening to their bodies with health care including in the anaesthetic environment. Can the patient have the opportunity to play an active role in decision-making and is there a place to practise this in the time and space that is available? Are outcomes of direct interest to patients reported in the relevant research?

The preanaesthetic consultation

The preanaesthetic consultation is a crucial time for someone who wants to have an interactive role in their health care. It is here they are able to discuss the process, risks and possible options for interventions and techniques and arrive at informed consent. It ideally takes place when an individual is not sedated, only minimally stressed or anxious, has support – for example with a carer – and in a suitable environment with adequate privacy and at an appropriate time. The consultation ideally provides sufficient time to ask any questions, consult notes and previous records and have the required medical examinations and tests to *ensure* safety and quality experience while promoting patient satisfaction.

The consultation is preferably conducted by the attending anaesthetist responsible for anaesthesia care. The aim is to ensure that the person feels comfortable that they are physically and mentally prepared for anaesthesia, for example by satisfying and reassuring them if they are already on medications, have an existing medical condition that may affect their response to an anaesthetic and a history of less than optimal previous anaesthetic experiences.

• The perspective that "the patient" brings away from the consultation is important for the comfort of the individual, the value of the informed consent and in improving communication.

Other relevant issues for consumers are: the place of care (or setting); duration of stay; the provision of care in terms of health providers available; whether the surgery is emergency or elective; how they can (or must) prepare for surgery and any precautions they can take, especially if they have co-existing conditions or disabilities; and the information that is made available to them. The purpose is to reassure, rather than alarm, and to be aware of possibilities so that an individual can better prepare physically, psychologically and emotionally for the episode of health care.

The immediate preanaesthesia period

The immediate preanaesthesia period is a time when it is important to confirm that informed consent (with awareness of risks and techniques to be used) has been given and that it is documented. Prophylactic anti-emetic treatment is given to individuals with a history of postoperative nausea and vomiting; adequate peri-operative management of current medications is confirmed; any adverse incidents relating to administration of preoperative medication recorded and given to the patient for future reference. These processes of care management can all involve the individual and serve to reassure the patient.

Surveys of patient perceptions of the quality of information and communication provided are important, as reflected in the following input from consumers.

"In our system they give you the information in advance when they do the pre-operation examinations, in order to get you to sign consent, but they again go over it all when you are on your operating theatre bed, 5 min just before the operation. They verify that you really do know what is about to happen and what the risks are – just to be sure! This is because sometimes the people that prepped you in advance are no longer the ones about to do the deeds, because the shift has changed. Every individual has to be sure that you have received the information. I can see the rationale from their point of view, but it is awful for the patient".

"Preadmission education seems to be the 'norm' now for anything other than emergency surgery given hospital stays, etc. Unfortunately, I think the level of information given varies greatly – even within the same institution iatrogenic errors and other errors are never mentioned in my experience in spite of the fact that both evidence and literature inform us that these are very, very common".

Furthermore, an e-mail was sent out (July 2005) to a number of different cancer survivors (ovarian, breast and colorectal cancer) in Canada asking them about the level of information or counselling on the risks of anaesthesia they had received before a surgical procedure. The response from 31 women indicated that more than half (61%) did not recall receiving such information either before or on the day of surgery (most experiences after the year 2000). A number of those who confirmed a "Yes" response indicated that they did not understand what they were being told (Sandi P, personal communication).

The intraoperative period

The intraoperative period is a "lost time" for the patient (hopefully but not always the case as is shown by legal actions in Victoria, Australia [29]). What is important is that a person is not aware of activities at any time when they are meant to be "under" a general anaesthetic (many people's nightmare) and that they are adequately monitored by appropriately trained staff. It is also important for the patient that an adequate record is kept and any untoward events (particularly life-threatening physiological events) recorded (perioperatively and during immediate postoperative recovery) and that these are available to the patient to inform future anaesthetic procedures; and that they are satisfied with the quality of their recovery.

The immediate postoperative period

The main trend today is to make the postoperative period as comfortable as possible for the patient and to facilitate the anaesthetist's workload. This is an attitude that also benefits the patient.

Pain management

Management of acute pain and any untoward reactions or events as a result of pain management (or lack of) are reflected in patient satisfaction. Patients benefit from effective pain management as they are more ready to actively participate in rehabilitation (e.g., with coughing, and physically moving about). Awareness by staff of pain intensity and provision of adequate attention and care has a large impact on a person's postoperative care.

Day surgery

Day surgery anaesthesia also requires consultation by an anaesthetist for medical assessment, at an appropriate time and in adequate consultation facilities. In this setting patients are required to meet specific discharge criteria prior to separation. It is important that these criteria are clear to and discussed with the patient – in a way that reassures patients about safety, patient care and efficiency of the health care facilities. Concerns for a patient include the waiting time from arrival to procedure; total fasting time; rushed and unexpected tests; cancellation of procedure and any adverse or unplanned events. The facility has a duty of care to the patient; this too needs to be explained to the patient and their carer ahead of time so that they are able to make appropriate arrangements with realistic expectations.

Return to normal daily function and optimising recovery

Areas that an individual may want information on and which are components of informed consent are age considerations; possible postanaesthetic effects; pain and anxiety management; any special care and considerations around aggravation of co-existing conditions.

What consumers want to know about anaesthesia

As an initial step in finding out more about what *the patient wants*, we asked members of The Cochrane Collaboration Consumer Network, best described as informed consumers, what their main concerns are about anaesthesia. This was possible through an e-mail discussion list with around 270 members (26 July 2005) of whom 25 responded (Figure 11.1). It is apparent from this informal e-mail survey that people do want to have relevant information conveyed to them. The purpose is to help them be informed in a way that facilitates mutual satisfaction and so that they know what to expect, both as part of coping and to plan social

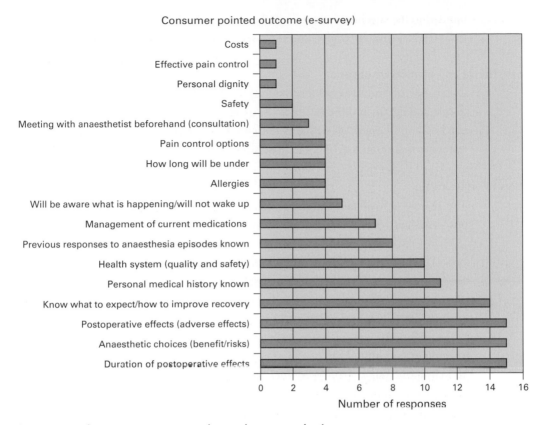

Figure 11.1 What consumers want to know about anaesthesia

support. An idea of the duration of possible postoperative effects, for example cognitive effects and the ability to be involved in choices about anaesthesia is important. These consumers were concerned about the postoperative recovery period, in terms of residual effects of the anaesthetic and how long these are likely to persist.

People also wanted to receive a report on their response to an anaesthetic. This was for future reference, to be able to gain the relevant information from an anaesthesia episode to inform future requirements for anaesthesia.

In the light of ever-increasing use of day surgery, laser and endoscopic techniques, consumer concerns are likely to increase in significance and the impact of anaesthesia to be more apparent to the individual and their carers.

Outcomes measured in Cochrane anaesthesia protocols

To investigate the outcomes looked at in research, the authors selected review protocols from the Cochrane Anaesthesia Review Group, Cochrane Library module, blinded to the specified outcomes. Other reviews in *The Cochrane Library* that relate to anaesthesia but are under condition-specific Review Groups were not considered.

Anaesthesia and medical diseases

Outcomes of the selected protocols [30,31] related strongly to cardiovascular events and death, and the safety of the drug interventions; quality of life was measured in both. Length of stay was measured in [31] and can be seen as a system's outcome that relates strongly to provision of beds, use of resources and costs.

Drugs in anaesthesia

The review of Walker et al. [32] related specifically to day surgery with system's outcomes aimed at the turnaround time of patients. The review of Delgado et al. [33] covered procedures (endoscopy, radiological) also without hospital admission. The outcomes had a strong emphasis on the providers, their ability to successfully carry out the procedure and safety considerations for the patient. Length of stay and costs were considered. The outcomes pain tolerance to procedure adverse effects (including low oxygen levels, amnesia) related strongly to the service provider and system outcomes. Patient satisfaction was an important patient-orientated outcome. One of the reviews in children [34] was in a related setting and similarly had a strong provider perspective in terms of tolerance of the children to the procedure and its successful completion and any adverse events or safety issues. Parent satisfaction was considered. The paediatric review by Cardwell et al. [35] sets out to specifically look at a potential side effect of the intervention being considered. These outcomes translated into length of stay.

Perianaesthetic

A paediatric review by Cyna et al. [36] used outcomes of effectiveness against pain; any complications or adverse effects and outcomes were set against system's outcomes of delayed discharge/readmission, use of equipment, length of stay and overall costs. Procedural time was particularly relevant to service provider as well as the health facilities. One outcome was specific to the procedure.

The protocol by Werawatganon and Charuluxanun [37] described outcomes relating to the effectiveness of the intervention work balanced by possible adverse effects, pain and failure of the intervention. System-orientated outcomes were opioid consumption and length of hospital stay. The outcomes listed in Price et al. [38] related specifically to "did the intervention work and were there any adverse effects or safety issues"?

The review by Lee and Done [39] related in practice to older people. Deaths and complications were important outcomes. Patient well-being and return of function were also listed as was cognitive dysfunction after anaesthesia, an important consideration for patients and their caregivers. Readmission was the system's outcome considered.

Postanaesthetic unit

Death was the primary outcome in the review by Müllner et al. [40]. Patients were considered in terms of levels of anxiety and depression and quality of life; other outcomes related to requirements from the health services and subsequent costs. The review by Khan et al. [41] was specific to a clinical event and its adverse consequences. Outcomes related to death, cardiovascular events and increased use of hospital facilities.

Practice points
- *What we know*: is that "consumers" could be much more involved in setting the research agenda, so that they are given the opportunity to say what they feel is relevant to them as "patients".
- *What we think we know*: is that consumers are starting to participate in studies with very interesting results. Consumers are even in the early stages of writing their own systematic reviews. We hope this will be a growing trend.
- *What we do not know*: consumer information needs to be widely publicised before it can become a powerful instrument. Consumers need to know how, and why, they are so important in the development of research.

Research agenda
- Individuals have the right to information about their health care in the context of their own medical history; physical and psychological characteristics; personal and social values. This information plays an important role in informed consent, reducing anxiety and optimising health outcomes and increasing patient and provider satisfaction. More attention needs to be paid to it when research is in the planning stage.
- The increased accessibility of information adds to the importance of involving consumers in research. Consumer participation helps make research results more readily understandable.

Closing comments

Outcomes specified in review protocols that are of direct relevance to an individual patient's concerns about anaesthesia are reflected in a very limited way in the CARG module of *The Cochrane Library*. Consumers, or users of health care, are, therefore, less able to contribute to a meaningful dialogue in shared evidence-based decision-making in this area of health care as it now stands and in a way that promotes human values. In anaesthesia, clinical governance and financial management are vital factors in the availability and practice of effective health care. Cochrane systematic reviews play an important part in directing research and a considered view of the outcomes that are measured is important.

With the development of electronic patient records patients will have access to their medical information. As an example, in Denmark a person who has a digital signature can go to the internet and find valuable personal information that they can utilise to prepare for their next meeting with the health care system.

We hope that future research will strive to firmly establish consumer perspectives. Quality of life is very difficult to use as an effective measure of individual well-being. Similarly length of stay is a complex issue. The circumstances around discharge from a health care organisation influence patient satisfaction as well as having system and economic implications. We look forward to collaboration on developing consumer-identified outcomes and patient indicators of satisfaction in the area of anaesthesia and recovery in the future.

REFERENCES

1 Gyte G, Grant-Pearce C, Henderson S, Horey D et al. Does Consumer Refereeing Improve the Quality of Systematic Reviews of Health Care Interventions? The Perspective of Editors and Authors. *Fifth International Congress on Peer Review*. Chicago: Biomedical Publication, September 16–18, 2005.

2 Ghersi D. Making it happen: approaches to involving consumers in Cochrane reviews. *Eval Health Prof* 2002; 25(3): 270–83.

3 Sakala C, Gyte G, Henderson S, Neilson JP, Horey D. Consumer-professional partnership to improve research: the experience of the Cochrane Collaboration's Pregnancy and Childbirth Group. *Birth* 2001; 28(2): 133–7.

4 Skoetz N, Weingart O, Engert A. A consumer network for haematological malignancies. *Health Expect* 2005; 8(1): 86–90.

5 Kravitz RL, Melnikow J. Engaging patients in medical decision making. *BMJ* 2001; 323(7313): 584–5.

6 Jadad AR, Rizo CA, Enkin MW. I am a good patient, believe it or not. *BMJ* 2003; 326(7402): 1293–5.

7 Tooth L, McKenna K, Maas F, McEniery P. The effects of pre-coronary angioplasty education and counselling on patients and their spouses: a preliminary report. *Patient Educ Couns* 1997; 32(3): 185–96.

8 Entwistle V. Trust and shared decision-making: an emerging research agenda. *Health Expect* 2004; 7(4): 271–3.

9 Charles C, Gafni A, Whelan T. Self-reported use of shared decision-making among breast cancer specialists and perceived barriers and facilitators to implementing this approach. *Health Expect* 2004; 7(4): 338–48.

10 Kraetschmer N, Sharpe N, Urowitz S, Deber RB. How does trust affect patient preferences for participation in decision-making? *Health Expect* 2004; 7(4): 317–26.

11 Thom DH, Campbell B. Patient-physician trust: an exploratory study. *J Fam Pract* 1997; 44(2): 169–76.

12 Roberts C. "Only connect": the centrality of doctor-patient relationships in primary care. *Fam Pract* 2004; 21(3): 232–3.

13 Bauman AE, Fardy HJ, Harris PG. Getting it right: why bother with patient-centred care? *Med J Aust* 2003; 179(5): 253–6.

14 Harrington J, Noble LM, Newman SP. Improving patients' communication with doctors: a systematic review of intervention studies. *Patient Educ Couns* 2004; 52(1): 7–16.

15 Rogers WA. Is there a tension between doctors' duty of care and evidence-based medicine? *Health Care Anal* 2002; 10(3): 277–87.

16 Thornton H, Edwards A, Elwyn G. Evolving the multiple roles of "patients" in health-care research: reflections after involvement in a trial of shared decision-making. *Health Expect* 2003; 6(3): 189–97.

17 Ågård A. Informed consent: theory versus practice. *Nat Clin Pract Cardiovasc* 2005; 2: 270.

18 Beresford N, Seymour L, Vincent C, Moat N. Risks of elective cardiac surgery: what do patients want to know? *Heart* 2001; 86(6): 626–31.

19 O'Connor AM, Stacey D, Entwistle V, Llewellyn-Thomas H, Rovner D, Holmes-Rovner M, Talt V, Tetroe J, Fiset V, Barry M, Jones J. Decision aids for people facing health treatment or screening decisions. *The Cochrane Database of Syst Rev* 2003, Issue 1. Art. No.: CD001431. DOI: 10.1002/14651858.

20 Holmes-Rovner M. Likely consequences of increased patient choice. *Health Expect* 2005; 8(1): 1–3.

21 Montgomery AA, Fahey T. How do patients' treatment preferences compare with those of clinicians? *Qual Health Care* 2001; 10(Suppl 1): i39–43.

22 Garretson S. Benefits of pre-operative information programmes. *Nurs Stand* 2004; 18(47): 33–7.

23 Greenhalgh T. Outside ivory towers: evidence-based medicine in the real world. *Br J Gen Pract* 1998; no. 48: 1448–9.

24 Corner J. Interface between research and practice in psycho-oncology. *Acta Oncol* 1999; 38(6): 703–7.

25 Lexchin J, Bero LA, Djulbegovic B, Clark O. Pharmaceutical industry sponsorship and research outcome and quality: systematic review. *BMJ* 2003; 326(7400): 1167–70.

26 Tallon D, Chard J, Dieppe P. Relation between agendas of the research community and the research consumer. *Lancet* 2000; 355(9220): 2037–40.

27 Boote J, Telford R, Cooper C. Consumer involvement in health research: a review and research agenda. *Health Policy* 2002; 61(2): 213–36.

28 Kelson MC. Consumer collaboration, patient-defined outcomes and the preparation of Cochrane Reviews. *Health Expect* 1999; 2(2): 129–35.

29 Cass NM. Medicolegal claims against anaesthetists: a 20 year study. *Anaesth Intensive Care* 2004; 32(1): 47–58.

30 Choi PT, Beattie WS, Bender JS, Wijeysundera DN. Nitrates for the prevention of cardiac morbidity and mortality in patients undergoing noncardiac surgery. (Protocol) *The Cochrane Database of Syst Rev* 2004, Issue 4. Art. No.: CD005141. DOI: 10.1002/14651858.

31 Wiesbauer F, Domanovits H, Schlager O, Wildner B, Schillinger M. Perioperative beta-blockers for preventing surgery related mortality and morbidity. (Protocol) *The Cochrane Database of Syst Rev* 2003, Issue 2. Art. No.: CD004476. DOI: 10.1002/14651858.

32 Walker KJ, Smith AF, Pittaway AJ. Premedication for anxiety in adult day surgery. *The Cochrane Database of Syst Rev* 2003, Issue 1. Art. No.: CD002192. DOI: 10.1002/14651858.

33 Delgado M, Gempeler F, Rodríguez N. Analgo-sedation for diagnostic and therapeutic endoscopic or radiologic procedures in adults. (Protocol) *The Cochrane Database of Syst Rev* 2003, Issue 4. Art. No.: CD004582. DOI: 10.1002/14651858.

34 Evered L, Klassen TP, Hartling L, Wiebe N, Rowe BH. Options for procedural sedation in paediatric patients requiring painful or anxiety provoking procedures outside the operating room. (Protocol) *The Cochrane Database of Syst Rev* 2001, Issue 2. Art. No.: CD003704. DOI: 10.1002/14651858.

35 Cardwell M, Siviter G, Smith A. Non-steroidal anti-inflammatory drugs and perioperative bleeding in paediatric tonsillectomy. *The Cochrane Database of Syst Rev* 2005, Issue 2. Art. No.: CD003591. DOI: 10.1002/14651858.

36 Cyna AM, Jha S, Parsons JE. Caudal epidural block versus other methods of postoperative pain relief for circumcision in boys. *The Cochrane Database of Syst Rev* 2003, Issue 2. Art. No.: CD003005. DOI: 10.1002/14651858.

37 Werawatganon T, Charuluxanun S. Patient controlled intravenous opioid analgesia versus continuous epidural analgesia for pain after intra-abdominal surgery. *The Cochrane Database of Syst Rev* 2005, Issue 1. Art. No.: CD004088. DOI: 10.1002/14651858.

38 Price JD, Sear JW, Venn RM. Perioperative fluid volume optimization following proximal femoral fracture. *The Cochrane Database of Syst Rev* 2004, Issue 1. Art. No.: CD003004. DOI: 10.1002/14651858.pub2.

39 Lee A, Done ML. Stimulation of the wrist acupuncture point P6 for preventing postoperative nausea and vomiting. *The Cochrane Database of Syst Rev* 2004, Issue 3. Art. No.: CD003281. DOI: 10.1002/14651858.pub2.

40 Müllner M, Urbanek B, Havel C, Losert H, Waechter F, Gamper G. Vasopressors for shock. *The Cochrane Database of Syst Rev* 2004, Issue 3. Art. No.: CD003709. DOI: 10.1002/14651858.pub2.

41 Khan F, Kantor G, Saleemullah H. Pharmacological agents for preventing morbidity associated with the haemodynamic response to tracheal intubation. (Protocol) *The Cochrane Database of Syst Rev* 2001, Issue 4. Art. No.: CD004087. DOI: 10.1002/14651858.

12

Evidence-based medicine in the Third World

Ruth Hutchinson

Harare Central Hospital, Harare, Zimbabwe

This chapter focuses firstly on the differences between the West and the Third World, such as poverty, age of the population, disease burden, lack of skilled staff and equipment. Is simple equipment the best for resource-poor countries?

The importance of teaching evidence-based medicine to medical students is discussed, and the difficulties for the teachers of non-physician anaesthetists due to the lack of studies on the outcome of anaesthesia from non-physicians.

The Third World has huge research potential, but the major Western journals carry few studies from Third World workers. However some excellent work has been done especially when Western funding and expertise has joined hands with local workers. This is illustrated by the studies in mother to child HIV transmission carried out in Sub-Saharan Africa.

Introduction

A BBC reporter was interviewing a highly trained chest surgeon at a chest hospital in Afghanistan. There was no water supply, and the now unused theatre was filthy. The supply of drugs in the dispensary was minimal. The reporter did not understand what they were, but noticed that one box of tablets was 14 years old. The surgeon told how she had returned from the West to help rebuild her country, but the supposedly millions of dollars worth of aid never reached their hospital, so what use was she? At this point the surgeon was called to see a casualty, a road accident victim with a lung perforation. She called for a chest drain. There were none. The suggestion was they could do nothing. I found myself shouting at the radio. "Use a condom, you fool". You make a small slit on the end. The air will come out but not go in. Every Third World doctor should know this. This surgeon was trained in the West [1].

We live in a global village indeed, and we will survive or go under from global warming together. But on the ground we do live in different worlds. Our priorities are different. Our practice of medicine is different. The patients we try to care for are different.

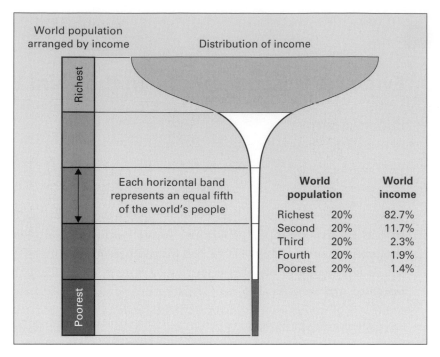

World population arranged by income

Distribution of income

Richest

Poorest

Each horizontal band represents an equal fifth of the world's people

	World population	World income
Richest	20%	82.7%
Second	20%	11.7%
Third	20%	2.3%
Fourth	20%	1.9%
Poorest	20%	1.4%

Figure 12.1   The champagne glass of world poverty. Work: Editor's choice *BMJ* 1999; 318 (10 April). Reproduced with kind permission from the BMJ Publishing Group

Each Third World country is unique. Each has its own problems and needs. The comments that follow focus on Africa, and more specifically Sub-Saharan Africa, and in particular Zimbabwe.

Poverty

Poverty is the first and most obvious difference. The patients who attend the government hospitals are poor, and much has been written in the last two decades about how this alone leads to an increase in ill health [2]. Because of their poverty especially in rural areas they are likely to present late to the hospital, or not at all. Transport may be an insuperable problem. My own gardener's wife ruptured an ectopic pregnancy in a rural homestead 4 km from the road. They pushed her to the bus stop in a wheelbarrow. But the bus driver thought she might die in his bus and refused to take her. They got a message to me, and after a 500-km drive, she had successful surgery. Her story is probably repeated daily all over rural Africa, but for most of the patients no rescue by landrover is available. The lucky ones reach hospital but with their condition far advanced. There may be further delays if the relatives do not have enough money for the admission fee, or are sent out to buy drugs.

Figure 12.1 illustrates the extent of global poverty [3].

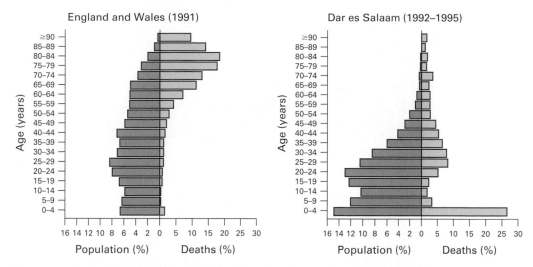

Figure 12.2   Outlook for survivors of childhood in Sub-Saharan Africa: adult mortality in Tanzania. Adult Morbidity and Mortality Project. Reproduced with kind permission from the BMJ Publishing Group

Age of population

The Third World has a predominantly young population. Birth rate is higher than in the West, but there is high mortality amongst the under 5 years old, and since the HIV/AIDS epidemic a high mortality in early middle life [4].

Distribution of age at death (percentage) and population structure in Dar es Salaam (Tanzania) was compared with distribution of age at death and population structure in England and Wales (Figure 12.2).

Life expectancy at birth in Zimbabwe has dropped to 37 years. It declined by 14 years between 1995 and 2001 [5]. There is a practical outcome of this range of population for anaesthetists. In Britain, paediatric anaesthesia is only administered by super-specialists. In Africa every trainee must learn quickly how to maintain a paediatric airway.

Disease burden

We see different diseases. There is an overlap of course. The killers in Sub-Saharan Africa are HIV/AIDS, TB, malaria and indeed road accidents, all of which occur in the West. There is plenty of diabetes, obesity and high blood pressure. We have the old age diseases and cancer too, but they take second place. The killers are infections predominantly HIV/AIDS [6].

It is important to remember that the collection of statistics in a Third World country may not have the accuracy of the West. Also many deaths are undiagnosed (Figure 12.3).

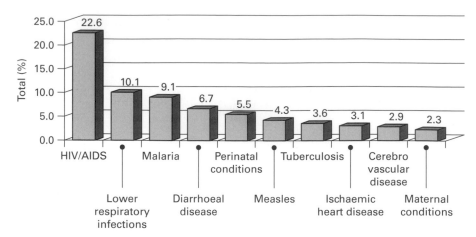

Figure 12.3 Leading causes of death in Africa 2000. *Source*: World Health Report (WHO) (2001), Zimbabwe Human Development Report (UNDP) (2003). Reproduced with kind permission from the University of Zimbabwe

Something must be said here about the disease burden of *pregnancy*. Where medical services are in short supply a higher percentage of work than in the West is with woman's problems. A study in Malawi showed that in rural hospitals in that country Caesarean section comprised 75% of all major surgery [7].

Maternal mortality in Britain is 13.1 per 100 000 [8]. In Zimbabwe maternal mortality is estimated to be 1100 [6]. Some of these are again AIDS related, but much stems from poor maternal care, late presentation and the unavailability of blood and the requisite drugs.

Trained health workers

Despite many efforts to train local students not only in medicine, but also to specialist medical standards, numbers of doctors are grossly inadequate (Table 12.1). Outside the main cities health care is usually provided by nurses and clinical officers. These too may be in short supply.

Inadequate training programmes may not be the main reason for these deficiencies.

There is an inevitable movement of skilled people from poor to rich countries, dubbed the brain drain. In 2005 it was reported that 100 of the first 203 graduates of Malawi's 12-year-old medical college were outside the country [10]. The poor country funds the training, but does not benefit from the product. A nurse trained to give anaesthetics will not be offered a job to do this in the West, but she will be a very useful member of an operating theatre team.

Table 12.1. Comparison of number of anaesthetists in First and Third Worlds [9]. (Figure 4 modified from the original generously supplied by Iain Wilson and reproduced with permission of *Anaesthesia News*; the newsletter of the Association of Anaesthetists of Great Britain and Ireland.)

Country	GDP US $	Physicians/100 000	Physician anaesthetists/population (million)
UK	29 600	164	12 000/64
Rwanda	1300	2	5/8.5
Eritrea	900	5	0/4.5
Afghanistan	800	19	10/28

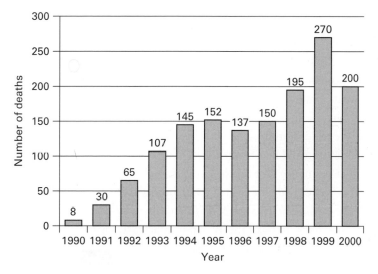

Figure 12.4   Statistics from Malawi [11]. Deaths from HIV/AIDS among health workers in Malawi, 1990–2000. Reproduced with kind permission from the WHO; from The World Health Report 2004 – changing history, Chapter 4: Health systems: finding new strength

A second reason for the shortage of health workers is the death of skilled health workers from the scourge of HIV/AIDS (Figure 12.4).

Equipment

Good medical care now requires first-class well-maintained tools. This is particularly so in anaesthesia. The advent of the pulse oximeter, the capnograph and other monitoring tools has impacted positively on anaesthetic mortality. Many Third World anaesthetists ask donors to give them the latest state of the art anaesthetic machines and monitoring devices. When the equipment fails it is realised that there is no technician with the skills to repair it, and no budget. This situation was appreciated as long ago as 1974 when the *Fourth Commonwealth Medical Conference* arranged a survey of medical technical training in a large number of developing countries. Only Papua New Guinea was reported to have a college with training in general electronics and medical instrument technology. It was part of the Posts and Telegraph Technical Training College. A novel and practical approach to the problem has been successfully introduced in East Africa by Dr Henry Bukwirwa [12]. Only the simplest of equipment, an oxygen concentrator and draw over vaporiser, is used. Anaesthetists are taught to carry out their own routine maintenance, releasing the technicians for more complex problems. The spin-off is that the technician skilled in giving a long life to an EMO ether vaporiser is not, sadly for him, marketable in the West.

Teaching evidence-based medicine

With this background should we be *teaching* medical students evidence-based medicine? We know that drugs and equipment shown to be the best are not available due to inadequate finance. "Inadequate finance" is preferable to "financial constraints". The latter has the suggestion that someone has produced a budget on the best way to spend the little money available. This is very unlikely as this has to be a trained "someone", supported by a trained staff able to implement his decisions. Such leaders and their teams are, like doctors, very thin on the ground.

Evidence-based medicine starts with a clinical problem, and with the formation of a question regarding optimal care. A literature review follows. In the Third World the search is more likely to be of the local pharmacies to see what is available. So should we teach students what should be done knowing that most of the time it cannot be done?

The answer is "yes". There are two reasons. Firstly, all medical students must be taught the principle of literature search to answer a clinical question. "We always do it this way here" is not always the best. Even if there is little chance of using the latest methods and drugs, a student needs to know the latest developments in medicine because these help him to a better understanding of the disease process. Only with this knowledge can he devise the best possible care for his own patients, and assess the cost effectiveness of his care. Later in his career he may be in the position to have input into the management of the available budget. Then he will need to be well informed.

A second reason for teaching evidence-based medicine is that most Third World countries have a smattering of rich people for whom private hospitals, often centres of excellence, are in place. The Steve Biko film was made in Zimbabwe. Before the contracts were signed the film company inspected the private medical facilities to make sure they were good enough should the actors or film team become ill. They were. At that time there were plenty of doctors trained up to the best Western standards.

The argument against training doctors to the highest possible standards is that they are then able to compete for employment all over the world. As we have shown the "brain drain" is a devastating reality in Third World countries. But in practice there is no way of holding back people of high intelligence if they decide to emigrate to greener pastures. Some, now with hands-on experience in Western medicine, will return home. Most will move into private practice staffing the available centres of excellence. A few will return to a career in teaching the next generation.

An important point to make here is that, though the teaching of anaesthetics to the highest standards to physicians should always be attempted, most anaesthetics in the Third World are given by non-physicians. These non-physicians may be trained nurse anaesthetists or clinical officers but could also be the theatre orderly. Training to the best of evidence-based Western standards is not an option. If you are working in rural Africa, often without electricity let alone a telephone line and a computer, a literature search is not possible. The best results are often obtained from training by rote. The commonest major operation is Caesarean section. Clearly the anaesthetic trainer must know what studies have shown the safest method of anaesthesia for this procedure. This is what he teaches.

So where does this trainer look for his evidence? Let us see him as an experienced doctor himself, with a sound education, and access to the Internet. He can consult the journals and follow the pyramid of evidence right up to the meta-analysis. But he then notices that all the papers he has found were written in the West. Are they applicable for his non-physician trainees? Fortunately for his lecture on anaesthesia for Caesarean section he has found one Third World study which corroborates what he has already found that spinal anaesthesia is safer than general anaesthesia for this procedure [13]. But what about the failed spinal? The trainee in the West is taught to put the mother on oxygen, and call for help if he now sees a difficult intubation ahead. No help is available for the clinical officer in rural Sub-Saharan Africa. Does the trainer teach general anaesthesia with a laryngeal mask if necessary, (if there is a laryngeal mask), or pure local anaesthesia? He would like to look for evidence, but can find none.

Research in Third World countries

Not many papers from the Third World find their way into the major journals.

Keiser et al. [14] found that only 5% of editorial and advisory board members from 12 referenced tropical medicine journals were from "countries with a low human development index", and only 13% of authors were from such countries. Raja and Singer [15] reviewed the contents of four leading medical journals and found that only 15% of articles were relevant to developing countries. *The Lancet* and *British Medical Journal* scored over 20%, but the *Journal of American Medical Association* and

New England Journal of Medicine only 5%. Priorities for pharmaceutical research, funded by the Dutch Government, were studied by WHO researchers Kaplan and Laing [16]. The detailed and scholarly report covers not only the common Third World killer diseases but also the rare "neglected" diseases like Huntingdon's chorea, and possible pandemic killers like severe acute respiratory syndrome (SARS). This report will be the basis for the European Union's research funding.

So our young doctor, trained in the principle of evidence-based medicine, even if he has electricity, a telephone line and a computer, may not find help for some of his clinical dilemmas. Fortunately this is not the case for the main condition he will be handling if he is practising in Sub-Saharan Africa. In Zimbabwe 30% of the population are HIV positive, but the percentage of the hospital population is much higher. Much research has been carried out on HIV/AIDS both in the West and in Third World countries.

Prevention of mother to child HIV infection

Prevention of mother to child HIV infection can be used as an example.

Mother to child transmission (MTCT) has been shown to occur in utero, during birth, and from breast milk. So in the West zidovudine during pregnancy, Caesarean section and no breastfeeding are de rigueur. Costly Caesarean section is not an option in the Third World, and all Mothers expect to breastfeed. The use of antiretroviral drugs (ARV) in pregnancy and around the time of delivery to reduce MTCT of HIV was first demonstrated in 1994 by the PACTG 076 Study Group [17] and evidence that short-course combination ARV treatment can be effective was demonstrated subsequently in both Thailand and West Africa [18,19]. However the study which led to real expansion of prevention of MTCT programmes was conducted in Uganda. This showed that a single dose of nevirapine given to mothers at the onset of labour followed by a single dose of the same drug to their babies within 72 hours of delivery reduced MTCT by 47% [20]. Similarly excellent studies clear up the question of what advice to give regarding breastfeeding to Mothers who do not have the facilities for safe formula feeding. If the baby *only* feeds on breast milk, the risk of HIV infection at six months is 1.3% [21]. There are many studies, and a meta-analysis is possible.

The MTCT studies for Sub-Saharan Africa can only be done in the Third World situation. They are now being implemented, and many lives will be saved. But they are irrelevant for the situation in the West. They show that evidence-based medicine is as essential for the poor countries as for the rich. But it must be based on research carried out in those countries. For HIV-related issues there has been much funding and other input from the West. But is it the same story for malaria, and what about Ebola? The marvellous opportunities and the need for research in the Third World are a clarion call.

> **Research agenda**
> - Research done in the West is often inappropriate for Third World conditions.
> - The potential for valuable work is enormous in the Third World.
> - Caesarean section is the commonest major procedure.
> - Many more mortality and morbidity studies are needed, focusing on areas where anaesthesia is given by non-physicians with no medical help available.
> - Should local anaesthesia be recommended for the failed spinal with a potentially difficult airway?
> - Does sophisticated equipment rather than the precordial stethoscope and sphygmomanometer improve outcome?
> - For hospitals with intensive care and qualified anaesthetists more work is needed on when to ventilate, and when not to ventilate patients with advanced AIDS.
> - In many fields excellent work has resulted from collaboration between local and Western workers, with Western funding.

Summary

The teaching of evidence-based medicine to medical students is just as important in the Third World as in the West, despite the fact that it is often impossible to implement due to lack of personnel and resources. The teaching of non-physician anaesthetists, who give the majority of anaesthetics in many countries, is often hampered by the absence of any studies as to what is the best in the conditions in which they are working. Studies from the West do not fit the situation and few of the wide circulation Western journals publish work from the Third World. The need for more research in many fields is enormous. Fortunately there is increasing evidence of successful collaboration between Western funding and expertise and local researchers.

Acknowledgement

The author gratefully thanks the help from Dr John Carlisle and residents in Ernie's Lane, Harare.

REFERENCES

1 BBC World Service 'From Our Own Correspondent' November 14, 2004.

2 Haines A, Smith R. Working together to reduce poverty's damage. *BMJ* 1997; 314: 529–30.

3 World Bank Development Report, 1992.

4 Kitange HM et al. Outlook for survivors of childhood in Sub-Saharan Africa: adult mortality in Tanzania. *BMJ* 1996; 312: 216–20.

5 Zimbabwe Human Development Report, 2003.

6 The State of the World's Children 2005, UNICEF Global Report.

7 Fenton PM. Epidemiology of District Surgery in Malawi: a 2 year study of surgical rates in rural Africa. *East Cent Afr J Surg* 1997; 3: 33–41.

8 Why Mothers Die. 2000–2001 Confidential Enquiry into Maternal and Child Health. RCOG Press.

9 Wilson, I. Editorial in Anaesthesia News, a publication of the AAGBI, Number 223 February 2006.

10 Thyoka. *BMJ* 2005; 330: 923.

11 Deaths form HIV/AIDS among health workers in Malawi, 1990–2000 WHO – World Health Report, 2004.

12 Bukwirwa Mbarara University of Science and Technology Anaesthesia Equipment Workshop Project (MAWP), 1999.

13 Fenton, Whitty and Reynolds. *BMJ* 2003; 327: 587–90.

14 Keiser J et al. Representation of authors and editors from countries with different Human Development Indexes in the leading literature on tropical medicine: survey of current evidence. *BMJ* 2004; 328: 1229–32.

15 Raja AJ, Singer P. *BMJ* 2004; 329: 1429.

16 Kaplan W, Laing R. Priority medicines for Europe and the world. Geneva: World Health Organisation, 1994. http://mednet3.who.int//mednet3.who.int/prioritymeds/report/index.htm

17 Connor EM, Sperling RS, Gleber R et al. Reduction of maternal-infant transmission of human immunodeficiency virus type 1 with zidovudine treatment. *New Engl J Med* 1994; 331(18): 1173–80.

18 Lallemant M, Jourdain G, Le Coeur S et al. Single dose perinatal nevirapine plus standard zidovudine to prevent mother-to-child transmission of HIV-1 in Thailand. *New Engl J Med* 2004; 351(3): 217–28.

19 Dabis F, Bequent L, Ekouevi DK et al. Field efficacy of zidovudine, lamivudine and single-dose nevirapine to prevent peripartum HIV transmission. *AIDS* 2005; 19(3): 309–18.

20 Guay LA, Musoke P, Fleming T et al. Intrapartum and neonatal single-dose nevirapine compared with zidovudine for prevention of mother-to-child transmission of HIV-1 in Kampala, Uganda: HIVNET 012 randomised trial. *Lancet* 1999; 354: 795–802.

21 Iliff PJ, Piwoz EG, Tavengwa NV et al. *AIDS* 2005; 19: 699–708.

13

Preoperative anaesthesia evaluation

Maurizio Solca

Anaesthesia and Intensive Care Medicine, Azienda Ospedaliera di Melegnano, Presidio Ospedaliero di Cernusco sul Naviglio, Ospedale "A. Uboldo", Cernusco sul Naviglio (MI), Italy

Preoperative assessment encompasses surgical and anaesthesia evaluation, preoperative testing, patients' preparation for surgery and obtaining informed consent. It is an everyday routine for anaesthesiologists, and sometimes it is taken as a boring and time-consuming chore, but it is vital for safe and appropriate patients' perioperative care. Scope of the present paper is to review available evidence on anaesthesia preoperative evaluation (who, when and how to conduct it) and its relevance to clinical practice, together with indications for future research.

Introduction

Preoperative assessment is a large and complex process, which includes multiple professional involvements: nursing, anaesthesiology, different surgical specialties, laboratory medicine, at times cardiology, pulmonology, radiology, and others. This results in a very large production of scientific literature (approximately 5000 papers over the past 10 years) [1]: unfortunately, from such a vast knowledge base very little evidence is available, leaving professionals with a large portion of uncertainty, even if we will limit to the anaesthesia preoperative evaluation for elective procedures, defined as "the process of clinical assessment that precedes the delivery of anaesthesia care for surgery and for non-surgical procedures" [2].

The intent of the present paper is not to be another systematic review of original research, but its scope is to present a summary of published evidence-based literature (systematic reviews, meta-analyses, clinical practice guidelines, health technology assessments) on the subject, which have been revised using the same methodology of the AGREE instrument [3].

Approximately 20 years ago, with expansion of surgical activities and growing concern over patients' safety, on one hand, and rising costs of health services and

Key words: Preoperative care, anaesthesia, evaluation.

Table 13.1. Summary of practice guidelines published by Anaesthesia National Societies, in chronological order of appearance

Country	Society	Year of publication	Reference
France	SFAR	1991, revised 1994	[13]
Germany	DIMDI	1998	[12]
Italy	SIAARTI	1998	[14]
Belgium	BSAR – BPASAR	1998	[15]
UK	AAGBI	2001	[16]
USA	ASA	2002, amended 2003	[2]
Canada	CAS/SAC	2004	[17]

limitation of available resources, on the other, a number of publications appeared in the western literature (I refer to "Western" world only for accessibility of published material) [4–9]. Their main focus was the identification of safe and effective clinical pathways in the process of preparation of patients to scheduled surgery, accompanied by stringent limitation to laboratory and instrumental investigations, at that time a major source of increasing costs in the preoperative phase.

During the following decade, health professionals' attention swung towards the appropriateness of the service provided to patients, and a few excellent health technology assessment reports were published [10–12]. Their goal was to further the cost-benefit ratio of ordering, and performing, preoperative testing of patients, avoiding at the same time inappropriate exposure of patients to the hazards of false-positive or -negative results.

Many national anaesthesia societies have published clinical recommendations and guidelines on the matter (Table 13.1), in order to help fellow anaesthesiologists improve their practice through the application of evidence-based criteria in performing preoperative patients' assessment.

What is the evidence?

All these documents, independently from the source, agree in affirming that an anaesthesia preoperative evaluation should be performed, even though systematic avoidance of such an evaluation versus performing it (as is the standard throughout the world) has never been studied. This is probably because not performing the evaluation would expose anaesthesiologists to legal and contractual issues.

Such an evaluation should involve review of available medical records, patient's interview(s) and history collection, and physical examination, which should comprise airway, pulmonary (including auscultation of the lungs), and cardiovascular examination [2]. The collection of anaesthesia history can be facilitated by a structured, ad hoc questionnaire [18]: its use is strongly encouraged by the *Italian* [14] and *British* [16] *Society Guidelines*.

Essential component of preanaesthesia evaluation is the assessment of patient's risk [2,13–17].

Who should perform it?

This is a highly controversial issue, and in real life economical and political reasons become clearly superimposed to scientific evidence. Properly trained nurses within anaesthesia departments are probably invaluable in performing at least a consistent portion of the evaluation [19–21], particularly in the psychological preparation to surgery [22]. Primary care physicians are also ideally fit to concur in the preoperative assessment of their patients [23], relieving anaesthesia departments of a heavy burden.

In any case, all anaesthesiological societies recommend that a physician anaesthesiologist would at least conclude this process [2,12–17].

When should it be performed?

There is no evidence of any influence of the timing of anaesthesia evaluation (performed either before or on the day of surgery) on outcome from anaesthesia. In clinical practice, the timing is influenced by customs, professional habits, regulations, and type of practice (prevalence of day surgery, which strongly favours assessment on the day of surgery). It is generally recommended [2,16] that the timing would be at minimum influenced by the invasiveness, hence the risk, of surgical procedure.

Preoperative testing

Preoperative tests should be ordered only after the patient's assessment, and only those relevant to the particular case [6,10,24–26]. Recently, a very exhaustive evaluation of the available evidence on the subject has been published by the National Institute for Clinical Excellence (NICE) in the UK [27].

It is suggested that in preoperative test ordering anaesthesiologists keep in consideration patient's age, physical status (Table 13.2), extension of planned procedure (Table 13.3) and presence of co-morbidity (particularly from cardiovascular, respiratory and renal disease).

Specific situations

Co-morbidity, particularly from cardiovascular disease, is a great concern to the clinical anaesthesiologist, leading to the preparation of specific recommendations [30].

Table 13.2. ASA physical status classification [28]

1	A normal healthy patient
2	A patient with mild systemic disease
3	A patient with severe systemic disease
4	A patient with severe systemic disease that is a constant threat to life
5	A moribund patient who is not expected to survive without the operation
6	A declared brain-dead patient whose organs are being removed for donor purposes

Table 13.3. Classification of surgical interventions in different intensity (and risk) categories; some examples for each category [29]

Grade 1 (minor)	Excision of lesion of skin; drainage of breast abscess; carpal tunnel release; nasal septum correction
Grade 2 (intermediate)	Primary repair of inguinal hernia; excision of varicose vein(s) of leg; tonsillectomy/adenotonsillectomy; knee arthroscopy; endoscopic bladder procedures; eye lens substitution
Grade 3 (major)	Total abdominal hysterectomy; endoscopic resection of prostate; lumbar discectomy; thyroidectomy; diaphragmatic hernia repair; operations on trachea; prosthetic femora head replacement
Grade 4 (major+)	Total joint replacement; lung operations; colonic resection; radical neck dissection; organ transplantation
Neurosurgery	
Cardiovascular surgery	

However, any coexisting disease or alteration of health status (i.e. acute respiratory illness) should be carefully evaluated, in order to assure the maximum safety to the patient with the minimum derangement of surgical activity [2,12–17].

Different age groups, particularly children, deserve specific attention. If there were little available evidence on the matter for adult preoperative evaluation, even less can be found on paediatric settings [31], and see specific appendix of Ref. [14].

Practice points
- All patients subject to anaesthesia should undergo anaesthesia preoperative evaluation.
- Patient assessment should consist of review of available medical records, patient's interview(s), physical examination and necessary additional testing.

- Any assessment should be concluded by an anaesthetist physician, but initial screening and in many cases the majority of the patient's work-up could be conducted by nurses or primary care physicians.
- Ideal timing of assessment is not defined; however, it should be performed earlier in the process as more compromised were the patient and/or more invasive were the procedure, in order to allow time for further necessary investigations.
- Additional tests should be ordered weighing the benefits of obtaining more detailed information about the health status of a single patient against the cost of performing them and the potential harm stemming from false-negative or -positive results; in any case the extent of additional testing should be guided by patient's age, physical status and co-morbidity, and by invasiveness of planned procedure.

Research agenda
- The value of nurses and primary care physician participation in the process of pre-operative assessment should be better defined.
- Further investigation is needed in defining the ideal timing of patient assessment.
- Ways for better decision making in ordering additional tests should be investigated, in order to reach a viable algorithm for the preparation of correct clinical pathways for specific patients' age and surgery class groups.

Conclusions

The abridged version of the *NICE Guidance* [32] presents possible combinations of the four dimensions (patients' age, physical status, grade of surgery and coexisting disease) as a series of lookout tables, in which appropriateness of a number of tests (Table 13.4) is evidenced, using the metaphor of the traffic light: the document is very compact, and easily accessible on the Internet.

Table 13.4. Examples of preoperative tests [32]

- Plain chest radiograph
- Resting electrocardiogram
- Full blood count
- Haemostasis including prothrombin time, activated partial thromboplastin time and international normalised ratio
- Renal function including tests for potassium, sodium, creatinine and/or urea levels
- Random blood glucose
- Urine dipstick tests for pH, protein, glucose, ketones, blood/haemoglobin
- Arterial blood gases
- Lung function including peak expiratory flow rate, forced vital capacity and forced expiratory volume

It is of invaluable help not only to the individual anaesthesiologist, but also in preparing clinical pathways for categories of patients and of type of surgery, an approach to the preoperative evaluation, which is favoured by a number of anaesthesia societies [2,14–17], in order to assure consistency and quality control to the process.

REFERENCES

1 US National Library of Medicine online database. September 2005; http://www.ncbi. nlm.nih.gov/entrez/query.fcgi?CMDZIndex&DBZpubmed

2 American Society of Anesthesiologists Task Force on Preanesthesia Evaluation. Practice Advisory for Preanesthesia Evaluation: a report by the American Society of Anesthesiologists Task Force on Preanesthesia Evaluation. *Anesthesiology* 2002; 96: 485–96. Amended October 2003; http://www.asahq.org/publicationsAndServices/preeval.pdf

3 The AGREE Collaboration. Appraisal of Guidelines for Research and Evaluation: AGREE Instrument. 2001; http://www.agreecollaboration.org/instrument

4 Kaplan ED, Sheiner LB, Boeckmann AJ, Roizen MF, Beal SL, Cohen SN et al. The usefulness of preoperative laboratory screening. *JAMA* 1985; 253: 3576–81.

5 American Society of Anesthesiologists. Basic Standards for Preanesthesia Care. 1987; http://www.asahq.org/publicationsAndServices/standards/03.pdf

6 Roizen MF. The compelling rationale for less preoperative testing. *Can J Anaesth* 1988; 35: 214–8.

7 Societé Belge de Anésthesie et Réanimation. Belgian standards for patient safety in anaesthesia. *Acta Anaesthesiol Belgica* 1989; 40: 231–8.

8 Qualitätssicherung in der Anästhesiologie. Richtlinien der Deutschen Gesellschaft für Anästhesiologie und Intensivmedizin. *Anästh Intensivmed* 1989; 30: 307–14.

9 SBU The Swedish Council on Technology Assessment in Health Care. Preoperative Routines. 1989; http://www.sbu.se/www/index.asp

10 Munro J, Booth A, Nicholl J. Routine preoperative testing: a systematic review of the evidence. *Health Technol Assess* 1997; 1: 1–62.

11 ANAES Agence National d'Accréditation et d'Evaluation en Santé. Recommendations et references médicales: les examens préopératoires systématiques. 1998; http://www.anacs.fr/ ANAES/ANAESparametrage.nsf/Page?ReadForm&Section=/ANAES/aproposdusite.ns/(ID)/ CD5AB88A93FA7428C1256E300042F7DC?opendocument

12 Röseler S, Duda L, Schwartz FW. Evaluation präoperativer Routinediagnostik (Röntgenthorax, EKG, Labor) vor elektiven Eingriffen bei Erwachsenen. Preoperative routine diagnostics (chest radiography, ECG, and laboratory tests) for elective surgery. In: Schwartz FW, Köbberling J, Raspe H, Schulenburg Graf von der JM (eds). *Schriftenreihe HTA des DIMDI (Medizinische Hochschule Hannover)*, Vol. 8. Baden-Baden: Nomos Verlagsgesellschaft, 1998, pp 1–152; http://gripsdb.dimdi.de/de/hta/hta_berichte/hta008_ bericht_de.pdf

13   SFAR Société FrançÁaise D'Anésthesie et de Réanimation. Recommandations concernant la période préanesthésique. 1991, revised 1994; http://www.sfar.org/recompreop.html

14   Gruppo di Studio SIAARTI per la Sicurezza in Anestesia e Terapia Intensiva. Raccomandazioni per la valutazione anestesiologica in previsione di procedure diagnostico-terapeutiche in elezione. Minerva Anestesiol 1998; 64: XVIII–XXVI; http://147.163.1.67/linee/pdf/valanest.pdf

15   Adriaensen H, Baele P, Camu F et al. Recommendations on pre-anaesthetic evaluation of patients put forward jointly with the BSAR and the BPASAR. The Belgian Society of Anesthesia and Reanimation and the Belgian Professional Association of Specialists in Anesthesia and Reanimation. *Acta Anaesthesiol Belg* 1998; 49: 47–50.

16   Association of Anaesthetists of Great Britain and Ireland. Pre-operative Assessment. *The Role of the Anaesthetist*, 2001; http://www.aagbi.org/pdf/pre-operative_ass.pdf

17   Canadian Anesthesiologists' Society. Guidelines to the Practice of Anesthesia. The Pre-anesthetic Period. Revised 2004; http://www.cas.ca/members/sign_in/guidelines/practice_of_anesthesia/default.asp?load=preanesthetic#top

18   McChesney J. Anaesthesia preadmission assessment using a screening questionnaire. *Can J Anaesth* 1998; 45: 596–7.

19   Girard N. Preoperative assessment. *Nurse Pract Forum* 1997; 8: 140–6.

20   Ziolkowski L, Strzyzewski N. Perianesthesia assessment: foundation of care. *J Perianesth Nurs* 2001; 16: 359–70.

21   Bramhall J. The role of nurses in preoperative assessment. *Nurs Times* 2002; 98: 34–5.

22   Fortner PA. Preoperative patient preparation: psychological and educational aspects. *Semin Perioper Nurs* 1998; 7: 3–9.

23   Clark E. Preoperative assessment. Primary care work-up to identify surgical risks. *Geriatrics* 2001; 56: 36–40.

24   Oliva G, Vilarasau J, Martín-Baranera M. *La valoración preoperatoria en los centros quirúrgicos catalanes: práctica y opinión de los profesionales implicados.* Barcelona: Agència d'Avaluació de Tecnologia i Recerca Mèdiques. Servei Català de la Salut. Departament de Sanitat i Seguretat Social. Generalitat de Catalunya. Abril de 2002; http:// www.gencat.net/salut/depsan/units/aatrm/pdf/in0203es.pdf

25   Calderini E, Adrario E, Petrini F et al. Indications to chest radiograph in preoperative adult assessment: recommendations of the SIAARTI-SIRM commission. *Minerva Anestesiol* 2004; 70: 443–51.

26   Agenzia per i Servizi Sanitari Regionali. Valutazione preoperatoria del paziente da sottoporre a chirurgia elettiva. Linee guida nazionali di riferimento. 2005; http://www.assr.it/plg/chirurgia_elettiva.pdf

27   National Institute for Clinical Excellence. Preoperative Tests. The use of routine preoperative tests for elective surgery. 2003; http://www.nice.org.uk/pdf/Preop_Fullguideline.pdf

28   American Society of Anesthesiologists. ASA Relative Value Guide. 2005; http://www.asahq.org/clinical/physicalstatus.htm

29   National Institute for Clinical Excellence. Preoperative Tests. The use of routine preoperative tests for elective surgery. Appendices, Guidelines & Information. http://www.nice. org.uk/pdf/PreopTests_Apps.pdf

30 Eagle KA, Berger PB, Calkins H et al. ACC/AHA Guideline Update for Perioperative Cardiovascular Evaluation for Noncardiac Surgery-Executive Summary. A report of the American College of Cardiology/American Heart Association Task Force on Practice Guidelines (Committee to Update the 1996 Guidelines on Perioperative Cardiovascular Evaluation for Noncardiac Surgery). *Anesth Analg* 2002; 94: 1052–64.

31 Maxwell LG. Age-associated issues in preoperative evaluation, testing, and planning: pediatrics. *Anesthesiol Clin N Am* 2004; 22: 27–43.

32 National Institute for Clinical Excellence. Preoperative Tests. The use of routine preoperative tests for elective surgery. Clinical Guideline 3. http://www.nice.org.uk/pdf/CG3NICEguideline.pdf

14

Regional anaesthesia versus general anaesthesia

Mina Nishimori[1] and Jane Ballantyne[2]

[1]Department of Anesthesia/Critical Care, Massachusetts General Hospital, Boston, MA, USA
[2]Department of Anesthesia, Massachusetts General Hospital, Pain Center, Boston, MA, USA

The question whether regional anaesthesia improves postoperative morbidity and mortality is complex. The answer would differ depending on the patient, the surgery, the method of regional and general anaesthesia, and the quality of perioperative care. We will start this chapter by discussing issues that construct the complexity of this question, such as heterogeneity and discrepancy between old and recent trials. Then we will assess current evidence of regional versus general anaesthesia on selected specific topics – hip fracture surgery, carotid endarterectomy, Caesarean section, ambulatory orthopaedic surgery, and postoperative cognitive dysfunction in elderly patients after non-cardiac surgery.

Introduction

The debate over the theoretical superiority of regional over general anaesthesia has persisted throughout most of the twentieth century, and there is still no satisfactory answer to the question of whether avoidance of general anaesthesia saves lives or reduces morbidity. But the answer eludes us only because the question is complex, and there is probably no simple answer. Multiple factors, including the patient's health status, the surgical procedure, choice of regional anaesthetic, whether regional is combined with general anaesthesia, and exact choice of general anaesthetic, influence outcome and effect the balance of benefits and risks. Moreover, changes occur in clinical practice over time that have an important effect on outcome, and often alter the balance of benefit between regional and general anaesthesia. It seems it will never be possible to state that one technique is better than another for all patients; only that for certain patients, the benefit versus risk analysis may favour one technique

Key words: Regional anaesthesia, general anaesthesia, heterogeneity, meta-analysis, randomised controlled trial, hip fracture, carotid endarterectomy, Caesarean section, ambulatory surgery, postoperative confusion.

over the other. This chapter reviews and analyses the evidence supporting an effect on surgical outcome of anaesthetic choice.

With different surgical procedures and patient populations, an effect or side effect of anaesthesia can be favourable or unfavourable. For example, sympathectomy and subsequent vasodilatation under spinal and epidural anaesthesia reduces venous return to the heart, which results in hypotension. This phenomenon can be devastating for frail elderly patients. The same phenomenon, however, reduces intraoperative blood loss by reducing local blood flow to the surgical site. Sometimes avoidance of general anaesthesia per se can be an advantage. The high risk of acid regurgitation and aspiration during general anaesthesia for Caesarean section [1] makes this a procedure for which regional anaesthesia is likely to be particularly beneficial. For carotid endarterectomy, using regional anaesthesia rather than general anaesthesia enables keeping patients awake during carotid artery clamping. This may reduce morbidity and mortality by early detection of the onset of intraoperative stroke. Choice of anaesthetic will inevitably fall on the characteristics of the patient and the operation, but the foundation for the choice will be currently available, best evidence.

Neuraxial versus general anaesthesia

Key evidence supporting advantages or disadvantages of intraoperative neuraxial anaesthesia on postoperative outcomes is summarised in Table 14.1. Here we will discuss some of the important issues in assessing and interpreting the results listed in this table.

Heterogeneity of the trials that compared regional versus general anaesthesia

The trials differ in various respects, including the populations under study, and the way in which the neuraxial anaesthesia is used. Sole neuraxial anaesthesia is not the same as neuraxial anaesthesia used as an adjunct to general anaesthesia in terms of likely benefits. First, the surgical procedures for which the two are indicated differ. The former is used for extremity, body surface surgery, and non-extensive intraabdominal and pelvic procedures, while adjunctive neuraxial anaesthesia is used for major intraabdominal and intrathoracic procedures and postoperative analgesia. The dense sympathetic blockade provided by intraoperative neuraxial anaesthesia will provide improved lower-extremity blood flow, diminished coagulability, and reduced cardiac work – incidences of deep venous thrombosis, pulmonary embolism, and cardiac events may thereby be reduced. On the other hand, postoperative epidural analgesia, using low-dose local anaesthetics with opioids, likely has different benefits, largely related to superior analgesia, continuous low-dose local anaesthetic effects, and avoidance of systemic opioids – improved bowel mobility,

Table 14.1. Summary of evidence supporting the benefits of intraoperative neuraxial anaesthesia

Outcome	Positive findings	Key references	Negative findings	Key references
Mortality	Neuraxial anaesthesia has been associated with decreased mortality in randomised controlled trials (RCTs) and meta-analyses. However, careful scrutiny of the studies reveals that the effect is mainly seen in studies with a high-control rate (i.e. death rate is high in the general anaesthesia group), and studies in which patients have not received thrombosis prophylaxis.	[2, 3][a], [4–6][b]	No differences in mortality are noted in the most recent studies.	[7–9][c], [10][d]
Length of hospital stay	The use of neuraxial anaesthesia for ambulatory surgery has been associated with shortened hospital stay.	[11][d]	In non-ambulatory surgery, the use of neuraxial anaesthesia has not been associated with shorter hospital stay.	[12,13][b], [14][d], [3][a], [15][e]
Thromboembolic events	Neuraxial anaesthesia has been shown to be associated with a lower incidence of thromboembolic events when compared to general anaesthesia. However, in the studies in which this benefit is shown, no thrombosis prophylaxis is used.	[2, 3][a], [5,6,16][b]	Neuraxial anaesthesia does not reduce thromboembolic events.	[7][c], [15][e]
Cardiac events	Reduced incidence of cardiac events has been associated with the use of neuraxial anaesthesia in some studies. The effect is most pronounced in patients with known coronary artery disease, undergoing major vascular and cardiac surgery, and receiving thoracic versus lumbar epidurals. Direct angiographic evidence of dilatation of stenotic vessels by neuraxial anaesthesia has also been demonstrated.	[7][c], [4,17][b], [18,19][d]	Other studies, including two large RCTs in high-risk patients, find few differences in cardiac morbidity, and no differences in cardiac mortality.	[7–9][c], [20–23][b]

Table 14.1. (*contd.*)

Outcome	Positive findings	Key references	Negative findings	Key references
Graft survival	Patients undergoing major vascular surgery under epidural anaesthesia achieve significant benefits (lower incidence of graft failure) compared with general anaesthesia.	[21,24][b]		
Perioperative blood loss	The use of neuraxial anaesthesia has frequently been associated with lower-blood loss when compared to general anaesthesia.	[2][a], [25][b]		
Activity levels and mobility	Neuraxial anaesthesia has been associated with increased activity and improved mobility in the immediate and the long-term postoperative period (up to 2 months postoperatively).	[26,27][b]	Time to first ambulation after surgery is not influenced by neuraxial versus general anaesthesia.	[28][e], [14][d]
Mental status	In the first few hours after surgery, cognitive function may be better after neuraxial anaesthesia than after general anaesthesia.	[29][b]	Beyond the first few hours after surgery, mental deterioration is not altered by selecting neuraxial rather than general anaesthesia.	[30–33][b]
Metabolic stress response	Full neural blockade using neuraxial anaesthesia can markedly attenuate or abolish the metabolic stress response to surgical trauma. The stress response is only partially altered by incomplete blockade, including neuraxial anaesthesia for intrathoracic and intraabdominal procedures.	[4][b], [34][d]		
Maternal morbidity and mortality	Maternal mortality and morbidity is reduced when cross-section is undertaken under neuraxial not general anaesthesia.	[35,36][d]		

[a]Meta-analysis, [b]RCT, [c]Large ($n > 800$) multicentre RCT, [d]other observational study, [e]non-RCT. Modified from table in *Journal of Clinical Anaesthesia.* 17(5), Ballantyne JC, Kupelnick B, McPeek B, Lau J. *Does the evidence support the use of spinal and epidural anesthesia for surgery?* 382–91, © 2005 Elsevier Inc with permission from Elsevier.

improved coughing and breathing, earlier ambulation, and consequently a lower incidence of thrombosis. The many studies that utilise intra- and postoperative epidural therapy do not allow any separation between the likely benefits arising from intraoperative epidural anaesthesia versus those arising from postoperative epidural analgesia.

A 2000 published meta-analysis strongly supports a reduction in mortality associated with use of intraoperative neuraxial anaesthesia. Rodgers et al. [2] used meta-analysis to assess the effect of intraoperative neuraxial blockade (with or without general anaesthesia) compared to general anaesthesia alone on postoperative mortality and morbidity. Based on their overall conclusion that neuraxial anaesthesia reduced postoperative mortality by about one third (33%), they recommended more widespread use of neuraxial anaesthesia. They drew this conclusion from a meta-analysis that included various kinds of patient populations with many different anaesthesia techniques and surgical procedures. They included studies of spinal and epidural anaesthesia, thoracic or lumbar catheter placements, used in combination with general anaesthesia or not, and many types of operations and patients. Their subgroup analyses showed, however, that significant reduction in mortality occurred only in specific patient populations with specific types of regional anaesthetic such as spinal anaesthesia for hip fracture surgery, and spinal or epidural anaesthesia for vascular surgery – both populations that seemed to do better in older studies, with no difference shown by newer studies. Therefore, applying their overall conclusion to every patient can be misleading. Benefit versus risk assessment should always be population and practice specific.

The discrepancy between recent and old trials

In 1987, Yeager et al. [4] found that epidural anaesthesia and postoperative epidural analgesia significantly reduced mortality and major morbidity in high-risk surgical patients when compared to general anaesthesia and postoperative parenteral opioid analgesia. However, recent large randomised controlled trials (RCTs) that tried to validate the findings of Yeager et al. failed to reproduce Yaeger's findings [7,8]. Recent improvements in the management of high-risk surgical patients such as short-acting drugs, high dependency and intensive care units, new standards of monitoring and vigilance, better preoperative optimisation, and less invasive surgical techniques, have all contributed to reductions in surgical mortality. These improvements may have overtaken epidural anaesthesia and analgesia in terms of improvement in serious morbidity. Moreover, even large trials may not have enough power to detect differences, as adverse events become increasingly rare.

In the following sections, we will discuss selected topics regarding postoperative outcome after sole regional anaesthesia versus general anaesthesia. Meta-analysis and systematic reviews are cited where available, and emphasis will be given to RCTs. Observational studies are cited when RCTs are not available, or not suitable for the research question and/or target population.

Regional anaesthesia versus general anaesthesia for hip fracture surgery

A systematic review [3] compared mortality and morbidity after hip fracture surgery between regional anaesthesia (spinal or epidural anaesthesia without general anaesthesia) and general anaesthesia. The primary outcome was mortality. Pooled results from eight trials [5,6,32,37–41] showed regional anaesthesia to significantly decrease mortality at 1 month (risk ratio, RR: 0.69, 95% confidence interval, CI: 0.50–0.95). At 3 months, mortality was also smaller in the regional anaesthesia group, but the result was not statistically significant (RR: 0.92, 95% CI: 0.71–1.21). Only two trials evaluated 1-year mortality, which was not significantly different between regional and general anaesthesia groups. Regional anaesthesia was associated with a reduced risk of deep venous thrombosis (RR: 0.64, 95% CI: 0.48–0.96), a decrease in operative blood loss (I-squared difference −85 mL, 95% CI: −162 to −9 mL), and a reduced risk of acute postoperative confusion (RR: 0.50, 95% CI: 0.26–0.95).

However, as the authors suggested, a weakness of this meta-analysis was that many of the included trials were old (seven out of eight studies were more than 15 years old). They may not represent current practice nor account for the advances in safety in the field of anaesthesia today, because of the reasons we discussed in the previous section. With the benefit of interventions such as pharmacological thromboprophylaxis and beta-blockade [42,43], the benefit of neuraxial anaesthesia in terms of improvement in serious morbidity seems to become less important. When the authors excluded the oldest trial with very high mortality in the general anaesthesia group [5], the difference in 1-month mortality was no longer significant.

There are several reports suggesting that better management of surgical patients contributes to improved surgical outcome. Parker et al. [44] prospectively observed 3025 patients who had acute hip fracture over a 1-year period to evaluate the effectiveness of their hip fracture service, in which they designated specific staff to treat hip fracture patients and encouraged early discharge with community nursing service. Mortality at 30 and 120 days after fracture decreased from 21% and 35% (year 1986) to 7% and 15% (year 1997). Unfortunately, they did not present data on the anaesthetic technique used or whether they used any method of thromboembolism prophylaxis.

According to a multicentre audit published in 1995 [10], only 46% of 580 patients admitted for femoral neck fracture received pharmacological thromboembolic prophylactic agents. A significant reduction in fatal pulmonary emboli was identified among patients who received thromboembolic prophylaxis. One of the hospitals included in this audit showed a higher-survival rate. This was thought to be due to the multidisciplinary team-based care, which utilises early assessment and surgery, routine thromboprophylaxis and early mobilisation; plans for discharge began almost immediately after surgery.

It is difficult to conduct large RCTs on a long-term basis. Carefully designed observational studies are valuable because this study design allows for the inclusion of a larger numbers of patients for longer time periods. Gilbert et al. [14] prospectively observed the effect of anaesthetic technique (spinal versus general anaesthesia) on long-term (2 years) morbidity and mortality in a large cohort ($n = 741$) of elderly (over 65) patients with acute hip fracture who had surgery from January 1990 to June 1991. After controlling the effect of demographics and baseline medical and surgical factors, there was no significant difference in mortality between patients who received spinal anaesthesia or general anaesthesia, or in the incidence of serious morbidity (pulmonary embolism, myocardial infarction, bowel obstruction, or pneumonia).

Current aggregated evidence suggests that intraoperative neuraxial anaesthesia reduces mortality and morbidity after hip fracture surgery during the first month after surgery. Yet the weight of evidence supporting this conclusion is old, and the overall conclusion may not be true of present-day practice. There is less support for improved morbidity and mortality in terms of long-term outcome. RCTs based on current standard of practice are needed. Such trials should clearly state what kind of thromboprophylaxis is used, and observe patients on a longer-term basis.

Regional anaesthesia versus general anaesthesia for carotid endarterectomy

Debate on the anaesthesia method for carotid endarterectomy raises several specific points. The advantage of regional anaesthesia is that it enables accurate neurological assessment during carotid clamping. Early detection and reversal of intraoperative brain ischemia may improve postoperative morbidity and mortality. However, being conscious during surgery may be stressful for both patients and surgeon, and the incidence of myocardial ischemia may increase as a result of increased distress and pain. Currently, most surgeons prefer general anaesthesia [45].

Rerkasem et al. [46] performed a systematic review on this topic. They included both non-randomised trials and randomised trials since not many randomized trials were found. They analysed randomised and non-randomised trials separately. The results from 41 non-randomized trials showed better outcomes among patients who received regional anaesthesia; significantly lower mortality (odds ratio, OR: 0.67,

95% CI: 0.46–0.97), significantly lower perioperative stroke (OR: 0.56, 95% CI: 0.44–0.70), and significantly lower risk of myocardial infarction within 30 days (OR: 0.55, 95% CI: 0.39–0.79). However, these results may overestimate the benefit of regional anaesthesia. Many of the trials were retrospective, and consecutive patients were not always included. Such trials are susceptible to publication bias and patient selection bias. On the other hand, the results from RCTs were underpowered. Only seven randomised trials including 554 operations were identified. None of the outcomes above were significant in the meta-analysis of randomised trials, and the results had wide 95% CIs. Because of the remaining uncertainty, a large multicentre RCT of 5000 patients is underway to determine whether the choice of anaesthesia (regional versus general) influences postoperative mortality and morbidity after carotid endarterectomy [47].

Regional anaesthesia versus general anaesthesia for Caesarean section

A large audit of obstetric anaesthesia between 1993–2003 including 377 159 deliveries in England was published recently [1]. It showed a significant increase in the Caesarean section rate from 13.6% (1993) to a high of 26.0% (2000). If the choice of anaesthesia affects outcome after Caesarean section, it can therefore affect many pregnant women and their babies. Both regional anaesthesia and general anaesthesia are used for Caesarean delivery with different advantages and disadvantages. Advantages and disadvantages must be considered both for the mother and the fetus.

The maternal risks of general anaesthesia include increased incidence of pulmonary aspiration of gastric contents and failed endotracheal intubation (the incidence was 1:238 in the previously mentioned audit) [1]. They are the major causes of maternal morbidity and mortality. Of course, maternal changes resulting from such outcomes as hypoxia and hypotension affect the outcome of the fetus. Use of halogenated volatile agents may be associated with a greater risk of maternal blood loss [48]. On the other hand, the advantage of general anaesthesia would be faster induction than regional anaesthesia in an emergency situation when fetal distress prompts urgent delivery.

The chief disadvantages of spinal and epidural anaesthesia are the potential for profound hypotension, and post-dural puncture headache (PDPH). Among parturient women, the risk of accidental dural puncture with epidural insertion is estimated as approximately 1.5%, of which half will result in PDPH. For spinal anaesthesia, the estimated incidence of PDPH is 1.7% [49]. From 1993 to 2003, significant decreases in the use of general anaesthesia for both elective (24.7–3.7% of total Caesarean sections) and emergency (43.6–11.1%) Caesarean sections were observed in the previously mentioned audit [1].

There are not many randomised trials of general versus regional anaesthesia for Caesarean section. A published meta-analysis therefore chose to include both randomised and non-randomised trials [50]. They conducted a meta-analysis on the effects of different anaesthesia methods (general, spinal, or epidural) on fetal/neonatal outcome. Their primary aim was to compare spinal anaesthesia with general anaesthesia. They performed two analyses: an analysis including all the trials, and an analysis including only RCTs. Umbilical artery pH was significantly lower and base deficit significantly higher in the group receiving spinal anaesthesia compared to the group receiving general anaesthesia in both analyses. This systematic review concluded that choice of spinal anaesthesia might not add advantage on fetal/neonatal outcome. Although significant heterogeneity and inclusion of non-randomised trials interfere with drawing solid conclusions, consistency between results from both randomised and non-randomised trials was seen, which strengthen the evidence. As they suggested, it is difficult to obtain consent from patients to randomly allocate them to very different anaesthesia methods – for example, sleeping or awake during the procedure. Careful evaluation of non-randomised trials therefore was inevitable and important in this situation.

Maternal outcome was not evaluated in the above systematic review. The advantage of spinal anaesthesia for maternal outcome may outweigh its possible advantage or disadvantage toward the fetus. A Cochrane systematic review is underway, which plans to evaluate both maternal and neonatal outcomes between using regional versus general anaesthesia [51].

Regional versus general anaesthesia for ambulatory orthopaedic surgery

Improvements in surgical and anaesthesia techniques over the past several years have led to an increase in the number and types of surgeries being performed in outpatient settings. Seventy percent of all surgical procedures performed in the United States are currently done on an ambulatory basis [52]. In ambulatory orthopaedic surgery, regional anaesthesia techniques are utilised extensively [53]. Regional anaesthesia provides excellent analgesia with reduced risk of opioid side effects such as nausea, vomiting, and drowsiness, which can frequently delay discharge or result in the patient being admitted [54,55].

Orthopaedic surgery has been shown to be one of the most painful procedures performed in ambulatory settings [56]. A recent study by Watt-Watson et al. [57] reported that 55% of ambulatory shoulder surgery patients had severe pain 7 days after discharge. The use of outpatient peripheral nerve blocks is frequently criticised, because intense pain may follow after the analgesic effect diminishes at home [58]. It is also suggested that long-acting peripheral nerve blockade results in elevated risk of injury as the result of loss of proprioception and the protective reflex of pain. In ambulatory surgery, substantial pain with limited function can still be a problem 7 days after discharge [59]. As Klein et al. reported, a large percentage of patients (17–27%) who receive regional anaesthesia with long-acting local anaesthetics, still used opioids at 7 days following upper or lower ambulatory orthopaedic surgeries [53].

Whether the type of anaesthesia affects long-term postoperative outcome such as pain and function after discharge is still unknown. Future study should look at outcomes after discharge from ambulatory surgery, with long-term basis.

Regional versus general anaesthesia: postoperative cognitive dysfunction in elderly patients after non-cardiac surgery

Postoperative cognitive dysfunction is common in elderly patients. Moller et al. prospectively observed 1218 elderly patients who underwent non-cardiac major surgery under general anaesthesia. They found that long-term cognitive dysfunction after surgery was common; the prevalence was 25.8% and 9.9% respectively at 1 week and 3 months after surgery [60]. They also suggested that long-term cognitive dysfunction correlated with decreased levels of activities of daily living.

It is believed that acute postoperative confusion and disorientation are less common after regional anaesthesia than after general anaesthesia. Parker et al. [3] showed a significant reduction in acute postoperative confusion in the regional anaesthesia group compared to the general anaesthesia group (RR: 0.50%, 95% CI: 0.26–0.95) in their meta-analysis of hip fracture patients. Current evidence does not support significant differences in longer-term cognitive dysfunction [30–33,61]. Rasmussen et al. [62] studied 438 patients over 60 years old undergoing major non-cardiac surgery. Participants were randomised to receive either general or regional anaesthesia (spinal or epidural, light sedation with propofol was permitted). The majority of participants underwent orthopaedic (hip and knee) and gynaecological procedures. The incidence of postoperative cognitive dysfunction was greater in the general anaesthesia group at 1 week after surgery. The difference was marginally significant. However, the difference did not exist after 3 months. A low-recruitment rate and poor adherence to the allocated anaesthetic by surgeons and anaesthetists underpowered and obscured the results.

For other trials, the sample size was small [30–57,61]. They used different methods for evaluating the level of cognitive dysfunction (use of different neuropsychological tests, comparing two treatment groups rather than looking at score change in individuals), which precluded combining data quantitatively. Moreover, the study population in these trials was almost exclusively orthopaedic, making it difficult to apply the result to other patient populations. Further study should pre-define postoperative cognitive dysfunction and include patients with various types of surgery.

Summary

The effect of regional anaesthesia on postoperative major morbidity and mortality is still unclear. Evidence suggests the possibility of reduced mortality among several specific patient populations such as hip fracture surgery under spinal anaesthesia. However the evidence supporting this is relatively old, and may not reflect outcomes of present-day practice. Evidence on long-term morbidity and mortality is too limited to draw any conclusions. There are not many RCTs comparing regional (without general anaesthesia) versus general anaesthesia, and most of them are small. Reasons may include the difficulty in obtaining consent from patients to randomly allocate them to very different anaesthesia methods – sleeping or awake during the procedure, and convince surgeons and anaesthetists to adhere to the allocated anaesthetic. Large, well-designed RCTs on a longer-term basis are necessary to draw solid conclusions. If it is not practical to perform such RCTs, carefully designed observational studies which address any possible confounding factors, and include large numbers of patients for longer time periods, would help evidence-based decision making.

Practice points

- A systematic review of trials assessing regional (versus general) anaesthesia for hip fracture surgery showed reduced risk of death and deep venous thrombosis. However, many included trials were old and may not represent current practice. For example: thromboembolism may have been a greater risk before modern thrombo-prophylaxis, with greater benefit from regional.
- Combined non-randomised trials of regional (versus general) anaesthesia for carotid endarterectomy show reduced incidences of death, perioperative stroke, and myocardial infarction. These differences are not shown by combined RCTs.
- Results of a systematic review of trials assessing fetal outcome after regional versus general anaesthesia for Caesarean section are inconclusive.
- For ambulatory orthopaedic surgery, regional (versus general) anaesthesia provides superior pain relief and opioid sparing early in the postoperative course.
- Immediate postoperative cognitive function in the elderly is improved by regional (versus general) anaesthesia, at least in orthopaedic cases. There is no evidence to support longer-term benefit.

Research agenda
- Trials of anaesthesia for hip fracture surgery should clarify the type of thrombo-prophylaxis used.
- A large multicentre RCT (5000 patients) assessing regional versus general anaesthesia for carotid endarterectomy is in progress.
- A Cochrane review is underway to assess the effect of regional versus general anaesthesia on both maternal and neonatal outcomes.
- Trials of anaesthetic options for ambulatory surgery should follow patients after discharge from hospital.
- Trials assessing postoperative cognitive dysfunction should predefine cognitive dysfunction, incorporate different surgical models, and include long-term assessments.
- Well-designed observational trials may be useful when randomisation is impractical.

REFERENCES

1 Rahman K, Jenkins JG. Failed tracheal intubation in obstetrics: no more frequent but still managed badly. *Anaesthesia* 2005; 60(2): 168–71.

2 Rodgers A, Walker N, Schug S, McKee A, Kehlet H, van Zundert A et al. Reduction of postoperative mortality and morbidity with epidural or spinal anaesthesia: results from overview of randomised trials. *BMJ* 2000; 321(7275): 1493.

3 Parker MJ, Handoll HHG, Griffiths R. Anaesthesia for hip fracture surgery in adults. *The Cochrane Database of Syst Rev* 2004, Issue 4. Art. No.: CD000521. DOI: 10.1002/14651858. pub2.

4 Yeager MP, Glass DD, Neff RK, Brinck-Johnsen T. Epidural anesthesia and analgesia in high-risk surgical patients. *Anesthesiology* 1987; 66: 729–36.

5 McLaren AD, Stockwell MC, Reid VT. Anaesthetic techniques for surgical correction of fractured neck of the femur. A comparative study of spinal and general anaesthesia in the elderly. *Anaesthesia* 1978; 33(1): 10–14.

6 McKenzie PJ, Wishart HY, Smith G. Long-term outcome after repair of fractured neck of femur. Comparison of subarachnoid and general anaesthesia. *Br J Anaesth* 1984; 56(6): 581–5.

7 Park YW, Thompson J, Lee K. Effect of epidural anesthesia and analgesia on perioperative outcome. A randomized, controlled Veterans Affairs Cooperative Study. *Ann Surg* 2001; 234: 560–71.

8 Rigg J, Jamrozik K, Myles P, Silbert B, Peyton P, Parsons R. Epidural anaesthesia and analgesia and outcome of major surgery: a randomised trial. *Lancet* 2002; 359(9314): 1276–82.

9 Peyton PJ, Myles PS, Silbert BS, Rigg JA, Jamrozik K, Parsons R. Perioperative epidural analgesia and outcome after major abdominal surgery in high-risk patients. *Anesth Analg* 2003; 96: 548–54.

10 Todd C, Freeman C, Camilleri-Ferrante C, Palmer C, Hyder A, Laxton C et al. Differences in mortality after fracture of hip: the East Anglican audit. *BMJ* 1995; 310: 904–8.

11 Williams BA, DeRiso BM, Figallo CM, Anders JW, Engel LB, Sproul KA et al. Benchmarking the perioperative process: III. Effects of regional anesthesia clinical pathway techniques on process efficiency and recovery profiles in ambulatory orthopedic surgery. *J Clin Anesth* 1998; 10: 570–8.

12 Norris EJ, Beattie C, Perler BA, Martinez EA, Meinert CL, Anderson GF et al. Double-masked randomized trial comparing alternate combinations of intraoperative anesthesia and postoperative analgesia in abdominal aortic surgery. *Anesthesiology* 2001; 95(5): 1054–67.

13 Priestley MC, Cope L, Halliwell R, Gibson P, Chard RB, Skinner M et al. Thoracic epidural anesthesia for cardiac surgery: the effects on tracheal intubation time and length of hospital stay. *Anesth Analg* 2002; 94: 275–82.

14 Gilbert TB, Hawkes WG, Hebel JR, Hudson JI, Kenzora JE, Zimerman SI et al. Spinal anesthesia versus general anesthesia for hip fracture repair: a longitudinal observation of 741 elderly patients during 2-year follow-up. *Am J Orthop* 2000; 29(1): 25–35.

15 Brinker MR, Reuben JD, Mull JR, Cox DD, Daum WJ, Parker JR. Comparison of general and epidural anesthesia in patients undergoing primary unilateral THR. *Orthopedics* 1997; 20(2): 109–15.

16 Modig J, Hjelmstedt A, Sahlstedt B, Maripuu E. Comparative influences of epidural and general anaesthesia on deep venous thrombosis and pulmonary embolism after total hip replacement. *Acta Chir Scand* 1981; 147(2): 125–30.

17 Scott NB, Turfrey DJ, Ray DAA, Nzewi O, Sutcliffe NP, Lal AB et al. A prospective randomized study of the potential benefits of thoracic epidural anesthesia and analgesia in patients undergoing coronary artery bypass grafting. *Anesth Analg* 2001; 93: 528–35.

18 Blomberg S, Emanuelsson H, Kwist H, Lamm C, Ponten J, Waagstein F et al. Effects of thoracic epidural anesthesia on coronary arteries and arterioles in patients with coronary artery disease. *Anesthesiology* 1990; 73: 840–7.

19 Turfrey DJ, Ray DAA, Sutcliffe NP, Ramayya P, Kenny GNC, Scott NB. Thoracic epidural anaesthesia for coronary artery bypass graft surgery. Effects on postoperative complications. *Anaesthesia* 1997; 52: 1090–4.

20 Baron J-F, Bertrand M, Barre E, Godet G, Mundler O, Coriat P et al. Combined epidural and general anesthesia versus general anesthesia for abdominal aortic surgery. *Anesthesiology* 1991; 75: 611–18.

21 Christopherson R, Beattie C, Frank SM, Norris EJ, Meinert CL, Gottlieb SO et al. Perioperative morbidity in patients randomized to epidural or general anesthesia for lower extremity vascular surgery. Perioperative ischemia randomized anesthesia trial study group. *Anesthesiology* 1993; 79(3): 422–34.

22 Bode RH, Lewis KP, Zarich SW, Pierce ET, Roberts M, Kowalchuk GJ et al. Cardiac outcome after peripheral vascular surgery: comparison of general and regional anesthesia. *Anesthesiology* 1996; 84: 3–13.

23 Garnett RL, MacIntyre A, Lindsay P, Barber GG, Cole CW, Hajjar G et al. Perioperative ischaemia in aortic surgery: combined epidural/general anaesthesia and epidural analgesia vs. general anaesthesia and IV analgesia. *Can J Anaesth* 1996; 43(8): 769–77.

24 Tuman KJ, McCarthy RJ, March RJ, DeLaria GA, Patel RV, Ivankovich AD. Effects of epidural anesthesia and analgesia on coagulation and outcome after major vascular surgery. *Anesth Analg* 1991; 73: 696–704.

25 Keith A. Anaesthesia and blood loss in total hip replacement. *Anaesthesia* 1977; 32: 444–50.

26 Williams-Russo P, Sharrock NE, Haas SB, Insall J, Windsor RE, Laskin RS et al. Randomized trial of epidural versus general anesthesia: outcomes after primary total knee replacement. *Clin Orthop* 1996; 331: 199–208.

27 Gottschalk A, Smith DS, Jobes DR, Kennedy SK, Lally SE, Noble VE et al. Preemptive epidural analgesia and recovery from radical prostatectomy. A randomized controlled trial. *JAMA* 1998; 279: 1076–82.

28 Koval KJ, Aharonoff GB, Rosenberg AD, Bernstein RL, Zucherman JD. Functional outcome after hip fracture. *Clin Orthopaed Relat Res* 1998; 348: 37–41.

29 Handley GH, Silbert BS, Mooney PH, Schwitzer SA, Aleen NB. Combined general and epidural anesthesia versus general anesthesia for major abdominal surgery: postanesthesia recovery characteristics. *Reg Anesth* 1997; 22(5): 435–41.

30 Riis J, Lomholt B, Haxholdt O, Kehlet H, Valentin N, Danielsen U et al. Immediate and long-term mental recovery from general versus epidural anesthesia in elderly patients. *Acta Anaesthesiol Scand* 1983; 27(1): 44–9.

31 Bigler D, Adelhoj B, Petring OU, Pederson NO, Busch P, Kalhke P. Mental function and morbidity after acute hip surgery during spinal and general anaesthesia. *Anaesthesia* 1985; 40(7): 672–6.

32 Berggren D, Gustafson Y, Eriksson B, Bucht G, Hansson LI, Reiz S et al. Postoperative confusion after anesthesia in elderly patients with femoral neck fractures. *Anesth Analg* 1987; 66(6): 497–504.

33 Williams-Russo P, Sharrock NE, Mattis S, Szatrowski TP, Charlson ME. Cognitive effects after epidural vs. general anesthesia in older adults. A randomized trial. *JAMA* 1995; 274(1): 44–50.

34 Hall GM, Ali W. The stress response and its modification by regional anaesthesia. *Anaesth* 1998; 53(Suppl 2): 10–2.

35 Tomkinson J, Turnbull A, Robson G, Dawson I, Cloake E, Adelstein AM et al. Report on Confidential enquires into Maternal Deaths in England and Wales. Department of Health and Social Security, 1976. UK: HMSO.

36 Hawkins J, Koonin L, Palmer S, Gibbs C. Anesthesia-related deaths during obstetric delivery in the United States, 1979–1990. *Anesthesiology* 1997; 86: 277–84.

37 Davis FM, Laurenson VG. Spinal anaesthesia or general anaesthesia for emergency hip surgery in elderly patients. *Anaesth Intens Care* 1981; 9(4): 352–8.

38 Davis FM, Woolner DF, Frampton C, Wilkinson A, Grant A, Harrison RT et al. Prospective, multi-centre trial of mortality following general or spinal anaesthesia for hip fracture surgery in the elderly. *Br J Anaesth* 1987; 59(9): 1080–8.

39 Juelsgaard P, Sand NP, Felsby S, Dalsgaard J, Jakobsen KB, Brink O et al. Perioperative myocardial ischaemia in patients undergoing surgery for fractured hip randomized to incremental spinal, single-dose spinal or general anaesthesia. *Eur J Anaesthesiol* 1998; 15(6): 656–63.

40 Racle JP, Benkhadra A, Poy JY, Gleizal B, Gaudray A. Comparative study of general and spinal anesthesia in elderly women in hip surgery. *Ann Fr Anesth Reanim* 1986; 5(1): 24–30.

41 Valentin N, Lomholt B, Jensen JS, Hejgaard N, Kreiner S. Spinal or general anaesthesia for surgery of the fractured hip? A prospective study of mortality in 578 patients. *Br J Anaesth* 1986; 58(3): 284–91.

42 Mismetti P, Laporte S, Darmon JY, Buchmuller A, Decousus H. Meta-analysis of low molecular weight heparin in the prevention of venous thromboembolism in general surgery. *Br J Surg* 2001; 88(7): 913–30.

43 Auerbach AD, Goldman L. Beta-blockers and reduction of cardiac events in non-cardiac surgery: clinical applications. *JAMA* 2002; 287(11): 1445–7.

44 Parker MJ, Pryor GA, Myles J. 11-year results in 2,846 patients of the Peterborough Hip Fracture Project: reduced morbidity, mortality and hospital stay. *Acta Orthop Scand* 2000; 71(1): 34–8.

45 Murie JA, John TG, Morris PJ. Carotid endarterectomy in Great Britain and Ireland: practice between 1984 and 1992. *Br J Surg* 1994; 81(6): 827–31.

46 Rerkasem K, Bond R, Rothwell PM. Local versus general anaesthesia for carotid endarterectomy. *The Cochrane Database of Syst Rev* 2004, Issue 2. Art. No.: CD000126. DOI: 10.1002/14651858.pub2.

47 GALA TRIAL home page. Available at: http://www.dcn.ed.ac.uk/gala/ (accessed on July/15, 2005).

48 Andrews WW, Ramin SM, Maberry MC, Shearer V, Black S, Wallace DH. Effect of type of anesthesia on blood loss at elective repeat Caesarean section. *Am J Perinatol* 1992; 9(3): 197–200.

49 Choi PT, Galinski SE, Takeuchi L, Lucas S, Tamayo C, Jadad AR. PDPH is a common complication of neuraxial blockade in parturients: a meta-analysis of obstetrical studies. *Can J Anaesth* 2003; 50(5): 460–9.

50 Reynolds F, Seed PT. Anaesthesia for Caesarean section and neonatal acid-base status: a meta-analysis. *Anaesthesia* 2005; 60(7): 636–53.

51 Afolabi BB, Lesi AFE. Regional versus general anaesthesia for caesarean section. (Protocol) *The Cochrane Database of Syst Rev* 2003, Issue 3. Art. No.: CD004350. DOI: 10.1002/14651858.

52 Capdevila X, Dadure C. Perioperative management for one day hospital admission: regional anesthesia is better than general anesthesia. *Acta Anaesthesiol Belg* 2004; 55(Suppl): 33–6.

53 Klein SM, Nielsen KC, Greengrass RA, Warner DS, Martin A, Steele SM. Ambulatory discharge after long-acting peripheral nerve blockade: 2382 blocks with ropivacaine. *Anesth Analg* 2002; 94(1): 65–70.

54 Mulroy MF, McDonald SB. Regional anesthesia for outpatient surgery. *Anesthesiol Clin N Am* 2003; 21(2): 289–303.

55 McGrath B, Chung F. Postoperative recovery and discharge. *Anesthesiol Clin N Am* 2003; 21(2): 367–86.

56 Chung F, Ritchie E, Su J. Postoperative pain in ambulatory surgery. *Anesth Analg* 1997; 85(4): 808–16.

57 Watt-Watson J, Chung F, Chan VWS, McGillion M. Pain management following discharge after ambulatory same-day surgery. *J Nurs Manage* 2004; 12: 153–61.

58 Klein SM. Beyond the hospital: continuous peripheral nerve blocks at home. *Anesthesiology* 2002; 96(6): 1283–5.

59 Beauregard L, Pomp A, Choiniere M. Severity and impact of pain after day-surgery. *Can J Anaesth* 1998; 45(4): 304–11.

60 Moller JT, Cluitmans P, Rasmussen LS, Houx P, Rasmussen H, Canet J et al. Long-term postoperative cognitive dysfunction in the elderly ISPOCD1 study. ISPOCD investigators. *Int Study Post-Oper Cogn Dysfunct* 1998; 351(9106): 857–61.

61 Casati A, Aldegheri G, Vinciguerra E, Marsan A, Fraschini G, Torri G. Randomized comparison between sevoflurane anaesthesia and unilateral spinal anaesthesia in elderly patients undergoing orthopaedic surgery. *Eur J Anaesthesiol* 2003; 20(8): 640–6.

62 Rasmussen LS, Johnson T, Kuipers HM, Kristensen D, Siersma VD, Vila P et al. Does anaesthesia cause postoperative cognitive dysfunction? A randomised study of regional versus general anaesthesia in 438 elderly patients. *Acta Anaesthesiol Scand* 2003; 47(3): 260–6.

15

Fluid therapy

Peter Choi[1] and J Mark Ansermino[2]

[1]Department of Anesthesia, Vancouver Hospital, University of British Columbia, Vancouver, British Columbia, Canada
[2]Department of Pediatric Anesthesia, British Columbia Children's Hospital, Vancouver, British Columbia, Canada

Despite hundreds of laboratory and clinical studies, the choice of intravenous (IV) fluid, the volume of fluid to be administered, and the timing of fluid administration remain controversial. Based on the evidence from clinical trials and meta-analyses, a statistically significant reduction in mortality or relevant adverse clinical outcomes amongst surgical or critically ill adult or paediatric patients has not been found with the use of any particular IV fluid.

Restrictive fluid regimens may decrease perioperative morbidity in adults undergoing elective intra-abdominal surgery but the results cannot be generalised to other populations or procedures. The effect of restricted versus liberal fluid regimens on clinical outcomes in patients undergoing minimally invasive or ambulatory procedures is still inconclusive.

Although there is a trend in fewer deaths with delayed fluid resuscitation of patients with penetrating trauma, the data are insufficient to draw guidelines. Large multicentre randomised controlled trials (RCTs) of fluid regimens with clinically relevant outcomes are still needed to address important questions in this field.

Introduction

The use of IV fluids for volume resuscitation and fluid replacement in the surgical or critically ill patient has been studied and practiced for nearly 90 years. Despite hundreds of laboratory and clinical studies, the choice of IV fluid, the volume of fluid to be administered, and the timing of fluid administration remain controversial. In this chapter, we have presented the evidence available to answer the following questions:

- Does the choice of IV fluid make a difference to clinical outcomes?
- Does the amount of IV fluid make a difference to clinical outcomes?
- Does the timing of IV fluid administration make a difference to clinical outcomes?

Key words: Colloid, crystalloid, randomised controlled trials, albumin.

We have focused on patients in the critical care or perioperative settings. This chapter discusses neither fluid therapy in the obstetrical setting (covered in Chapter 18) nor alternatives to allogeneic blood transfusions. Some details regarding patients undergoing abdominal surgery and critically ill patients can be found also in Chapters 19 and 25, respectively.

Whenever possible, we have presented the evidence from specific populations (e.g. paediatrics, trauma, burns, cardiac surgery). We have relied on the evidence from systematic reviews and meta-analyses. When such evidence was unavailable, the results from RCTs have been presented.

Does the choice of IV fluid affect clinical outcomes?

Nineteen systematic reviews [1–19] compared different IV fluids with regard to clinical outcomes. Of these, two [1,2] were older versions of updated systematic reviews. With the exception of one review of the data from animal studies of trauma [3], all systematic reviews focused on human data. Ten systematic reviews [4–13] included children, but only two [4,5] were exclusive to the paediatric population. Adult populations that have been studied include critically ill patients (especially those with burns, trauma, or hypoalbuminaemia) and surgical patients (including patients undergoing cardiopulmonary bypass). The results from the meta-analyses are summarised in Table 15.1.

Isotonic crystalloids versus colloids

Four systematic reviews [1,14–16] have pooled data from RCTs comparing isotonic crystalloids to colloids in clinically heterogeneous populations. Statistically significant differences in mortality [1,14–16] or pulmonary oedema [16] were not detected regardless of the manner in which the data were pooled.

Hypertonic crystalloids versus isotonic crystalloids

One systematic review [7] pooled data from 14 RCTs comparing hypertonic crystalloids to isotonic crystalloids in 654 trauma patients (six RCTs), 72 burn patients (three RCTs), and 230 surgical patients (five RCTs). Hypertonic saline was compared to Ringer's lactate and normal saline in 11 and three RCTs, respectively. All-cause mortality rates were not significantly different between hypertonic crystalloids and isotonic crystalloids.

Hypertonic crystalloids versus colloids

One systematic review [6] has examined the data from three RCTs comparing hypertonic crystalloids to albumin, hydroxyethyl starch (HES), or gelatin. Only one RCT [20] reported any deaths amongst its 38 patients and the numbers (3, albumin

Table 15.1. Meta-analyses of RCTs of different IV fluids and their effect on clinical outcomes

Reference	Population	Number of patients (studies; years)	Outcome	Effect size (95% CI)[a]
Colloids versus isotonic crystalloids				
Schierhout and	All critically ill	1315 (19; 1966–1996)	All-cause mortality	RR: 1.19 (0.98, 1.45)
Roberts [1]	Trauma	636 (6; 1977–1993)	All-cause mortality	RR: 1.30 (0.95, 1.77)
	Burns	416 (4; 1966–1983)	All-cause mortality	RR: 1.21 (0.88, 1.66)
	Surgery	191 (7; 1979–1996)	All-cause mortality	RR: 0.55 (0.18, 1.65)
Choi et al. [16]	All critically ill	180 (6; 1979–1990)	Pulmonary oedema	RR: 0.84 (0.28, 2.45)
	Trauma	86 (2; 1981–1983)	Pulmonary oedema	RR: 3.66 (0.59, 22.8)
	Non-trauma	94 (4; 1979–1990)	Pulmonary oedema	RR: 0.47 (0.19, 1.19)
	Surgery	68 (3; 1979–1990)	Pulmonary oedema	RR: 0.74 (0.26, 2.07)
Hypertonic crystalloids versus isotonic crystalloids				
Bunn et al. [7]	Trauma	651 (6; 1992–2004)	All-cause mortality	RR: 0.84 (0.69, 1.04)
	Burns	89 (3; 1978–1996)	All-cause mortality	RR: 1.49 (0.56, 3.95)
	Surgery	230 (5; 1987–1992)	All-cause mortality	RR: 0.51 (0.09, 2.73)
Albumin versus isotonic crystalloids				
Alderson	All critically ill	8452 (32; 1973–2004)	All-cause mortality	RR: 1.04 (0.95, 1.13)
et al. [10]	Hypovolaemia	7652 (19; 1977–2004)	All-cause mortality	RR: 1.01 (0.92, 1.10)
	Burns	163 (3; 1978–1995)	All-cause mortality	RR: 2.40 (1.11, 5.19)
	Hypoalbuminaemia	637 (10; 1973–1997)	All-cause mortality	RR: 1.38 (0.94, 2.03)
Russell	Cardiopulmonary bypass	353 (7; 1989–2002)	Platelet drop on bypass	WMD −23.8 (−42.8, −4.7)[b]
et al. [13]	Cardiopulmonary bypass	410 (9; 1981–2002)	COP drop on bypass	WMD −3.6 (−4.8, −2.3)[c]
	Cardiopulmonary bypass	276 (7; 1981–1993)	COP drop postoperative	WMD −2.0 (−2.9, −1.1)[c]
	Cardiopulmonary bypass	514 (10; 1981–2002)	On-bypass fluid balance	WMD −584 (−819, −348)[d]
	Cardiopulmonary bypass	219 (4; 1985–2001)	24 h weight gain	WMD −1.0 (−0.6, −1.3)[e]
HES versus isotonic crystalloids				
Roberts et al. [6]	All critically ill	374 (10; 1983–2001)	All-cause mortality	RR: 1.16 (0.68, 1.96)
Dextran versus isotonic crystalloids				
Roberts et al. [6]	All critically ill	834 (9; 1978–1997)	All-cause mortality	RR: 1.24 (0.94, 1.65)
Gelatin versus isotonic crystalloids				
Roberts et al. [6]	All critically ill	346 (7; 1993–2001)	All-cause mortality	RR: 0.54 (0.16, 1.85)

(Continued)

Table 15.1. (Continued)

Reference	Population	Number of patients (studies; years)	Outcome	Effect size (95% CI)[a]
Hypertonic saline/dextran versus isotonic crystalloids				
Roberts et al. [6]	Trauma	1238 (8; 1990–1994)	All-cause mortality	RR: 0.88 (0.74, 1.05)
Wade et al. [17]	Trauma	1233 (8; 1990–1994)	Survival rate	OR: 1.20 (0.94, 1.57)
Wade et al. [19]	Traumatic brain injury	223 (6; 1990–1994)	24 h survival rate	OR: 1.93 (0.97, 3.84)
	Traumatic brain injury	223 (6; 1990–1994)	Survival to discharge	OR: 2.12 (1.01, 4.49)
Albumin versus HES				
Bunn et al. [11]	All critically ill	1029 (20; 1982–1997)	All-cause mortality	RR: 1.17 (0.91, 1.50)
Wilkes et al. [12]	Cardiopulmonary bypass	653 (16; 1982–1998)	Postoperative bleeding	SMD −0.24 (−0.40, −0.08)
Albumin versus gelatin				
Bunn et al. [11]	All critically ill	542 (4; 1987–1996)	All-cause mortality	RR: 0.99 (0.69, 1.42)
Gelatin versus HES				
Bunn et al. [11]	All critically ill	945 (11; 1994–2001)	All-cause mortality	RR: 1.00 (0.78, 1.28)

CI: confidence interval; COP: colloid oncotic pressure; OR: odds ratio; RR: relative risk; SMD: standardised mean difference; WMD: weighted mean difference.

[a] For ORs and RRs, a value <1 indicates the outcome is lower in the first group; a value >1 indicates the outcome is higher in the first group. For standardised and weighted mean differences, a value <0 indicates the outcome is lower in the first group and a value >0 indicates the outcome is higher in the first group. The effect size is statistically significant ($P < 0.05$) if the 95% CI does not include 1 for OR and RR and does not include 0 for SMD and WMD.

[b] Units are in $\times 10^9 L^{-1}$.

[c] Units are in mmHg.

[d] Units are in mL.

[e] Units are in kg.

group; 0, hypertonic saline group) were too small to detect a statistically significant difference.

Albumin or plasma protein fraction

Human albumin has received the most attention and controversy amongst IV fluids. Nine meta-analyses [2,5,6,8–10,13] have reviewed the data from RCTs [11–13] comparing albumin or plasma protein fraction to crystalloids or other colloids. Reviewers from the Cochrane Injuries Group had initially found a statistically significant increase in mortality amongst critically ill patients with hypovolaemia, burns, or hypoalbuminaemia from the use of albumin or plasma protein fraction compared to crystalloids [2], but this effect was not statistically significant after the results of a large multicentre RCT, the Saline versus Albumin Fluid Evaluation (SAFE) Study [10], was included in a subsequent update of their meta-analysis. Reviewers from Hygeia Associates have found similar results for mortality when data were pooled from studies of surgery, trauma, burns, hypoalbuminaemia, ascites, or high-risk neonates [8].

One qualitative systematic review [9] has reported decreased fluid requirements and pulmonary and intestinal oedema amongst patients undergoing non-cardiac surgery from the use of albumin compared to crystalloids. Morbidity was also decreased amongst patients with hypoalbuminaemia, ascites, sepsis, or burns [9].

In cardiac surgery, pump priming with albumin reduced the on-bypass drop in platelet counts, the decline in colloid oncotic pressure, the on-bypass positive fluid balance, and the postoperative weight gain compared to pump priming with crystalloids [13]. Postoperative bleeding was statistically lower amongst patients receiving albumin compared with HES during cardiopulmonary bypass although the difference in pooled mean blood loss was not clinically significant between patients receiving albumin (693 ± 350 mL) and patients receiving HES (789 ± 487 mL) [12].

Despite similar results, the recommendations from different reviewers have been discordant. The reviewers from the Cochrane Injuries Group have suggested that "albumin should only be used within the context of [sic] well concealed and adequately powered randomised controlled trial" [10]. In contrast, the reviewers from Hygeia Associates, who were funded by the Plasma Protein Therapeutics Association and the American Red Cross, concluded that their "findings should allay concerns about the safety of albumin" [8]. The opposing conclusions, based on fairly similar findings on mortality, are confusing. Furthermore, critics have pointed out the clinical heterogeneity of the patient populations, the interventions, and the co-interventions (including changes in practice over time) amongst the RCTs pooled in the various systematic reviews [21], the potential of publication bias, and the risk of false-positive findings when data from small studies are pooled; all of these threaten the validity and applicability of using meta-analysis in this situation.

The lack of a clear answer regarding the effect of albumin on mortality amongst critically ill patients led to a large, multicentre, double-blind RCT, the Saline versus Albumin Fluid Evaluation (SAFE) Study [22]. The SAFE Study randomised 6997 patients who had been admitted to the intensive care unit (ICU) to receive either human albumin (3497 patients) or normal saline (3500 patients) for intravascular fluid resuscitation during the 28 days after randomisation. The study had 90% power to detect an absolute difference of 3% from a baseline mortality of 15%. There were no significant differences between the two groups in 28-day all-cause mortality (primary outcome) or in length of ICU stay, hospital stay, mechanical ventilation, or renal-replacement therapy (Table 15.2). The results suggested that any potential

Table 15.2. RCTs of fluid therapy that have not been pooled in meta-analyses

Reference	Population	Interventions	Outcome, Results, and Effect Size (95% CI)[a]
Albumin versus isotonic crystalloids			
SAFE Study [22]	Critically ill adult patients requiring fluid resuscitation	4% albumin versus 0.9% saline	*28-day mortality rate* 726/3497 (albumin) versus 729/3500 (saline) RR: 0.99 (0.91, 1.09)[b]
Liberal versus restrictive fluid administration			
Fortune et al. [27]	Trauma patients with class III–IV haemorrhage	Blood transfusion to maintain haematocrit at 0.30 versus 0.40	*3-day mortality rate*
Dunham et al. [28]	Hypotensive adult trauma patients	RBC, FFP, platelets, and crystalloids: large volumes versus small volumes	*In-hospital mortality rate* 5/20 (liberal) versus 5/16 (restrictive) RR: 0.80 (0.28, 2.29) PT: 14.8 s (liberal) versus 13.9 s (restrictive) PTT: 47.3 s (liberal) versus 35.1 s (restrictive)
Dutton et al. [29]	Hypotensive trauma patients	RBC, FFP, and plasmalyte to maintain SBP of 100 mmHg versus 70 mmHg	*In-hospital mortality rate* 4/55 (liberal) versus 4/55 (restrictive) RR: 1.00 (0.26, 3.81)
Brandstrup et al. [31]	Adult patients undergoing elective colorectal resection with epigeneral anaesthesia	Liberal intraoperative fluid therapy: 0.5 L HES preload +0.5 L NS maintenance +NS 7 mL kg^{-1}h^{-1} (0–1 h), 5 mL kg^{-1}h^{-1} (>1–3 h), 3 mL kg^{-1}h^{-1} (>3 h) third space replacement +1 −1.5 L NS (EBL $\leq$ 0.5 L), HES (EBL > 0.5 L), blood transfusion (EBL > 1.5 L) versus restrictive intraoperative fluid therapy: 0.5 L 5% glucose in water	*30-day postoperative complication rate* 44/72 (liberal) versus 28/69 (restrictive)[c] RR: 1.51 (1.07, 2.12)

(Continued)

Table 15.2. (Continued)

Reference	Population	Interventions	Outcome, Results, and Effect Size (95% CI)[a]
		maintenance + volume-for-volume HES up to 0.5 L + blood transfusion (EBL > 1.5 L)	
Holte et al. [32]	Adult patients undergoing elective laparoscopic cholecystectomy	Intraoperative fluid therapy: 40 mL kg^{-1} LR versus 15 mL kg^{-1} LR	*Pulmonary function over first 24 h after surgery* FVC and FEV$_1$ better in liberal group at 2 h postoperatively; FVC better in liberal group at 4 h postoperatively Readiness for hospital discharge on day of surgery 23/24 (liberal) versus 16/24 (restrictive)[d]
Nisanevich et al. [33]	Adult patients undergoing elective intra-abdominal surgery	Intraoperative fluid therapy: 10 mL kg^{-1} bolus +12 mL kg^{-1} h^{-1} LR versus 4 mL kg^{-1} h^{-1} LR	*In-hospital postoperative complication rate* 23/75 (liberal) versus 13/77 (restrictive)[e]

Early versus delayed fluid resuscitation

Reference	Population	Interventions	Outcome, Results, and Effect Size (95% CI)[a]
Blair et al. [34]	Patients with acute gastrointestinal haemorrhage and hypotension	Early versus delayed blood transfusion	*In-hospital mortality rate* 2/24 (early) versus 0/26 (delayed) RR: 5.4 (0.3, 107.1) PTT: 48 s (early) versus 41 s (delayed) WMD 7.0 s (6.0, 8.0)
Bickell et al. [35]	Adult patients with penetrating trauma and hypotension	Pre-hospital early versus delayed crystalloid fluid resuscitation	*In-hospital mortality rate* 116/309 (early) versus 86/289 (delayed) RR: 1.26 (1.00, 1.58) PT: 14.1 s (early) versus 11.4 s (delayed) WMD 2.7 s (0.9, 4.5)

(Continued)

Table 15.2. (Continued)

Reference	Population	Interventions	Outcome, Results, and Effect Size (95% CI)[a]
Turner et al. [36]	Hypotensive adult trauma patients	Early versus delayed fluid resuscitation	PTT: 31.8 s (early) versus 27.5 s (delayed) WMD 4.3 s (1.7, 6.9) *6-month mortality rate* 73/699 (early) versus 60/610 (delayed) RR: 1.06 (0.77, 1.47)

CI: confidence interval; EBL: estimated blood loss; FEV_1: forced expiratory volume in 1 s; FFP: fresh frozen plasma; FVC: forced vital capacity; LR: lactated Ringers; NS: normal saline; PT: prothrombin time; PTT: partial thromboplastin time; RBC: red blood cells; RR: relative risk; SBP: systolic blood pressure; WMD: weighted mean difference.

[a] For RRs, a value <1 indicates the outcome is lower in the first group; a value >1 indicates the outcome is higher in the first group; and a value of 1 indicates no difference. For weighted mean differences, a value <0 indicates the outcome is lower in the first group and a value >0 is higher in the first group. The effect size is statistically significant ($P < 0.05$) if the 95% CI does not include 1 for RR and does not include 0 for WMD.

[b] $P = 0.87$.

[c] $P = 0.013$.

[d] $P < 0.02$.

[e] $P = 0.046$.

difference in all-cause mortality between the two IV fluids would be less than 3%. The study was not powered to draw conclusions on potential subgroups of critically ill patients who may benefit either from albumin or from normal saline.

Hydroxyethyl starch

HESs are synthetic IV colloids derived from modification of amylopectin [23]. Commercial products in North America have molecular weights (MW) that are either high (450–480 kDa; e.g. hetastarch) or medium (130–200 kDa; e.g. pentastarch). Products in Europe are more varied and include HES with low MW (40–70 kDa) [23]. A number of RCTs have compared high- or medium-MW HES with other IV fluids. The pooled data did not show any significant differences in mortality when HES was compared with crystalloids [6], albumin or plasma protein fraction [11], or gelatins [11]. As noted earlier, in patients undergoing cardiopulmonary bypass, there was a significantly larger difference in bleeding with HES compared with albumin but the difference in pooled mean blood loss was not clinically significant [12].

Dextrans

Dextrans are glucose polymers with a mean MW of either 40 kDa (dextran 40) or 70 kDa (dextran 70); however, only dextran 70 is used in fluid resuscitation. As of November 2005, dextran 70 will no longer be available in Europe. Pooled data from nine RCTs [6] did not show any significant differences in mortality when dextran 70 was compared with isotonic crystalloids amongst critically ill patients.

Wade and colleagues have pooled most of the mortality data on 7.5% hypertonic saline –6% dextran 70 (HSD) in trauma patients [17–19]. There was no difference in survival rates after fluid resuscitation using HSD compared with isotonic crystalloids. When data from individual patients of the eight RCTs were obtained and pooled (individual patient meta-analysis), the survival rate to hospital discharge was significantly higher in the HSD group compared with the isotonic crystalloid group, but the results were based on data from only 604 of the original 1233 patients [18]. Similarly, individual patient meta-analysis [19], based on data from 223 patients (103 in HSD group; 120 in isotonic crystalloid group) in six RCTs, revealed no difference in the 24 h survival rate between HSD and isotonic crystalloid. Relative to isotonic crystalloids, HSD increased the survival rate to discharge [19]. For both outcomes, the Glasgow Coma Scale score (>8 versus ≤ 8) was the most important factor to influence survival [19].

Amongst patients with penetrating injuries requiring surgery, initial fluid resuscitation with HSD, compared with isotonic crystalloids, appears to increase the survival rate to hospital discharge; however, this result was based on a subgroup analysis of an individual patient analysis [18]. A subsequent evaluation of the efficacy of HSD for fluid resuscitation in patients with penetrating injuries was reported as a meta-analysis [24], but the results are based on the individual patient data from a subgroup of patients in a previous RCT [25]. Overall, there was no difference between the survival rate of patients receiving HSD (99/120) and the survival rate of patients receiving 0.9% saline (83/110; $P = 0.189$) [24].

Gelatins

The effect of gelatins on all-cause mortality has been examined in two systematic reviews [6,11]. No difference was seen in mortality between gelatins and crystalloids [6], albumin or plasma protein fraction [11], or HES [11]. Two RCTs have compared gelatin with dextran 70, but there were no deaths [11].

Does the amount of IV fluid make a difference to clinical outcomes?

Kwan et al. [26] reviewed the effect of volume of fluid administration (blood products with or without crystalloids) for trauma patients with bleeding but were unable to pool the data due to the heterogeneity between the three RCTs [27–29]. There was no significant difference in mortality between the group administered larger volumes compared with the group administered smaller volumes in all three RCTs (Table 15.2). The small number of patients precluded any conclusions.

Holte and Kehlet evaluated the effect of compensatory fluid administration for preoperative dehydration in a qualitative review [30]. In nine RCTs with 1390 patients undergoing elective surgery, <1 L oral fluid (150–500 mL) versus none or little oral fluid (10 mL) was studied: preoperative thirst was reduced in the former group but there was insufficient data to draw conclusions on nausea, vomiting, headache, or pain. In eight RCTs with 1046 patients undergoing minor surgery, >1 L IV fluid (1–2 L) versus no or little IV fluid (2 mL kg^{-1}) was studied: postoperative drowsiness and dizziness were reduced in the former group but the effect on nausea, vomiting, and thirst remained unclear [30].

Since Holte and Kehlet's review, three other RCTs have compared liberal versus restricted fluid administration [31–33]. In a multicentre, assessor-blinded RCT, Brandstrup et al. allocated 172 adult patients undergoing elective colorectal resection with epigeneral anaesthesia to either a "standard" fluid regimen (>2 L IV crystalloids and >500 mL IV HES) or a restricted fluid regimen (500 mL oral fluids and ≤500 mL IV HES). One hundred and forty-one patients completed the RCT. Restricted fluid administration significantly reduced postoperative complications but did not affect mortality significantly (Table 15.2) [31]. Similarly, in a single-centre, assessor-blinded RCT, Nisanevich et al. randomised 152 adult patients undergoing elective intra-abdominal surgery, excluding liver resection, with general anaesthesia and epidural analgesia to a liberal fluid regimen (IV lactated Ringer's 10 mL kg^{-1} bolus followed by 12 mL kg^{-1}h^{-1} infusion) or a restricted fluid regimen (IV lactated Ringer's 4 mL kg^{-1}h^{-1} infusion without an initial bolus). Restricted fluid administration resulted in fewer perioperative complications than liberal fluid therapy; no deaths were seen in this RCT (Table 15.2) [33].

In contrast, Holte et al. randomised 48 adult patients undergoing elective laparoscopic cholecystectomy to either liberal (40 ml kg^{-1}) or restrictive (15 mL kg^{-1}) fluid administration. Liberal fluid administration improved postoperative pulmonary function at 2 and 4 h after surgery; decreased the stress response, nausea, thirst, dizziness, drowsiness, and fatigue; and increased the chance of meeting discharge criteria on the day of surgery (Table 15.2) [32].

The discordant results amongst the RCTs may be due to differences in their surgical populations, surgical procedures, durations of follow-up, and study outcomes. At this time, the evidence suggests that restrictive fluid administration may be beneficial for elective major intra-abdominal surgery. Whether liberal fluid therapy improves clinical outcomes amongst patients undergoing minimally invasive or ambulatory procedures is still uncertain.

Does the timing of IV fluid administration make a difference to clinical outcomes?

Kwan et al. [26] reviewed the timing of fluid administration for patients with bleeding but were unable to pool the data due to the heterogeneity between the three RCTs [34–36]. There was no significant difference in mortality between the group receiving early fluid resuscitation compared with the group receiving delayed fluid resuscitation in all three RCTs although the trends favoured delayed fluid therapy (Table 15.2). Differences in coagulation times were not statistically significant in either of the two RCTs in which haematological parameters were examined (Table 15.2) [34,35]. The small number of patients studied to date precluded any con·lusions.

Paediatric IV fluid resuscitation

Children are different from adults in a number of important ways: absence of myocardial disease and atherosclerosis, faster rates of biotransformation, relatively increased volumes of distribution per unit of body weight or surface area, and greater diversity in haemodynamic response to fluid resuscitation are just a few examples. Much of the management of paediatric fluid resuscitation is based on experience and research from adult populations. RCTs done in the paediatric population have either been excluded from consideration in systematic reviews [16] or indiscriminately included with adult data [6].

With the exception of early volume resuscitation or albumin administration for low serum albumin in preterm infants [4,5], high-level evidence is not available for guiding fluid administration in infants and children. The lack of high-level evidence does not necessarily indicate the absence of any evidence. For example, the risk of perioperative cerebral injury associated with hyponatraemic encephalopathy as a consequence of perioperative hyponatraemic fluids is well described and is much more likely to occur in prepubertal children than adults [37,38]. With the multitude of IV fluids available, we do not need to await the outcome of RCTs before restricting the use of hyponatraemic fluids to avoid the risks of perioperative cerebral injury associated with hyponatraemia in children in the perioperative setting.

Neonates

Two systematic reviews [4,5] have summarised the evidence in neonates from RCTs. One [4] pooled the data from RCTs comparing early volume expansion with normal saline, fresh frozen plasma, albumin, plasma substitutes, or blood versus no treatment or another form of volume expansion in preterm infants less than 32 weeks gestation or less than 1500 g. The evidence did not support the routine use of early volume expansion in very preterm infants without cardiovascular compromise.

There was insufficient evidence to determine whether infants with cardiovascular compromise benefit from volume expansion in the prevention of respiratory distress syndrome, mitigation of asphyxia, or treatment of hypotension. The other systematic review [5] assessed the effect of albumin infusions in preterm neonates with low serum albumin and did not find sufficient evidence to support its routine use.

Children

Studies in any of the reviews that included children were few and often impossible to analyse separately from the adult data (Table 15.3). Studies during surgery and post-cardiopulmonary bypass [39–41] did not show any difference between albumin compared to HES on coagulation or outcome or any benefit of albumin over saline. Four RCTs [20,42–44] compared colloid or hypertonic saline to crystalloids or lower doses of colloid in the treatment of children with burns. Increased doses of colloid and hypertonic saline reduced the amount of weight gain but did not affect outcome. One study [45] did show lower intracranial pressure, fewer complications, and reduced ICU stay in children treated with hypertonic saline compared to Ringer's lactate.

Current limitations and future research

A large number of RCTs have been conducted in the field of fluid therapy; however, most of them have been small and not powered to detect differences in clinical outcomes. Attempts to pool the data have been thwarted by the clinical heterogeneity amongst the studies even in the absence of statistical heterogeneity. As well, the risk of false-positive findings, when studies with small sample sizes are pooled, limits the strength of the findings of meta-analyses in fluid therapy. For example, the initial conclusion, from one meta-analysis, that albumin increased mortality compared to crystalloids has not been borne out by a subsequent large multicentre RCT. To date, a paucity of high-level evidence exists to guide our fluid management in surgical and critically ill patients (see Research box). Our decisions will continue to depend mainly on our understanding of the pharmacology of fluids, the physiological state of the patient, economic considerations, and clinical and patient preferences.

In spite of the gaps that remain in our knowledge, the advances in this millennium are promising. Recent RCTs on fluid therapy have been more rigorous and tended to address clinical outcomes. The publication of the SAFE Study has demonstrated the feasibility of conducting large multicentre RCTs to answer questions on fluid therapy. Currently, there are several other RCTs in progress in Europe and North America that may provide answers to questions in this field.

Table 15.3. RCTs of fluid therapy in children

Reference	Population	Intervention	Result
Surgery			
Hausdörfer et al. [39]	Children ≤16 year of age undergoing surgery	Volume replacement with albumin 14 mL kg^{-1} versus HES 14 mL kg^{-1} (15 patients per group)	No differences in serum creatinine, PTT, or thromboelastogram
Boldt et al. [40]	Children <3 year of age undergoing primary repair of congenital heart lesions	Pre-cardiopulmonary bypass volume loading with 6% HES 12 mL kg^{-1} versus 20% albumin 8.5 mL kg^{-1} (15 patients per group)	No differences in antithrombin-III, fibrinogen, platelet count, postoperative blood loss, or COP
Brutocao et al. [41]	Children ≥1 year of age undergoing elective repair of congenital heart lesions	Post-cardiopulmonary bypass volume replacement with 5% albumin ($n = 18$) versus 6% HES in 0.9% saline ($n = 20$)	No differences in coagulation parameters (PT, PTT, TT, fibrinogen, platelet count) or amount of replacement fluids required
Burns			
Hall and Sørensen [42]	Adults with >15% BSA and children with >10% BSA thermal/corrosive burns (mean age 20 year)	Fluid resuscitation with dextran 70 versus LR	No difference in mortality: 18/86 (dextran 70) versus 16/86 (LR)
Caldwell and Bowser [43]	Paediatric patients (mean age 9.5 year) with ≥30% BSA thermal burns	IV HS 2 mL kg^{-1} % BSA burn^{-1} in first 24 h + IV HS 0.6 mL kg^{-1} % BSA burn^{-1} and oral Haldane's solution in second 24 h versus IV LR 2 mL kg^{-1} % BSA burn^{-1} and IV 5% dextrose replacement fluid in first 24 h + IV LR 1 mL kg^{-1} % BSA burn^{-1} and IV 5% dextrose in second 24 h	HS resulted in significantly lower water load over first 48 h post-burn; no difference in sodium balance. No difference in mortality: 1/17 (HS) versus 1/20 (LR)
Bowser-Wallace and Caldwell [20]	Patients 5 months – 21 year of age with ≥30% BSA	IV HS 2 mL kg^{-1} % BSA burn^{-1} in first 24 h + IV HS 0.6 mL kg^{-1} % BSA	LR colloid resulted in significantly higher fluid balances and more weight gain than HS

(Continued)

Table 15.3. (Continued)

Reference	Population	Intervention	Result
	thermal burns	burn^{-1} and oral Haldane's solution in second 24 h versus IV LR mL kg^{-1} % BSA burn^{-1} in first 24 h + IV Plasmanate 0.5 mL kg^{-1} % BSA burn^{-1} and IV 5% dextrose in second 24 h	No difference in mortality: 3/19 (LR colloid) versus 0 /19 (HS)
Greenhalgh et al. [44]	Children 1–18 year of age with >20% BSA burns	25% albumin to maintain serum albumin between 25 and 35 g L^{-1} (high) versus 25% albumin to maintain serum albumin >15 g L^2 (low)	Maintenance of high serum albumin was expensive: US$ 51,115 (high) versus US$ 2,470 (low) No difference in mortality: 7/34 (high) versus 3/36 (low) No difference in length of stay 45.7 ± 6.2 d (high) versus 48.7 ± 7.3 d (low)
Other critically ill patients			
Simma et al. [45]	Children (age <16 year) with severe traumatic brain injury and Glasgow Coma Scale score <8	72 h fluid therapy with LR versus HS to keep ICP ≤15 mmHg	HS increased serum sodium and decreased ICP. No difference in mortality: 2/17 (LR) versus 0/15 (HS) Trend towards fewer complications with HS: 14/17 (LR) versus 7/15 (HS)[a] ICU length of stay was shorter with HS: 11.6 ± 6.1 d (LR) versus 8.0 ± 2.4 d (HS)[b]
Ngo et al. [46]	Children 1–15 year of age with dengue haemorrhagic fever ± circulatory failure (tachycardia, and pulse pressure ≤20 mmHg)	Fluid therapy with dextran 70 ($n = 55$) versus 3% gelatin ($n = 56$) versus LR ($n = 55$) versus normal saline ($n = 56$)	Colloid therapy showed a trend towards more rapid recovery in patients with low pulse pressures.

BSA: body surface area; HS: hypertonic saline; ICP: intracranial pressure; LR: lactated Ringer's; PT: prothrombin time; PTT: partial thromboplastin time; TT: thrombin time.
[a] $P = 0.08$.
[b] $P = 0.04$.

> **Research box**
> - RCTs in fluid therapy require a sufficiently large sample size to detect biologically plausible differences in clinically relevant outcomes such as all-cause mortality, perioperative morbidity (by organ system), and fluid-related adverse events.
> - Study populations need to be homogeneous (e.g. specific critically ill populations and surgical populations). Studies need to focus on adults and children.
> - With the exception of albumin, studies on the type of IV fluid are still needed.
> - Studies comparing restrictive versus liberal fluid therapy are still needed.
> - Studies comparing early versus delayed fluid therapy are still needed.

Summary

- A statistically significant reduction in mortality or relevant adverse clinical outcomes amongst surgical or critically ill adult or paediatric patients has not been found with the use of any particular IV fluid.
- Current evidence suggests that restricted fluid regimens may decrease perioperative morbidity in adults undergoing elective intra-abdominal surgery but the results cannot be generalised to other populations or procedures.
- The effect of restricted versus liberal fluid regimens on clinical outcomes in patients undergoing minimally invasive or ambulatory procedures is still inconclusive.
- Although there is a trend in fewer deaths with delayed fluid resuscitation of patients with penetrating trauma, the data is insufficient to draw guidelines.
- Large multicentre RCTs of fluid regimens with clinically relevant outcomes are still needed to address important questions in this field.

REFERENCES

1 Schierhout G, Roberts I. Fluid resuscitation with colloid or crystalloid solutions in critically ill patients: a systematic review of randomised trials. *BMJ* 1998; 316: 961–4.

2 Cochrane Injuries Group Albumin Reviewers. Human albumin administration in critically ill patients: systematic review of randomised controlled trials. *BMJ* 1998; 317: 235–40.

3 Mapstone J, Roberts I, Evans P. Fluid resuscitation strategies: a systematic review of animal trials. *J Trauma* 2003; 55: 571–89.

4 Osborn DA, Evans N. Early volume expansion versus inotrope for prevention of morbidity and mortality in very preterm infants. *The Cochrane Database Syst Rev* 2001, Issue 2, Art No.: CD002056. DOI: 10.1002/14651858.pub2.

5 Jardine LA, Jenkins-Manning S, Davies MW. Albumin infusion for low serum albumin in preterm newborn infants. *The Cochrane Database Syst Rev* 2004, Issue 3, Art No.: CD004208. DOI: 10.1002/14651858.pub2.

6 Roberts I, Alderson P, Bunn F, Chinnock P, Ker K, Schierhout G. Colloids versus crystalloids for fluid resuscitation in critically ill patients. *The Cochrane Database Syst Rev* 2004, Issue 4, Art No.: CD000567. DOI: 10.1002/14651858.pub2.

7 Bunn F, Roberts I, Tasker R. Hypertonic versus near isotonic crystalloid for fluid resuscitation in critically ill patients. *The Cochrane Database Syst Rev* 2004, Issue 3, Art No.: CD002045. DOI: 10.1002/14651858.pub2.

8 Wilkes MM, Navickis RJ. Patient survival after human albumin administration: a meta-analysis of randomized, controlled trials. *Ann Intern Med* 2001; 135: 149–64.

9 Haynes GR, Navickis RJ, Wilkes MM. Albumin administration – what is the evidence of clinical benefit? A systematic review of randomized controlled trials. *Eur J Anaesthesiol* 2003; 20: 771–93.

10 The Albumin Reviewers (Alderson P, Bunn F, Li Wan Po A, Li L, Roberts I, Schierhout G). Human albumin solution for resuscitation and volume expansion in critically ill patients. *The Cochrane Database Syst Rev* 2004, Issue 4, Art No. CD001208. DOI: 10.1002/14651858.

11 Bunn F, Alderson P, Hawkins V. Colloid solutions for fluid resuscitation. *The Cochrane Database Syst Rev* 2003, Issue 1, Art. No.: CD001319. DOI: 10.1002/14651858.

12 Wilkes MM, Navickis RJ, Sibbald WJ. Albumin versus hydroxyethyl starch in cardiopulmonary bypass surgery: a meta-analysis of postoperative bleeding. *Ann Thorac Surg* 2001; 72: 527–34.

13 Russell JA, Navickis RJ, Wilkes MM. Albumin versus crystalloid for pump priming in cardiac surgery: meta-analysis of controlled trials. *J Cardiothorac Vasc Anesth* 2004; 18: 429–37.

14 Velanovich V. Crystalloids versus colloid fluid resuscitation: a meta-analysis of mortality. *Surgery* 1989; 105: 65–71.

15 Bisonni RS, Holtgrave DR, Lawler F, Marley DS. Colloids versus crystalloids in fluid resuscitation: an analysis of randomized controlled trials. *J Fam Pract* 1991; 32: 387–90.

16 Choi PT-L, Yip G, Quinonez LG, Cook DJ. Crystalloids vs. colloids in fluid resuscitation: a systematic review. *Crit Care Med* 1999; 27: 200–10.

17 Wade CE, Kramer GC, Grady JJ, Fabian TC, Younes RN. Efficacy of hypertonic 7.5% saline and 6% dextran-70 in treating trauma: A meta-analysis of controlled clinical studies. *Surgery* 1997; 122: 609–16.

18 Wade C, Grady J, Kramer G. Efficacy of hypertonic saline dextran (HSD) in patients with traumatic hypotension: meta-analysis of individual patient data. *Acta Anaesthesiol Scand Suppl* 1997; 110: 77–9.

19 Wade CE, Grady JJ, Kramer GC, Younes RN, Gehlsen K, Holcroft JW. Individual patient cohort analysis of the efficacy of hypertonic saline/dextran in patients with traumatic brain injury and hypotension. *J Trauma* 1997; 42(Suppl) 61S–5S.

20 Bowser-Wallace BH, Caldwell Jr FT. A prospective analysis of hypertonic lactated saline v. Ringer's lactate-colloid for the resuscitation of severely burned children. *Burns* 1986; 12: 402–9.

21 Boldt J. The good, the bad, and the ugly: should we completely banish human albumin from our intensive care units? *Anesth Analg* 2000; 91: 887–95.

22 The SAFE Study Investigators. A comparison of albumin and saline for fluid resuscitation in the intensive care unit. *N Engl J Med* 2004; 350: 2247–56.

23 Treib J, Baron J-F, Grauer MT, Strauss RG. An international view of hydroxyethyl starches. *Intens Care Med* 1999; 25: 258–68.

24 Wade CE, Grady JJ, Kramer GC. Efficacy of hypertonic saline dextran fluid resuscitation for patients with hypotension from penetrating trauma. *J Trauma* 2003; 54(Suppl) S144–8.

25 Mattox KL, Maningas PA, Moore EE et al. Prehospital hypertonic saline/dextran infusion for post-traumatic hypotension. The USA Multicenter Trial. *Ann Surg* 1991; 213: 482–91.

26 Kwan I, Bunn F, Roberts I, on behalf of the WHO Pre-Hosptial Trauma Care Steering Committee. Timing and Volume of fluid administration for patients with bleeding. *The Cochrane Database Syst Rev* 2003, Issue 3, Art. No.: CD002245. DOI: 10.1002/14651858.

27 Fortune JB, Feustel PJ, Saifi J, Stratton HH, Newell JC, Shah DM. Influence of the hematocrit on cardiopulmonary function after acute hemorrhage. *J Trauma* 1987; 27: 243–9.

28 Dunham CM, Belzberg H, Lyles R et al. The rapid infusion system: a superior method for the resuscitation of hypovolemic patients. *Resuscitation* 1991; 21: 207–27.

29 Dutton RP, MacKenzie CF, Scalea TM. Hypotensive resuscitation during active haemorrhage: impact on in-hospital mortality. *J Trauma* 2002; 52: 1141–6.

30 Holte K, Kehlet H. Compensatory fluid administration for preoperative dehydration – does it improve outcome? *Acta Anaesthesiol Scand* 2002; 46: 1089–93.

31 Brandstrup B, Tønnesen H, Beier-Holgersen R et al. Effects of intravenous fluid restriction on postoperative complications: comparison of two perioperative fluid regimens. A randomized assessor-blinded multicenter trial. *Ann Surg* 2003; 238: 641–8.

32 Holte K, Klarskov B, Christensen DS et al. Liberal versus restrictive fluid administration to improve recovery after laparoscopic cholecystectomy. A randomized, double-blind study. *Ann Surg* 2004; 240: 892–9.

33 Nisanevich V, Felsenstein I, Almogy G, Weissman C, Einav S, Matot I. Effect of intraoperative fluid management on outcome after intraabdominal surgery. *Anesthesiology* 2005; 103: 25 32.

34 Blair SD, Janvrin SB, McCollum CN, Greenhaigh RM. Effect of early blood transfusion on gastrointestinal haemorrhage. *Br J Surg* 1986; 73: 783–5.

35 Bickell WH, Wall MJ, Pepe PE et al. Immediate versus delayed fluid resuscitation for hypotensive patients with penetrating torso injuries. *New Engl J Med* 1994; 331: 1105–9.

36 Turner J, Nicholl J, Webber L, Cox H, Dixon S, Yates D. A randomised controlled trial of pre-hospital intravenous fluid replacement therapy in serious trauma. *Health Technol Assessment* 2000; 4(31).

37 Arieff AI, Ayus JC, Fraser CL. Hyponatraemia and death or permanent brain damage in healthy children. *BMJ* 1992; 304: 1218–22.

38 Arieff AI. Postoperative hyponatraemic encephalopathy following elective surgery in children. *Pediatr Anaesth* 1998; 8: 1–4.

39 Hausdörfer J, Hagemann H, Heine J. Vergleich der volumeenersatzmittel humanalbumin 5% und hydroxyäthylstärke 6% (50.000/0,5) in der kinderanästhesie. *Anästh Intensivether Notfallmed* 1986; 21: 137–42.

40 Boldt J, Knothe C, Schindler E, Hammermann H, Dapper F, Hempelmann G. Volume replacement with hydroxyethyl starch solution in children. *Br J Anaesth* 1993; 70: 661–5.

41 Brutocao D, Bratton SL, Thomas R, Schrader PF, Coles PG, Lynn AM. Comparison of hetastarch with albumin for postoperative volume expansion in children after cardiopulmonary bypass. *J Cardiothorac Vasc Anesth* 1996; 10: 348–51.

42 Hall KV, Sørensen B. The treatment of burn shock: results of a 5-year randomized, controlled clinical trial of Dextran 70 *v*. Ringer lactate solution. *Burns* 1978; 5: 107–12.

43 Caldwell FT, Bowser BH. Critical evaluation of hypertonic and hypotonic solutions to resuscitate severely burned children: A prospective study. *Ann Surg* 1979; 189: 546–52.

44 Greenhalgh DG, Housinger TA, Kagan RJ et al. Maintenance of serum albumin levels in pediatric burn patients: A prospective randomized trial. *J Trauma* 1995; 39: 67–74.

45 Simma B, Burger R, Falk M, Sacher P, Fanconi S. A prospective, randomized, and controlled study of fluid management in children with severe head injury: Lactated Ringer's solution versus hypertonic saline. *Crit Care Med* 1998; 26: 1265–70.

46 Ngo TN, Cao XTP, Kneen R et al. Acute management of dengue shock syndrome: A randomized double-blind comparison of 4 intravenous fluid regiments in the first hour. *Clin Infect Dis* 2001; 32: 204–13.

16

Antiemetics

John Carlisle

Department of Anaesthetics, NHS Torbay Hospital, Torquay, Devon, UK

Introduction

In this chapter I will discuss three groups of interventions that reduce the number of people who experience postoperative nausea or vomiting (PONV). The first group is changing the anaesthetic method to reduce risk. The second group is giving preventative drugs or acupoint P6 stimulation to reduce risk. The third group is drug treatment to shorten the duration or reduce the severity of established nausea or vomiting.

It is obvious that if no one experiences PONV there is no benefit in either changing anaesthetic technique or giving drugs to prevent PONV. It is also obvious that if everyone experiences PONV then everyone has a chance of benefiting from either intervention. The majority of people in a population in which less than 50% have PONV cannot benefit from prophylaxis. It is therefore crucial to know the incidence of PONV to calculate the risks and benefits of antiemetic prophylaxis.

We know the likelihood of reducing PONV for many drugs. We know the likelihood of common minor side effects. We do not know the likelihood of rare serious side effects.

Reducing emetic stimuli

Perioperative emetic stimuli are usually assumed to operate through particular characteristics of: the patient, the surgery and the anaesthetic. Only a few factors, in just a few studies, have been shown to independently predict PONV: sex, history of smoking, motion sickness or PONV, duration of operation, opioid administration [1–3]. Few of these predictors can be modified in randomised controlled trials (RCTs). Surgical technique has rarely been assessed in RCTs that report PONV.

Although anaesthetic factors are not included in risk scores, meta-analyses of RCTs show that modification of anaesthetic technique can reduce PONV.

Key words: Nausea, vomiting, antiemetic, postoperative.

Fasting and nasogastric tubes

There is no convincing evidence from meta-analyses that the duration and type of perioperative fast, or the insertion of nasogastric tubes, affect PONV [4–9].

General anaesthetic agents

Induction

There is no meta-analysis that compares all intravenous induction agents. One meta-analysis showed that the incidence of PONV is less after induction with propofol than with sevoflurane [10]. One other meta-analysis combined all studies that assessed various induction agents versus propofol so the meaning of the result is unclear [11]. These analyses did not adequately explore heterogeneity and publication bias. The relative risk (RR) for PONV after propofol compared to sevoflurane may be about 0.8.

Maintenance

There is no meta-analysis for the RCTs that compare the maintenance of anaesthesia with different inhalational agents.

There is no meta-analysis for the RCTs that compare the maintenance of anaesthesia with different intravenous agents.

Maintenance of anaesthesia with intravenous propofol decreases PONV compared to an amalgam of inhalational agents. It is unclear what the size and uncertainty of the effect is for each inhalational agent versus toropofol because they are all analysed together: both analyses compare propofol with a composite of all inhalational agents [11,12]. A conservative estimate of the RR of PONV following maintenance with propofol compared with one of the inhalational agents is possibly about 0.50. A thorough assessment of publication bias might suggest that the difference between propofol and inhalational agents is less than this; that is, the RR may be more. The meta-analyses report the effect as odds ratios (ORs) and numbers needed to treat (NNTs) rather than RRs. It is possible to derive the RR from the OR, but I was unable to determine the incidence in the control group that would have allowed me to make this calculation.

Two more meta-analyses with similar limitations review the effect on PONV of nitrous oxide (N_2O) [13,14]. The RR of PONV after general anaesthesia that omits N_2O may be about 0.85 compared to a general anaesthetic that includes it.

Analgesia

Regional techniques

Three Cochrane meta-analyses report no difference in the RR of PONV between epidural and systemic analgesia [15–17]. One Cochrane meta-analysis reported a reduction in nausea with epidural (caudal) analgesia but commented that this result is unreliable [18].

One meta-analysis assessed the effect of adding epidural opioid and one assessed the effect of adding intrathecal fentanyl [19,20]. Both are limited by few included studies and methodological limitations. There was no evidence that intrathecal fentanyl affected PONV and limited evidence that epidural morphine increases PONV, perhaps with an RR of about 1.3.

Oral analgesics

A series of 11 Cochrane meta-analyses assessed the effect of oral analgesics given for postoperative pain [21–31]. Rofecoxib was associated with a reduction in post-operative vomiting but not nausea: if there is a difference the RR would possibly be between 0.8 and 1 [28]. Oxycodone was associated with an increase in PONV with an RR of between 1 and 1.6 [29].

Cholinesterase inhibitors (with or without antimuscarinic agents)

Two meta-analyses [32] assessed the effect on PONV of combinations of a cholinesterase inhibitor (edrophonium or neostigmine) and an antimuscarinic (atropine or glycopyrrolate). Our meta-analysis assessed these combinations and each drug alone. Neither meta-analysis provides evidence that any of these drugs, either alone or in combination, reliably alter PONV. The earlier meta-analysis presented a

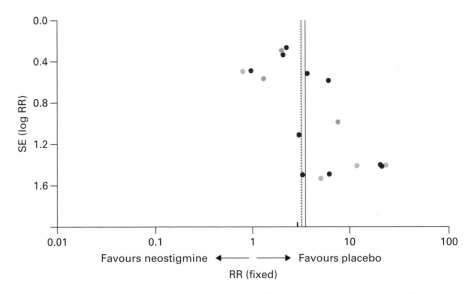

Figure 16.1 Each dot is an outcome from one study. Nausea: • (RR 3.80; 0.95–15.16). Vomiting: • (RR 3.89; 0.79–18.99). Nausea or vomiting: • (RR 3.19; 1.71–5.93). The outcomes of dots closer to the top (SE 0.0) are more certain.

composite outcome for neostigmine from studies that combined it with atropine or glycopyrrolate, compared to either placebo or no treatment [33]. We identified funnel plot asymmetry (possible publication bias) for studies of neostigmine that makes the calculated emetogenic effect of neostigmine an overestimate (Figure 16.1). Neostigmine may increase the chance of PONV with an RR of between 1 and 2. The decision to administer cholinesterase inhibitors should be determined by the need to reverse neuromuscular blockade, not by concerns about PONV.

Counteracting emetic symptoms: prevention of PONV

I will concentrate on the eight drugs that reliably reduced PONV from the 60 we assessed in our Cochrane Systematic Review. I will list the drugs in order, with the drug that has the most certain antiemetic effect first and the drug that has the least certain antiemetic effect last. Please note, we found substantial asymmetry in the funnel plots for comparison of one drug with another (probably due to publication bias). This means that there is no reliable evidence that one of these drugs is more effective than any other. This contrasts with the conclusions of previous meta-analyses that did not rigorously explore this bias, that sometimes indirectly compared the effects of one drug versus another rather than directly comparing them, and that often used composite comparators (for instance all $5\text{-}HT_3$ receptor antagonists). I quote the results of our systematic review and I have also referenced other systematic reviews of each drug.

Drugs versus placebo

Droperidol [34–37]

The RR for PONV after droperidol is probably between 0.65 and 0.70 after publication bias is taken into account.

Metoclopramide [36–38]

Metoclopramide showed the least funnel plot asymmetry (Figure 16.2). The RR is probably between 0.75 and 0.85.

Ondansetron [36,39–44]

The funnel plot asymmetry for ondansetron was similar to the severity that we plotted for droperidol. The adjusted RR possibly exceeds 0.65.

Tropisetron

The RR for PONV is probably between 0.70 and 0.80.

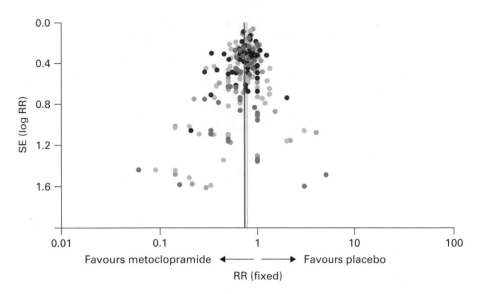

Figure 16.2   Each dot is an outcome from one study. Nausea: ● (RR 0.82; 0.76–0.88). Vomiting: ● (RR 0.75; 0.70–0.81). Nausea or vomiting: ● (RR 0.76; 0.70–0.82). Rescue antiemetic: ● (RR 0.78; 0.69–0.88). Vertical lines mark the summative RR for each outcome. The outcomes of dots closer to the top (SE 0.0) are more certain.

Dolasetron

The funnel plot was very asymmetric – the RR for PONV is probably between 0.80 and 0.90.

Dexamethasone [36,39,45–47]

The RR for PONV is probably between 0.55 and 0.65.

Cyclizine

The data for cyclizine are sparse, but the RR is probably between 0.70 and 0.85.

Granisetron [48]

The RR is probably between 0.65 and 0.75. Figure 16.3 shows severe funnel plot asymmetry and compares the majority of studies authored by Fuji et al with studies published by other authors.

We identified 12 other drugs that have uncertain antiemetic effects: alizapride, diazepam, dimenhydrinate, dixyrazine, ginger, hyoscine, lorazepam, midazolam, perphenazine, prochlorperazine, promethazine and ramosetron.

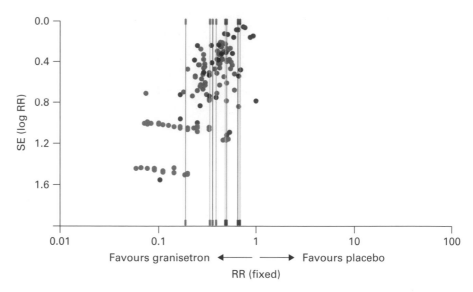

Figure 16.3 Each dot is an outcome from one study. RRs are coloured grey from studies authored by
Fujii and black from other authors. Vertical lines mark the summative RR for each
outcome, those calculated for Fujii always being less than those for other authors: nausea
0.39 (0.31–0.49) compared with 0.68 (0.62–0.75); vomiting 0.34 (0.29–0.40) compared
with 0.49 (0.43–0.55); nausea or vomiting 0.36 (0.31–0.42) compared with 0.65
(0.58–0.74); rescue 0.19 (0.14–0.25) compared with 0.50 (0.41–0.61). The outcomes of
dots closer to the top (SE 0.0) are more certain.

Dose

We found that the assumption that "more drug is more effective" is probably true
for droperidol, dexamethasone and ondansetron, and possibly true for metoclopramide. Halving the dose of each drug reduces antiemetic effect by about 1.2. A
maximum dose above which there is no further antiemetic effect was not reliably
demonstrated for any drug.

Side effects

We found only a few minor side effects in our meta-analysis: droperidol was slightly
sedative (RR about 1.3) and prevented headache (RR about 0.8); ondansetron
increased the incidence of headache slightly (RR 1.1). Between two and four
people in every hundred will be affected.

Context sensitivity

We performed a subgroup analysis of studies that gave one of these drugs alone
and studies that gave a drug with another antiemetic drug. We found that the
antiemetic effect (RR) of a drug was not affected by co-administration with another

antiemetic drug. The IMPACT study [50] similarly failed to find synergy or antagonism between antiemetic drugs. We also did not find an effect of age (adults versus children), sex (males versus females), surgery (11 subgroups) or timing of drug administration (preoperative, induction, intraoperative, postoperative).

- Drugs act independently. In combination the RRs of drugs multiply – for instance dexamethasone (RR about 0.65) and metoclopramide (RR about 0.75) given together will reduce the risk of PONV by 0.65 times 0.75, which is about 0.5.

Drug versus drug

There are 28 possible head-to-head comparisons of two drugs from the eight we listed. Eleven of these comparisons have been assessed in RCTs. Three comparisons have been assessed in numerous studies. We found no reliable differences in the efficacy of these eight drugs.

Droperidol versus metoclopramide

Twenty-six studies compared these two drugs. The calculated difference in effect depends upon the asymmetry in the funnel plot (probably publication bias). There is no reliable difference between these two drugs.

Droperidol versus ondansetron

Forty-five studies compared these two drugs. The calculated difference in effect depends on the asymmetry in the funnel plot. There is no reliable difference between these two drugs.

Metoclopramide versus ondansetron

Forty-two studies compared these two drugs. The calculated difference in effect depends upon the asymmetry in the funnel plot. There is no reliable difference between these two drugs (Figure 16.4).

P6 acupoint stimulation

Two published meta-analyses by the same authors assessed prevention of PONV by stimulation (skin puncture, skin pressure, injection, electrical current, laser light) of the P6 acupoint on the wrist [51,52]. The asymmetric funnel plot suggests that the calculated antiemetic effect versus sham is an overestimate, the adjusted RR being about 0.9 (Figure 16.5). There were insufficient studies comparing P6 stimulation with individual drugs to draw reliable conclusions.

Counteracting emetic symptoms: treatment of PONV

The only treatments that have been assessed in a meta-analysis for nauseated or vomiting postoperative patients are drugs [53]. There is less known about the

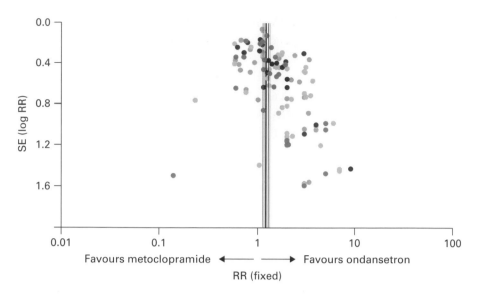

Figure 16.4   Each dot is an outcome from one study. Nausea: • (RR 1.22; 1.01–1.47). Vomiting: • (RR 1.48; 1.23–1.77). Nausea or vomiting: • (RR 1.28; 1.03–1.58). Rescue antiemetic: • (RR 1.12; 0.99–1.27). Vertical lines mark the summative RR for each outcome. The outcomes of dots closer to the top (SE 0.0) are more certain.

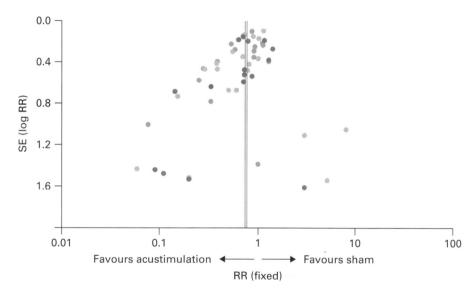

Figure 16.5   Each dot is an outcome from one study. Nausea: • (RR 0.72; 0.59–0.89). Vomiting: • (RR 0.71; 0.56–0.91). Rescue antiemetic: • (RR 0.77; 0.60–0.99). Vertical lines mark the summative RR for each outcome. The outcomes of symbols closer to the top (SE 0.0) are more certain.

effects of drugs used to treat PONV than there is about drugs used to prevent PONV. For instance, 1091 participants were recruited into RCTs that assessed the ability of ondansetron to stop PONV, but 17 958 participants have been recruited into RCTs that assessed the ability of ondansetron to prevent PONV. In addition multiple publications of the same data distort results in favour of drugs. This is apparent for both the treatment and prevention of PONV by drugs.

Practice points

- Informed patients should help to decide what type of anaesthetic and drugs they have.
- Maintain a current database of the incidences of PONV in your patients to estimate the likelihood of PONV for various subgroups, for instance women having laparoscopic cholecystectomies, and to formally recalibrate published scoring systems.
- The incidences of important rare side effects caused by interventions are not available from RCTs and available observational evidence provides uncertain causation and incidences.
- Maintenance of anaesthesia with propofol rather than a volatile agent probably halves the incidence of PONV. The PONV risk after inhalational anaesthetics maintained with N_2O is about 1.15 times the incidence without N_2O. Techniques that avoid opioid administration may reduce PONV although the evidence for this is sparse.
- If you give an antiemetic drug to a population in which the incidence of PONV would otherwise be 5/100, 2 people will benefit and 98 will not. If you give two drugs 3 people will benefit (97 will not).
- If you give an antiemetic drug to a population in which the incidence of PONV would otherwise be 50/100, 17 people will benefit and 83 will not. If you give two drugs 29 will benefit (71 will not) (Figure 16.6).
- If you stimulate acupoint P6 for all 100 people in the second population you will increase the number who benefit from 29 to 31 (and reduce the number who do not from 71 to 69).
- The incidence of side effects will increase with more antiemetics. It is not known whether drugs interact to increase the incidence or severity of side effects more than expected (synergism) or less than expected (antagonism). It is unclear to what extent some people may suffer from side effects more than others.
- The cost of preventing PONV depends on: the incidence of PONV without drug(s); the cost of the drug(s); the interaction between increasing effect and increasing cost with combinations of drugs.
- The most cost-efficient preventative antiemetic is metoclopramide followed in order by: cyclizine and metoclopramide combined; cyclizine alone; dexamethasone and metoclopramide combined; cyclizine, dexamethasone and metoclopramide combined; dexamethasone alone; cyclizine and dexamethasone combined; ondansetron; granisetron.

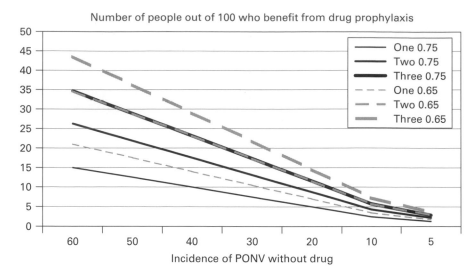

Figure 16.6   There are two series on this graph: three drugs with an RR of 0.75 for PONV; three drugs with an RR of 0.65 for PONV

- Therefore every patient given PONV drug prophylaxis should receive metoclopramide unless there is a specific contraindication (Figure 16.7).
- Treatment cannot reduce the incidence of PONV although it may reduce the duration and severity of PONV.
- We do not know how many patients can expect to benefit from treatment.
- An economic evaluation of the best strategy (prophylaxis, treatment or both) would have to use all costs (not just drugs) associated with nausea and vomiting and would require reliable data on the efficacy of treatment that is not currently available.

Research points
- You should collaborate in multinational research to determine the incidences and severities of important side effects of antiemetic prevention and treatment, drug and non-pharmacological.
- Although there may be minor differences in the effectiveness of prophylactic antiemetic drugs these are not important. If research shows that important side effects are not synergistically increased by co-administration of antiemetic drugs then PONV can be best prevented by the combination of two or more antiemetics.

Summary

All strategies used to limit and reduce the burden of PONV have other effects, some wanted and some unwanted. The decision to use anaesthetic techniques that

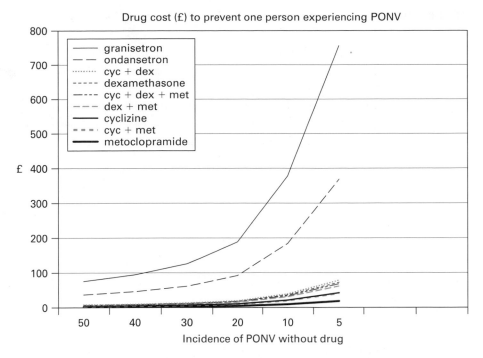

Figure 16.7 Drug prices listed in the British National Formulatory (March 2005) for the following intravenous doses: metoclopramide 10 mg; cyclizine 50 mg; dexamethasone 10 mg; granisetron 1 mg; ondansetron 4 mg.

limit PONV, drugs and non-pharmacological methods to prevent PONV, and drugs to treat established PONV must take into account all of these effects.

Omission of N_2O from the inhalational maintenance of anaesthesia reduces PONV. Maintenance of general anaesthesia with intravenous propofol instead of a volatile agent reduces the risk of PONV. Eight drugs reliable reduce the risk of PONV to about 0.7: droperidol, metoclopramide, ondansetron, tropisetron, dolasetron, dexamethasone, cyclizine and granisetron. There is no reliable direct evidence for differences in the efficacy of these eight drugs. The more drugs given the less the risk of PONV. Acupoint P6 stimulation reduces the risk of PONV by about 0.9.

There is less direct evidence for using regional analgesia instead of systemic analgesia and reducing opioid use, although there is substantial indirect evidence that this limits PONV. It is unclear what the dose-responses are for the eight antiemetic drugs, both for the wanted reduction in PONV and the unwanted increase in side effects.

REFERENCES

1 Van den Bosch JE, Kalkman CJ, Vergouwe Y, Van Klei WA, Bonsel GJ, Grobbee DE, Moons KGM. Assessing the applicability of scoring systems for predicting postoperative nausea and vomiting. *Anaesthesia* 2005; 60: 323–31.

2 Rüsch D, Eberhart L, Biedler A, Dethling J, Apfel CC. Prospective application of a simplified risk score to prevent postoperative nausea and vomiting. *Can J Anaesth* 2005; 52(5): 478–84.

3 Apfel CC, Kranke P, Eberhart LHJ, Roos A, Roewer N. Comparison of predictive models for postoperative nausea and vomiting. *Br J Anaesth* 2002; 88(2): 234–40.

4 Brady M, Kinn S, Stuart P. Preoperative fasting for adults to prevent perioperative complications. *The Cochrane Database of Syst Rev* 2003, Issue 4. Art. No.: CD004423. DOI: 10.1002/14651858.

5 Brady M, Kinn S, O'Rourke K, Randhawa N, Stuart P. Preoperative fasting for preventing perioperative complications in children. *The Cochrane Database of Syst Rev* 2005, Issue 2. Art. No.: CD005285. DOI: 10.1002/14651858.

6 Mangesi L, Hofmeyr GJ. Early compared with delayed oral fluids and food after caesarean section. *The Cochrane Database of Syst Rev* 2002, Issue 3. Art. No.: CD003516. DOI: 10.1002/14651858.

7 Lewis SJ, Egger M, Sylvester PA, Thomas S. Early external feeding versus "nil by mouth" after gastrointestinal surgery: systematic review and meta-analysis of controlled trials. *BMJ* 2001; 323: 773–6.

8 Cheatham ML, Chapman WC, Key SP, Sawyers JL. A meta-analysis of selective versus routine nasogastric decompression after elective laparotomy. *Ann Surg* 1995; 221(5): 469–78.

9 Nelson R, Edwards S, Tse B. Prophylactic nasogastric decompression after abdominal surgery. *The Cochrane Database of Syst Rev* 2004, Issue 3. Art. No.: CD004929. DOI: 10.1002/14651858.

10 Joo HS, Perks WJ. Sevoflurane versus propofol for anaesthetic induction: a meta-analysis. *AnesthAnalg* 2000; 91: 213–9.

11 Tramèr M, Moore A, McQuay H. Propofol anaesthesia and postoperative nausea and vomiting: quantitative systematic review of randomized controlled studies. *Br J Anaesth* 1997; 78: 247–55.

12 Sneyd JR, Carr A, Byrom WD, Bilski AJT. A meta-analysis of nausea and vomiting following maintenance of anaesthesia with propofol or inhalational agents. *Eur J Anaesthesiol* 1998; 15: 433–45.

13 Divatia JV, Vaidya JS, Badwe RA, Hawalder RW. Omission of nitrous oxide during anesthesia reduces the incidence of postoperative nausea and vomiting. *Anesthesiology* 1996; 85: 1055–62.

14 Tramèr M, Moore A, McQuay H. Omitting nitrous oxide in general anaesthesia: meta-analysis of intraoperative awareness and postoperative emesis in randomized controlled trials. *Br J Anaesth* 1996; 76: 186–93.

15 Choi PT, Bhandari M, Scott J, Douketis J. Epidural analgesia for pain relief following hip or knee replacement. *The Cochrane Database of Syst Rev* 2003, Issue 3. Art. No.: CD003071. DOI: 10.1002/14651858.

16 Jørgensen H, Wetterslev J, Møiniche S, Dahl JB. Epidural local anaesthetics versus opioid-based analgesic regimens for postoperative gastrointestinal paralysis, PONV and pain after abdominal surgery. *The Cochrane Database of Syst Rev* 2001, Issue 1. Art. No.: CD001893. DOI: 10.1002/14651858.

17 Werawatganon T, Charuluxanun S. Patient controlled intravenous opioid analgesia versus continuous epidural analgesia for pain after intra-abdominal surgery. *The Cochrane Database of Syst Rev* 2005, Issue 1. Art. No.: CD004088. DOI: 10.1002/14651858.

18 Cyna AM, Jha S, Parsons JE. Caudal epidural block versus other methods of postoperative pain relief for circumcision in boys. *The Cochrane Database of Syst Rev* 2003, Issue 2. Art. No.: CD003005. DOI: 10.1002/14651858.

19 Curatolo M, Petersen-Felix S, Scaramozzino P, Zbinden AM. Epidural fentanyl, adrenaline and clonidine as adjuvants to local anaesthetics for surgical analgesia: meta-analyses of analgesia and side-effects. *Acta Anaesth Scand* 1998; 42(8): 910–20.

20 Dahl JB, Jeppesen IS, Jorgensen H, Wetterslev J, Moiniche S. Intraoperative and post-operative analgesic efficacy and adverse effects of intrathecal opioids in patients undergoing Cesarean section with spinal anesthesia: a qualitative and quantitative systematic review of randomized controlled trials. *Anesthesiology* 1999; 91(6): 1919–27.

21 Collins SL, Edwards JE, Moore RA, McQuay HJ. Single dose dextropropoxyphene, alone and with paracetamol (acetaminophen), for postoperative pain. *The Cochrane Database of Syst Rev* 1999, Issue 1. Art. No.: CD001440. DOI: 10.1002/14651858.

22 Edwards JE, McQuay HJ, Moore RA. Single dose dihydrocodeine for acute postoperative pain. *The Cochrane Database of Syst Rev* 2000, Issue 2. Art. No.: CD002760. DOI: 10.1002/14651858.

23 Edwards JE, Meseguer F, Faura CC, Moore RA, McQuay HJ. Single dose dipyrone for acute postoperative pain. *The Cochrane Database of Syst Rev* 2001, Issue 1. Art. No.: CD003227. DOI: 10.1002/14651858.

24 Barden J, Edwards J, Moore RA, McQuay HJ. Single dose oral diclofenac for postoperative pain. *The Cochrane Database of Syst Rev* 2004, Issue 2. Art. No.: CD004768. DOI: 10.1002/14651858.

25 Collins SL, Moore RA, McQuay HJ, Wiffen PJ, Edwards JE. Single dose oral ibuprofen and diclofenac for postoperative pain. *The Cochrane Database of Syst Rev* 1999, Issue 1. Art. No.: CD001548. DOI: 10.1002/14651858.

26 Mason L, Edwards JE, Moore RA, McQuay HJ. Single dose oral naproxen and naproxen sodium for acute postoperative pain. *The Cochrane Database of Syst Rev* 2004, Issue 4. Art. No.: CD004234. DOI: 10.1002/14651858.

27 Barden J, Edwards J, Moore A, McQuay H. Single dose oral paracetamol (acetaminophen) for postoperative pain. *The Cochrane Database of Syst Rev* 2004, Issue 1. Art. No.: CD004602. DOI: 10.1002/14651858.

28 Barden J, Edwards J, Moore RA, McQuay HJ. Single dose oral rofecoxib for postoperative pain. *The Cochrane Database of Syst Rev* 2005, Issue 1. Art. No.: CD004604. DOI: 10.1002/14651858.

29 Edwards JE, Moore RA, McQuay HJ. Single dose oxycodone and oxycodone plus paracetamol (acetaminophen) for acute postoperative pain. *The Cochrane Database of Syst Rev* 2000, Issue 2. Art. No.: CD002763. DOI: 10.1002/14651858.

30 Moore A, Collins S, Carroll D, McQuay H, Edwards J. Single dose paracetamol (acetaminophen), with and without codeine, for postoperative pain. *The Cochrane Database of Syst Rev* 1998, Issue 4. Art. No.: CD001547. DOI: 10.1002/14651858.

31 Edwards JE, Loke YK, Moore RA, McQuay HJ. Single dose piroxicam for acute postoperative pain. *The Cochrane Database of Syst Rev* 2000, Issue 2. Art. No.: CD002762. DOI: 10.1002/14651858.

32 Carlisle J, Stevenson C. Drugs for preventing postoperative nausea and vomiting. *The Cochrane Database of Syst Rev* 2006, Issue 3.

33 Tramèr MR, Fuchs-Buder T. Omitting antagonism of neuromuscular block. Effect on postoperative nausea and vomiting and risk of residual paralysis: a systematic review. *Br J Anaesth* 1999; 82(3): 379–86.

34 Tramèr MR, Walder B. Efficacy and adverse effects of prophylactic antiemetics during patient-controlled analgesia therapy: a quantitative systematic review. *Anesth Analg* 1999; 88(6): 1354–61.

35 Henzi I, Sonderegger T, Tramèr MR. Efficacy, dose-response, and adverse effects of droperidol for prevention of postoperative nausea and vomiting. *Can J Anesth* 2000; 47(6): 537–51.

36 Hirayama T, Ishii F, Yago K, Ogata H. Evaluation of the effective drugs for the prevention of nausea and vomiting induced by morphine used for postoperative pain: a quantitative systematic Yakugaku Zasshi. *J Pharm Soc Jpn* 2001; 121(2): 179–85.

37 Tramèr M, Moore A, McQuay H. Prevention of vomiting after paediatric strabismus surgery: a systematic review using the numbers-needed-to-treat method. *Br J Anaesth* 1995; 75(5): 556–61.

38 Henzi I, Walder B, Tramèr MR. Metoclopramide in the prevention of postoperative nausea and vomiting: a quantitative systematic review of randomized, placebo-controlled studies. *Br J Anaesth* 1999; 83(5): 761–71.

39 Gupta A, Wu CL, Elkassabany N, Krug CE, Parker SD, Fleisher LA. Does the routine prophylactic use of antiemetics affect the incidence of postdischarge nausea and vomiting following ambulatory surgery: a systematic review of randomized controlled trials. *Anesthesiology* 2003; 99(2): 488–95.

40 Tramèr MR, Reynolds JM, Moore RA, McQuay HJ. Efficacy, dose-response, and safety of ondansetron in prevention of postoperative nausea and vomiting: a quantitative systematic review of randomized placebo-controlled trials. *Anesthesiology* 1997; 87(6): 1277–89.

41 Figueredo ED, Canosa LG. Ondansetron in the prophylaxis of postoperative vomiting: a meta-analysis. *J Clin Anesth* 1998; 10(3): 211–21.

42 Figueredo E, Canosa L. Prophylactic ondansetron for post-operative emesis: meta-analysis of its effectiveness in patients with and without a previous history of motion sickness. *Eur J Anaesthesiol* 1999; 16(8): 556–64.

43 Figueredo E, Canosa L. Prophylactic ondansetron for postoperative emesis: meta-analysis of its effectiveness in patients with previous history of postoperative nausea and vomiting. *Acta Anaesth Scand* 1999; 43(6): 637–44.

44 Tramèr MR, Reynolds DJ, Moore RA, McQuay HJ. Impact of covert duplicate publication on meta-analysis: a case study. *BMJ* 1997; 315: 635–40.

45 Steward DL, Welge JA, Myer CM. Steroids for improving recovery following tonsillectomy in children. *The Cochrane Database of Syst Rev* 2002, Issue 1. Art. No.: CD003997. DOI: 10.1002/14651858.

46 Henzi I, Walder B, Tramèr MR. Dexamethasone for the prevention of postoperative nausea and vomiting: a quantitative systematic review. *Anesth Analg* 2000; 90(1): 186–94.

47 Goldman AC, Govindaraj S, Rosenfeld RM. A meta-analysis of dexamethasone use with tonsillectomy. *Otolaryng Head Neck Surg* 2000; 123(6): 682–6.

48 Kranke P, Apfel CC, Eberhart LH, Georgieff M, Roewer N. The influence of a dominating centre on a quantitative systematic review of granisetron for preventing postoperative nausea and vomiting. *Acta Anaesth Scand* 2001; 45(6): 659–70.

49 Apfel CC, Korttila K, Abdalla M, Kerger H, Turan A, Vedder I et al. (for the IMPACT Investigators). A factorial trial of six interventions for the prevention of postoperative nausea and vomiting. *New Eng J Med* 2004; 350(24): 2441–51.

50 Lee A, Done ML. Stimulation of the wrist acupuncture point P6 for preventing postoperative nausea and vomiting. *The Cochrane Database of Syst Rev* 2004, Issue 3. Art. No.: CD003281. DOI: 10.1002/14651858.pub2.

51 Lee A, Done ML. The use of nonpharmacologic techniques to prevent postoperative nausea and vomiting: a meta-analysis. *Anesth Analg* 1999; 88: 1362–9.

52 Kazemi-Kjellberg F, Henzi I, Tramèr MR. Treatment of established postoperative nausea and vomiting: a quantitative systematic review. *BMC Anesthesiol* 2001; 1(2): www.biomedcentral.com/1471-2253/1/2.

17

Anaesthesia for day-case surgery

Kevin Walker and Andrew Smith

Department of Anaesthetics, Royal Lancaster Infirmary, Lancaster, UK

The practice of day-case surgery has grown substantially over the last 20 years. It presents some clinical and organisational challenges, as patients are discharged home promptly after surgery. This chapter summarises the results of a systematic literature search published between the dates of 1990 and July 2005. We have concentrated on clinical aspects of day surgery, which we feel are most relevant to anaesthetic personnel. Whilst we have attempted to concentrate on practice specific to day surgery, we have reported on studies which have included inpatients when we felt this was either relevant or the only evidence available. We have made it clear throughout which work is not restricted to day surgery.

When day surgery was first introduced, it was felt that only healthy patients without systemic disease were suitable. The evidence which we have summarised suggests that although patients with systemic illness have a higher incidence of minor intraoperative events, they are not at increased risk of unexpected hospital admission or major morbidity and mortality.

Otherwise healthy patients are often subjected to a series of preoperative tests. We have found that routine testing, even when abnormal results are found, is unlikely to alter clinical management or improve outcome. We have suggested simple guidelines for testing in patients who are elderly or have systemic disease.

There is a lot of published work looking for the ideal anaesthetic agent for day surgery. Particular concerns include speed of recovery and prevention of postoperative nausea and vomiting (PONV). We found propofol to be the intravenous (IV) induction agent of choice for day surgery, with induction agents having a greater influence on awakening than maintenance agents. Early and intermediate recovery were faster with sevoflurane or desflurane compared with isoflurane or propofol, however the clinical differences are small.

Postoperative pain is a common problem following day surgery and a multi-modal approach to analgesia is recommended. The oral route is effective, comparable to parenteral administration and should be used where possible. Wound infiltration and peripheral nerve blocks are useful adjuncts.

Although PONV is frequent in day surgery, routine prophylaxis is not effective. The emphasis should be on choosing a technique which keeps the risk of a PONV to a minimum, and providing effective treatment when it occurs. Prophylaxis is, however, warranted in high-risk cases and should consist of a multi-modal approach.

Discharge criteria should be in place to allow effective discharge from day surgery units (DSUs). Numerical scoring systems can be used and may allow safe delegation to other members of staff.

Introduction

Day-case surgery – known as ambulatory surgery in North America – has grown substantially in the last 20 years. (The two terms are used interchangeably in this chapter.) The prospect of spending less time in hospital tends to be popular with patients, and the associated reduction in costs is popular with those who fund health care. However, it presents some clinical and organisational challenges.

The fact that patients must be discharged home promptly throws postoperative problems into sharper relief. In particular, postoperative pain and nausea need to be controlled before discharge and provision must be made for continuing treatment at home where necessary.

As day-case surgery is a relatively new development, there is a fair amount of published evidence on clinical aspects. Organisational issues tend to be less closely evaluated, springing as they do from experience. Many are published as guidelines by professional and managerial bodies [1,2]. In this chapter we focus only on the clinical aspects of day-case surgery most relevant to anaesthetic personnel.

The chapter summarises the results of a systematic literature search of The Cochrane Database, Medline and EMBASE for material published between 1990 and July 2005, with scrutiny of reference lists of retrieved papers for further relevant work.

We have also tried to be explicit not only about the nature and strength of the evidence we have found but also about practice contexts, as practices vary between hospitals and between countries. This is shown even in the definition of a "day case", which can vary from a patient who spends less than 4 h in hospital to one who may stay overnight but whose total stay is less than 24 h. It is important to bear such definitional differences in mind as they can affect the extent to which research evidence gleaned from one setting can be applied to another.

Patient selection

Despite increasing demand for day-case surgery and advances in surgical technique, patient selection remains important to reduce postoperative complications. Medical, surgical and social factors influence suitability for day-case surgery.

Originally only patients graded I or II on the ASA (American Society of Anesthe-siologists) physical status classification were considered suitable. However, sys-temic disease is no longer thought to contraindicate day-case admission.

Evidence

We found a number of studies tracking the progress of patients with co-existing medical disease through day-case surgery. These are summarised in Table 17.1. Note that we have assumed that the conditions are optimally treated before the patient is admitted for surgery. Where risk is increased, each case should be dealt with on its individual merits.

Table 17.1. Co-existing medical conditions in day surgery

Condition	Studies	Conclusion
Physical Status (ASA grade)	1 In a retrospective case-controlled study of 896 ASA III day-surgery patients, there was no significant increase in unexpected admissions compared with ASA I and II controls (admission rate 2.6% ASA III; 1.9% ASA I–II) [3] 2 In a prospective study of 38 598 ambulatory patients, incidence of severe morbidity (myocardial infarction, central nervous system deficit, pulmonary embolism and respiratory failure) was distributed equally between ASA grades I–III. 24% of cohort were ASA III [4]	No increase in admission rate of major morbidity with ASA III patients.
Obesity	1 In a cohort of 17 683 patients, 2779 patients were defined as obese (BMI >30). No increase in cardiovascular events. Increased risk of respiratory events (OR: 3.89; 99.9% CI: 1.14–13.3)[5] 2 Increased risk of lower respiratory events in cohort of 6914 patients (RR: 5.4; $P < 0.01$) [6]	Increased risk of perioperative respiratory events
Hyper-reactive airway disease	1 In a prospective cohort of 17 683 ambulatory patients, there was an increased risk of postoperative respiratory events in asthmatics (OR: 4.61; 99.9% CI: 1.18–18.0) and smokers (OR: 3.84; 95% CI: 1.11–13.3) [5] 2 A cohort of 6914 ambulatory patients found increased risk of perioperative lower airway events in patients with asthma (RR: 7.2; $P < 0.01$) and COPD (RR: 10.1; $P < 0.01$) [6] 3 A retrospective analysis of 16 411 ambulatory patients showed no association between respiratory disease and length of stay in recovery [7]	Increased risk of perioperative and postoperative respiratory events
Diabetes	1 Diabetes not an independent predictor of morbidity following ambulatory surgery [5]	No increased risk of perioperative events

(Continued)

Table 17.1. (Continued)

Condition	Studies		Conclusion
	2	Diabetics increased risk of unanticipated admission following ambulatory surgery (OR: 2.0; 95% CI: 1.3–2.2). However, was not significant when other variables accounted [8]	
	3	A Cochrane Review of 176 RCTs showed no episodes of lactic acidosis in over 35 000 patient-years of treatment with metformin [9]	
Smoking	1	In a cohort of 489 ambulatory patients, Smokers had increased risk of respiratory complications (OR: 1.71; 95% CI: 1.03–2.84) and wound complications (OR: 16.3; 95% CI: 1.58–175). Smoking cessation <4 weeks preoperatively resulted in adverse effects similar to non-smokers [10]	Smokers are at increased risk of respiratory and wound complications. This risk falls if smoking stopped at least 4 weeks preoperatively
	2	An RCT of 120 patients undergoing joint arthroplasty showed smoking cessation 6–8 weeks preoperatively reduced wound complications (number needed to treat: 4; 95% CI: 2–8) [10] (not ambulatory)	
Coronary artery disease	1	A prospective study of complications in 38 598 ambulatory patients, 14 had a myocardial infarction within 1 month (rate 1:3220). No details about incidence of coronary artery disease in study population [4]	Low risk of adverse intraoperative or postoperative events
	2	In a prospective cohort of 17 683 patients, when corrected for age, sex, duration and type of surgery, history of angina or myocardial infarction were not predictors of intraoperative or postoperative adverse events [5]	
Hypertension	1	In a prospective cohort of 17 683 patients, increase in cardiovascular events (OR: 2.47; 95% CI: 1.37–3.58) and all intraoperative events (OR: 2.21; 99.9% CI: 1.37–3.58) [5]	Increased risk of perioperative cardiovascular complications
	2	No prediction of postoperative events in cohort study of 544 patients >70 years for non-cardiac surgery (not ambulatory) [12]	
Cardiac failure	1	12% increase in postoperative stay (relative length of stay 1.11; 99.9% CI: 1.0–1.23) [13]	Increased risk of postoperative complications
	2	In a prospective cohort of 17 683 patients there is 11.1% incidence of intraoperative adverse cardiovascular events, but not significant predictor when corrected for age, sex, duration and type of surgery [5]	
Gastroesophageal reflux	1	In a prospective cohort of 17 683 patients, eight fold increase in intubation related adverse effects (OR: 8.0; 99.9% CI: 1.17–54.6) [5]	Increased risk of intubation complications

OR: odds ratio; RR: relative risk; CI: confidence interval.

> **Practice points**
> - Patients with pre-existing medical conditions need not be excluded from day surgery.
> - Patients of ASA physical status grade III do not appear to be at greater risk of unanticipated hospital admission, mortality or major morbidity than those of grade I or II.
> - Patients with systemic disease do, however, have a higher incidence of minor intra-operative adverse events and we suggest that these more challenging patients be cared for by experienced anaesthetic personnel.

Preoperative testing

Preoperative testing may be divided into tests which are "routine", where they are used as a screening tool in all patients, and "indicated", where the decision to test is directed by findings from clinical history or examination. Test results are assumed to show a statistically normal distribution. As reference ranges usually include ± 2 standard deviations around the mean, some normal healthy people will, by definition, have results which fall outside those reference ranges. The usefulness of a test must be questioned when an abnormal result is unlikely to influence clinical management.

Evidence

The role of routine tests in otherwise asymptomatic patients in the absence of any specific clinical indication has been considered in a systematic review (search date 1996) [14]. All studies included were results of case series as no randomised trials have been published. This review was not specific to day-case surgery and the studies included a variety of surgical specialities. The results are summarised in Table 17.2.

In 2003, the UK National Institute for Clinical Excellence (NICE) published guidelines for routine preoperative testing [15]. A systematic search was conducted for evidence published since the search conducted for the above review. The results from the systematic review confirmed the previous work's conclusion that there is no evidence that routine preoperative testing either improves or worsens outcome. However, the resulting guidance does not reflect this entirely, as the guidelines were drawn up by a consensus of interested stakeholders. They are comprehensive and detailed and attempt to stratify patients by ASA grade, type of operative procedure and cardiovascular, respiratory or renal disease. Table 17.3 shows some of the document's suggestions for testing in healthy older patients and patients with some medical conditions, though it must be emphasised that there is no evidence that testing healthy patients of any age improves outcome.

Table 17.2. Value of routine preoperative tests [14]

Test	Percentage with abnormal findings	Percentage of tests where result changed clinical management	Reviewers' interpretation of evidence for routine use of test	Studies included
Chest X-ray	2.5–37% (increases with age)	0–2.1%	Limited evidence about effect on clinical outcomes. Limited evidence about predictive value about postoperative respiratory complications	28 reports (18 913 CXRs). Only six studies assessed change in management after routine CXR
ECG	4.6–31.7% (increases with age)	0–2.2%	No evidence to support routine preoperative ECG. Evidence suggests benefit of "baseline" ECG. Predictive value of postoperative cardiac complications is low	16 reports (8889 ECGs). Seven studies considered change in management after routine test
Full blood count	Hb: <10–10.5 upto 5%; platelet count: low <1.1%; WCC: abnormal <1%	Hb: 0.1%–2.7%; platelet count: Rare; WCC: Rare	Evidence suggests abnormal results rarely alter clinical management	23 (20 807 blood tests)
Clotting	Bleeding time: 3.8%; Prothrombin time: 4.8%; Partial thromboplastin time: 15.6%	Rare	No evidence to support routine use	23 (12 944 blood tests)
Biochemistry	Serum sodium and potassium: 1.4%; Urea/creatinine: 2.5%; Glucose: 5.2%	Rare	No evidence to support routine use	8 (4185 blood tests)
Urinalysis	1–34.1%	0.1–2.8%	Evidence suggests no predictive value about postoperative complications in non-urinary tract surgery. Results in treatment for urinary tract infection around 1:40	11 (6740 urine tests)

ECG: electrocardiogram; Hb: haemoglobin; WCC: white cell count.

Table 17.3. Suggested **routine** preoperative investigations [15]

	Full blood count	Renal function	Electrocardiogram	Chest X-ray
ASA I	>60 years	No	>80 years	No
ASA II–III				
Cardiovascular	>60 years	Yes	Yes	No
Respiratory	>60 years	No	>60 years	No
Renal	>60 years	Yes	>60 years	No

Practice points
- We suggest that healthy patients should not be submitted to routine preoperative tests as the results, even if abnormal, are unlikely to alter clinical management and testing has not been shown to improve outcome.
- Older patients, or those with systemic disease, may warrant specific tests and simple guidelines are shown above.

Preoperative fasting and premedication

It has been shown in one study that day-case patients have a higher preoperative gastric volume than inpatients [16]. However, six studies gathered by a qualitative non-systematic review found no difference in residual gastric volumes between ambulatory patients and inpatients [17]. There also may be reluctance to give anxiolytic premedication to day-surgery patients for fear of delaying recovery or discharge.

Evidence

A Cochrane systematic review of randomised controlled trials (RCTs) has assessed fasting before surgery (search date 2003) [18]. This was not restricted to day-case anaesthesia and included 22 trials, generally in healthy adults not at risk of regurgitation or aspiration. The trials used surrogate outcomes rather than the incidence of aspiration or regurgitation. There was no evidence of difference in volume or pH of gastric contents when a shortened fluid fast was compared with a standard fast. Patients allowed water preoperatively had statistically but not clinically significant lower gastric volumes (weighted mean difference 2.5 ml, 95% CI: 0.42–4.6). While this review is well conducted, it relies, of necessity, on the outcome measures of the primary studies on which it is based. As none featured clinical outcomes, the evidence is at best supportive of shortened fluid fasting rather than conclusive.

A Cochrane review has considered anxiolytic premedication in adult patients undergoing day-case surgery (search date 2002) [19]. Fifteen RCTs published since

1990 were included. The primary outcome used was time to discharge; most studies were designed to assess the sedative effect of the premedicants preoperatively using psychomotor tests and where these tests were repeated postoperatively, this was used as a secondary outcome for the review. A wide range of drugs was used, including benzodiazepines, beta-blockers and opiates. Premedication was not found to delay time to discharge in any study. Out of four studies which used psychomotor tests to assess recovery, three showed impaired recovery after premedication with benzodiazepines. However, in the studies which used a combination of clinical criteria and psychomotor tests, none showed a delay in discharge.

A task force of the ASA reviewed the evidence on the use of pharmacological agents to reduce the risk of pulmonary aspiration [20]. The studies were performed on healthy patients undergoing elective procedures and are not exclusive to ambulatory procedures. Whilst there was evidence to support reduced gastric acidity and volume with H_2 receptor antagonists and proton pump inhibitors, there was insufficient evidence to support routine use to reduce frequency of aspiration or reduce morbidity/mortality following aspiration.

> **Practice points**
> - Day-case patients should be fasted for 6 h following light meal (8 h following fatty meal) and allowed clear fluids up to 2 h preoperatively.
> - We do not recommend routine use of acid prophylactic medication preoperatively in day-case patients with no risk factors for regurgitation or aspiration.
> - Anxiolytic premedication can be given to day-surgery patients and does not delay discharge.

Anaesthetic technique

The ideal anaesthetic for day-case surgery would provide rapid recovery, quick return to "street fitness" and be free of side-effects. Other considerations include turnover times and cost-effectiveness.

Recovery can be defined as a three-stage process – Phase I: extends from end of anaesthesia until maintenance of protective reflexes and motor function; Phase II: return to home readiness; Phase III: full recovery to preoperative status. In the context of day surgery, Phase I usually occurs in the postanaesthesia care unit (PACU), Phase II in the DSU and Phase III at home. Stages of recovery following general anaesthesia can also be described as Early (eye opening or tongue protrusion to command); Intermediate (orientation) and Late (walk unaided, discharge). Psychomotor recovery and unwanted side-effects (PONV, pain and anxiety) can also be measured.

Evidence

General anaesthesia

We found two systematic reviews comparing recovery from different anaesthetic agents in ambulatory surgery [21,22]. We found a further four meta-analyses assessing recovery profiles [23–26], although these included both day cases and inpatients.

A systematic review of clinical outcomes after different anaesthetic techniques for day-surgery patients (search date 2000) was published in 2002 [21]. Eighty-nine primary studies, mostly of high quality, were included. Recovery was assessed in stages as described above (early/intermediate/late/psychomotor/unwanted side-effects). A further systematic review (search date 2002) found an additional 27 studies [22]. The studies are summarized in Table 17.4. The "practice points" box draws practical recommendations (see below).

These findings are supported by a further four meta-analyses which also included inpatient studies [23–26].

Regional anaesthesia

We found no systematic reviews comparing regional and general anaesthesia. One RCT compared general anaesthesia with spinal anaesthesia for inguinal hernia repair [27]. Thirty-four patients were included in the study, which randomised patients to general anaesthesia with propofol or spinal anaesthesia with hyperbaric lignocaine. Total time to discharge was a little longer in the spinal anaesthetic group (average 285.4 min; 95% CI: 251–317 min) compared with general anaesthesia (261.7 min; 95% CI: 223–293 min). Patients in the spinal group spent less time in the operating room and in Phase I recovery (159 min versus 188 min), but longer in Phase II recovery (129 min versus 78 min). Patient and surgeon satisfaction with anaesthetic technique was high in both groups. A further RCT compared general anaesthesia with desflurane and spinal anaesthesia for outpatient knee arthroscopy [28]. The study included 64 patients who were randomly allocated into two groups. Patients in the spinal group received 4 mg (0.8 ml) of hyperbaric bupivacaine and were positioned in a lateral decubitus position. Spinal anaesthesia was inadequate in two patients who were converted to general anaesthesia and excluded from the study. Time to home readiness was similar in both groups (spinal anaesthesia: median 114 min, range 31–174; general anaesthesia: 129 min, range 28–245).

Monitoring

A meta-analysis compared Bispectral Index (BIS) monitoring and standard practice in ambulatory surgery patients (search date 2004) [29]. Eleven RCTs were included involving 1380 patients. The use of BIS monitoring reduced anaesthetic consumption by 19%, reduced nausea and vomiting (32% versus 38%) and

Table 17.4. Anaesthetic agents in day surgery

Comparison		Number of studies (number of patients)	Findings	Quality of studies
IV induction agents	Propofol versus thiopentone	16 (883)	11 trials propofol superior (early, intermediate, late and psychomotor recovery); five trials no difference	Only six studies kept maintenance of anaesthesia constant in both study groups; eight studies blinded
	Propofol versus etomidate	2 (70)	One trial early recovery better with etomidate; one trial early/intermediate recovery better with propofol	Methods of randomisation not given; not blinded
	Propofol versus methohexitone	3 (240)	Recovery better with propofol	Methods of randomisation not given
IV versus inhalational induction	Propofol versus sevoflurane	5 (348)	No difference in recovery in four trials (two sevoflurane maintenance; two TIVA versus total sevoflurane); Early, intermediate and late recovery more rapid in one trial comparing TIVA with total sevoflurane technique	Two trials blinded; methods of randomisation given in two trials
	Thiopentone versus sevoflurane	1 (78)	Recovery time better with sevoflurane	Not blinded; method of randomisation not given
	Propofol versus desflurane	5 (323)	One trial showed improved early/intermediate recovery with desflurane; No difference in recovery in four trials	Four trials blinded; four trials method of randomisation not given; one trial crossover volunteers
	Thiopentone versus desflurane	1 (80)	Intermediate recovery delayed with thiopentone	Blinded; method of randomisation not given
Inhalational induction agents	Isoflurane versus sevoflurane	1 (50)	No difference early/intermediate/late/ psychomotor recovery	Not blinded; method of randomisation not given

(Continued)

Table 17.4. (Continued)

Comparison		Number of studies (number of patients)	Findings	Quality of studies
IV versus inhalational maintenance	Propofol versus isoflurane	23 (1910)	No difference in early/intermediate/late/ psychomotor recovery when propofol used for induction in both groups	Seven trials blinded; 16 trials randomisation method not given; 14 trials kept induction drug same in both groups; four trials not known
	Propofol versus sevoflurane	14 (1071)	Early recovery: sevoflurane better eight trials; no difference five trials; propofol better one trial Intermediate recovery: sevoflurane better five trials; no difference seven trials; propofol better two trials Late recovery: sevoflurane better one trial; propofol better one trial; no difference three trials Psychomotor recovery: sevoflurane better two trials; propofol better one trial; not examined 11 trials	Two trials blinded; seven trials method of randomisation not given
	Propofol versus desflurane	19 (1179;	Early recovery better with desflurane nine trials; intermediate recovery better with desflurane in three trials Early recovery better with propofol two trial and late recovery better with propofol in two trials	Five trials blinded; eight method of randomisation not given; one crossover volunteer study. Quality not given 10 trials
	Propofol versus enflurane	3 (660)	No difference in early/intermediate/late/ psychomotor recovery when propofol induction used	Two trials blinded; two method of randomisation not given

	Propofol versus halothane	2 (92)	No difference in early/intermediate/late/psychomotor recovery in one trial. Psychomotor recovery faster with propofol in one trial	One trial blinded; both trials method of randomisation not given
Inhalational maintenance	Sevoflurane versus desfluarne	6 (306)	Two trials showed faster early recovery with desflurane. No difference in late recovery in any study	One trial not randomised; one trial blinded; two trials method of randomisation not given; three trials not known
	Isoflurane versus desfluarne	5 (267)	Desflurane better in early recovery in four trials; desflurane better in intermediate recovery in three trials. No difference in late recovery	Two trials blinded; three trials method of randomisation not given; two trials not known
	Sevoflurane versus isoflurane	5 (455)	Early/intermediate/psychomotor recovery better with sevoflurane when propofol used for induction. No difference in late recovery. No difference with thiopentone induction	One trial blinded; four trials method of randomisation not given
	Halothane versus isoflurane	2 (92)	No difference in psychomotor recovery	One trial not blinded; both trials method of randomisation not given
	Enflurane versus halothane	3 (144)	Two trials found early/intermediate recovery better with enflurane. one trial found no difference	Two trials not blinded; method of randomisation not given in any
	Enflurane versus isoflurane	3 (753)	No difference in recovery	Two trials not blinded; one trial method of randomization not given
	N20 versus air	10 (2157)	No difference in early, intermediate or late recovery when nitrous oxide omitted from a volatile technique; early recovery better when nitrous oxide omitted from propofol TIVA in two out of four trials	Six trials blinded; six trials method of randomisation not given

reduced time in the recovery area by 4 min (45.2 min versus 49.1 min). There was no significant difference between groups in time to hospital discharge. Cost analysis showed that minor savings in anaesthetic agents, time in PACU and prevention of PONV were offset by the costs of the BIS electrode.

> **Practice points**
> - Propofol is the IV induction agent of choice in day-case anaesthesia and has more influence on awakening than the choice of maintenance agent.
> - Sevoflurane and desflurane provided faster early and intermediate recovery when compared to propofol or isoflurane. The differences are small and clinical advantages will be dependant on infrastructure of the DSU (see "fast-tracking" below).
> - When interpreting these results it is important to remember the structured protocol for each anaesthetist in a trial does not allow clinical experience to influence how a drug is used. Careful timing in ending anaesthesia may greatly influence awakening times regardless of what agent is used.
> - Recovery from spinal anaesthesia compares well with general anaesthesia in the day-case setting, though more work is needed to establish the best technique for day surgery.
> - Whilst BIS monitoring reduces anaesthetic drug consumption, it does not improve time to discharge or reduce costs of anaesthesia.

Analgesia

Postoperative pain is one of the most frequently occurring adverse events after day-case surgery. A prospective study of 10 008 day-surgery patients found the incidence of severe pain was 5.3% in the PACU, 1.7% in the DSU and 5.3% at 24 h despite standard analgesia [30]. Increased body mass index and greater duration of anaesthesia were predictive factors for severe pain. In another study of ambulatory surgical patients, the procedures most associated with severe pain at 24 h were orchidectomy/hydrocele repair (26.3%), shoulder arthroscopy (22.3%), laproscopic cholecystectomy (18%), microdiscectomy (17.9%) and knee arthroscopy (15.5%) [31]. Uncontrolled pain was cited as the reason for 12.1% unanticipated admissions following day surgery [32].

Evidence

Pre-emptive analgesia

One systematic review was found concerning pre-emptive analgesia (search date 2000) [33]. Eighty studies were included and involved both minor and major surgical procedures. No distinction was made about day surgery. There was no evidence of additional benefit from pre-emptive non-steroidal anti-inflammatory drugs (NSAIDs), opioids or preincisional wound infiltration.

Postoperative analgesia

A systematic review of oral analgesia attempted to compare the effects of commonly used oral analgesics with morphine and with each other. This was not restricted to the day-case setting but as oral analgesia is the mainstay of postoperative analgesia in ambulatory surgery it is highly relevant [34]. This is summarised in Table 17.5.

One meta-analysis was found reviewing incisional local anaesthesia for abdominal operations (search date 1997) [35]. Twenty-six studies were included with 1211 patients which were separated into inguinal herniotomy (five RCTs), hysterectomy (four), open cholecystectomy (eight) and a variety of procedures (nine). Following inguinal herniotomy pain scores were consistently lower from 2–7 h postoperatively. One study found reduced pain scores up to 24 h and one found a difference up to 48 h. Four of the studies found a significant reduction in time to first analgesic request.

Table 17.5. Summary of recommendations from systematic review of analgesia in day surgery [34]

Interventions of proven value	1 Includes standard oral analgesics (standard doses) – paracetamol; ibuprofen; diclofenac; tramadol; dextropropoxyphene
	2 Single dose oral NSAIDs are effective and provide comparable analgesia to 10 mg intramuscular morphine (NNT 50% pain relief: Ibuprofen 400 mg 2.7 (95% CI: 2.5–3.0); diclofenac 50 mg 2.3 (95% CI: 2.0–2.7); morphine 10 mg intramuscular 2.9 (95% CI: 2.6–3.6)
	3 Paracetamol and codeine combinations appear effective (NNT 50% pain relief): paracetamol 1000 mg 4.6 (95% CI: 3.9–5.4); paracetamol 600 mg/Codeine 60 mg 3.1 (95% CI: 2.6–3.9); Paracetamol 1000 mg/Codeine 60 mg 1.9 (95% CI: 1.5–2.6)
Interventions of doubtful value	1 Injecting morphine into knee joint – has small analgesic effect lasting up to 24 h but no evidence of clinical value
	2 Pre-emptive analgesia – no more effective than standard methods
	3 Injectable or rectal NSAIDs in patients which can swallow – are no more effective
	4 Administering codeine in single dose – has poor analgesic efficacy
Ineffective interventions	1 TENS (transcutaneous electric nerve stimulator) in acute postoperative pain
	2 Local injections of opioids at sites other than knee joint
	3 Dihydrocodeine 30 mg

NNT: number needed to treat; CI: confidence interval

Intra-articular techniques for analgesia following knee arthroscopy have been considered in two systematic reviews [36,37]. A systematic review of intra-articular local anaesthesia for analgesia following knee arthroscopy (search date 1998) included 20 studies; 12 of the studies showed improved pain parameters and in 10 studies pain scores were significantly lower (reduction in visual analogue score of 10–35 mm). Most studies only showed an early postoperative effect, from 1–4 h. The effect of intra-articular morphine was considered in a systematic review (search date 2004). Out of the nine studies which were included in analysis, seven showed no benefit from intra-articular morphine; 23 RCTs were excluded due to low scientific quality.

No systematic reviews or large RCTs were found evaluating peripheral nerve blocks in day surgery. Three randomised trials were found, however the number of patients in each was small (30–55), and will just be mentioned in summary. The addition of ilioinguinal and hypogastric nerve blocks to patients having inguinal hernia repair under local anaesthesia resulted in lower pain scores in PACU and less oral analgesia after discharge [38]. In another study, paravertebral nerve blocks provided equivalent analgesia to ilioinguinal–hypogastric nerve blocks, but no comparison was made to a control group [39]. Following outpatient arthroscopic anterior cruciate repair, femoral nerve block with 0.25% or 0.5% bupivacaine provided up to 24 h of analgesia [40].

Practice points
- There appears to be no additional benefit from pre-emptive analgesia, although preoperative timing of analgesia may be convenient for short procedures and allow oral route of administration.
- Oral analgesia should be used whenever possible. Oral NSAIDs are as effective as injectable or rectal NSAIDs and give equivalent analgesia to intramuscular morphine.
- Wound infiltration is effective at reducing early postoperative pain and should be used where possible. It may "buy time" to establish effective oral analgesia postoperatively.
- Peripheral nerve blockade may help with postoperative analgesia but there is insufficient evidence to comment on its efficacy.

Postoperative nausea and vomiting

PONV is an important cause of morbidity following day surgery and along with pain is a major cause of unexpected admission. One systematic review found the incidence of nausea to be 17% (0–55%) and vomiting to be 8% (0–16%) [41].

Evidence

PONV was included in a systematic review of anaesthetic agents [20]. Out of 48 studies involving propofol TIVA (total IV anaesthesia), 21 showed a lower incidence of PONV in the propofol group. PONV was less after induction with propofol when compared with thiopentone or inhalational agents. PONV was greater with TIVA in only two studies and in the remaining 25 there was no difference. Four studies considered PONV following nitrous oxide. Three found no difference and one found increased PONV with nitrous oxide.

A systematic review including 22 studies assessed PONV prophylaxis in day surgery [42]. Overall incidence of post-discharge nausea was 32.6% and post-discharge vomiting 14.7%. Prophylactic metoclopramide and droperidol were no different to placebo in preventing post-discharge nausea and vomiting. Ondansetron, dexamethasone and combination treatment reduced post-discharge nausea (number needed to treat: ondansetron 4 mg: 12.9; dexamethasone: 12.2). The total incidence of postoperative vomiting in the treatment group was 14.6% compared with 26.5% in the placebo group.

In general, management of PONV should be directed towards reducing the risk (by using propofol for maintenance and by omitting nitrous oxide). Specific prophylaxis of PONV is likely to be less worthwhile that treating the symptoms when they occur [43]. For patients at high risk of PONV, baseline risk should be reduced as above and a combination of antiemetics should be used as single agents are not effective. Although these studies were not restricted to day-case patients, we suggest that the results are largely transferable.

Practice points
- Routine PONV prophylaxis is not effective and day surgery is not in itself a valid reason for routine prophylaxis.
- Emphasis should be focused on reducing baseline risk of PONV (consider using propofol TIVA and omitting nitrous oxide) and effective treatment of symptoms when they do occur.
- No single agent is effective in prophylaxis for PONV and in high risk patients a balanced combination approach should be followed.

Discharge criteria

Criteria which must be satisfied before patients can be allowed home have been developed in many day-case units. Some have been published. One well-known set of criteria is shown below (see Table 17.6).

Table 17.6. Guidelines for safe discharge after ambulatory surgery [49]

Vital signs must have been stable for at least 1 h

The patient must be:
  Orientated to person, place and time
  Able to retain orally administered fluids
  Able to void urine
  Able to dress
  Able to walk without assistance

The patient must not have:
  More than minimal nausea and vomiting
  Excessive pain
  Bleeding

The patient must be discharged by both the person who administered anaesthesia and the person who performed surgery, or by their designates. Written instructions for the postoperative period at home including a contact place and person must be reinforced

The patient must have a responsible "vested" adult to escort them home and stay with them at home

Numerical scoring systems have also been developed, which assign values to such criteria and allow progression from one phase of recovery to the next when certain scores have been reached [44,45].

Although scoring systems are widely used to help decide when it is suitable to transfer a patient from one phase to the next, they have never been formally evaluated. There are some differences between them, the main one being the need to keep oral fluids down, and void urine before being allowed home.

Fast-tracking involves bypassing the PACU, with early recovery occurring in the operating theatre then the patient being transferred directly to the DSU. It is dependent on the use of anaesthetic drugs with short duration of action and fast offset [46].

Evidence

No systematic reviews were found comparing different discharge criteria.

We found one RCT comparing fast-tracking to a standard day-surgery technique [47]. Patients in the fast-tracking group were awakened in the operating theatre and transferred directly to the DSU, thus bypassing the PACU. A scoring system was used to assess sufficient recovery to allow fast-tracking. Patients in the standard group were not transferred to PACU until they opened their eyes to command. Two hundred and seven day-surgery patients undergoing hysteroscopy, arthroscopy or laparoscopy were randomised. The mean time to discharge was less in the fast-tracking group (17 min less) but there was a significant difference between the different surgical groups (hysteroscopy 43 min; arthroscopy 35 min; laparoscopy 2 min). They found little difference between nursing workload, measured by nursing interventions and care hours, or significant cost savings between the two groups. There were differences between the surgical groups in both success in meeting fast-track criteria and reduced time to discharge and certain procedures may be more suited to this technique.

A prospective observational study assessed anaesthetic and non-anaesthetic factors which influenced discharge times in 1088 day-surgery patients [48]. After anaesthetic technique, the most influential factor was found to be the nurse administrating Phase II care (13% variability in discharge time). System factors accounted for the majority of delays in Phase II discharge (41%) and of these, 53% were due to lack of an immediate escort for the patient.

Practice points

- Patients should meet defined criteria before discharge from DSU. Numerical scoring systems may allow safe delegation to other members of staff but there is insufficient evidence that they allow safer or more effective discharge than simple guidelines.
- 'Fast-Tracking' reduces, but does not remove, the need for a PACU and has not been shown to offer clear advantages in terms of work load or costs. Releasing the potential of 'fast-tracking' will depend heavily on structure and practice of individual day-case units.

Research agenda

Although differences between general anaesthetic agents have been well studied, RCT evidence using important clinical outcomes is lacking for many aspects of day-case anaesthesia. In particular, preoperative fasting, the use of preoperative tests, and the application of discharge criteria have not been formally tested.

List of abbreviations

ASA:	American Society of Anesthesiologists
BIS:	Bispectral index monitoring
CI:	Confidence interval
COPD:	Chronic obstructive pulmonary disease
DSU:	Day-surgery unit
NNT:	Number needed to treat
NSAIDs:	Non-steroidal anti-inflammatory drugs

OR: Odds ratio
PACU: Postanaesthesia care unit
PONV: Postoperative nausea and vomiting
RCT: Randomised controlled trial
RR: Relative risk
TENS: Transcutaneous electrical nerve stimulation
TIVA: Total intravenous anaesthesia

REFERENCES

1 Department of Health. Day Surgery: Operational guide (2002). http://www.dh.gov.uk/PublicationsAndStatistics/Publications/fs/en (accessed 27th June 2006)

2 The Association of Anaesthetists of Great Britain and Ireland. Day Surgery (revised 2005). http://www.aagbi.org/guidelines.html (accessed 27th June 2006)

3 Ansell G, Montgomery J. Outcome of ASA III patients undergoing day case surgery. *Br J Anaesth* 2004; 92: 71–4.

4 Warner M, Shields S, Chute C. Major morbidity and mortality within 1 month of ambulatory surgery and anesthesia. *JAMA* 1993; 270: 1437–41.

5 Chung F, Mezei G, Tong D. Pre-existing medical conditions as predictors of adverse events in day-case surgery. *Br J Anaesth* 1999; 83: 262–70.

6 Duncan PG, Cohen MM, Tweed WA, Biehl D, Pope WD, Merchant RN, DeBoer D. The Canadian four-centre study of anaesthetic outcomes. III. Are anaesthetic complications predictable in day surgical practice? *Can J Anesth* 1992; 39: 440–8.

7 Chung F, Mezei G. Factors contributing to a prolonged stay after ambulatory surgery. *Anesth Analg* 1999; 89:1352–9.

8 Fortier J, Chung F, Su J. Unanticipated admission after ambulatory surgery – a prospective study. *Can J Anesth* 1998; 45: 612–9.

9 Salpeter S, Greyber E, Pasternak G, Salpeter E. Risk of fatal and nonfatal lactic acidosis with metformin use in type 2 diabetes mellitus. *The Cochrane Database Syst Rev* 2003; Issue 3, Art. No.: CD002967. DOI: 10.1002/14651858.

10 Myles PS, Iacono GA, Hunt JO, Fletcher F, Morris J McIlroy D, Fritschi L. Risk of respiratory complications in wound infection in patients undergoing ambulatory surgery: smokers versus nonsmokers. *Anesthesiology* 2002; 97: 842–7.

11 Møller AM, Villebro N, Pedersen T, Tonnesen H. Effect of preoperative smoking intervention on postoperative complications: a randomized clinical trial. *Lancet* 2002; 359: 114–7.

12 Leung JM, Dzankic S. Relative importance of preoperative health status versus intraoperative factors in predicting postoperative adverse outcomes in geriatric surgical patients. *J Am Geriatric Soc* 2001; 49: 1080–5.

13 Chung F, Mezei G. Factors contributing to a prolonged stay after ambulatory surgery. *Anesth Analg* 1999; 89: 1352–9.

14 Munro J, Booth A, Nicholl J. Routine preoperative testing: A systematic review of the evidence. *Health Technol Assess* 1997; 1(12).

15 *Preoperative Testing. The Use of Routine Preoperative Tests for Elective Surgery. Evidence, Methods and Guidance.* The National Collaborating Centre for Acute Care. Available from www.nice.org.uk

16 Ong BY, Palahniuk RJ, Cumming M. Gastric volume and pH in out-patients. *Can Anaesth Soc J* 1978; 25: 36–9.

17 Kallar SK, Everett LL. Potential risks and preventive measures for pulmonary aspiration: new concepts in preoperative fasting guidelines. *Anesth Analg* 1993; 77: 171–82.

18 Brady M, Kinn S, Stuart P. Preoperative fasting for adults to prevent perioperative complications. *The Cochrane Database Syst Rev* 2003, Issue 4. Art. No.: CD004423. DOI: 10.1002/ 14651858.

19 Walker KJ, Smith AF, Pittaway AJ. Premedication for anxiety in adult day surgery. *The Cochrane Database Syst Rev* 2003; Issue 1. Art. No.: CD002192. DOI: 10.1002/14651858.

20 Practice guidelines for preoperative fasting and the use of pharmacological agents to reduce the risk of pulmonary aspiration: application to healthy patients undergoing elective procedures. A Report by the American Society of Anesthesiologists Task Force on Preoperative Fasting. *Anesthesiology* 1999; 90: 896–905.

21 Elliot RA, Payne K, Moore JK, Davies LM, Harper NJN, St Leger AS et al. Which anaesthetic agents are cost-effective in day surgery? Literature review, national survey of practice and randomised controlled trial. *Health Technol Assess* 2002; 6(30).

22 Gupta A, Stierer T, Zuckerman R, Sakima N, Parker S, Fleisher L. Comparison of recovery profile after ambulatory anesthesia with propofol, isoflurane, sevoflurane and desflurane: a systematic review. *Anesth Analg* 2004; 98: 632–41.

23 Dexter F, Tinker J. Comparisons between desflurane and isoflurane or propofol on time to following commands or time to discharge: a meta-analysis. *Anesthesiology* 1995; 77: 77–82.

24 Ebert T, Robinson B, Uhrich T, Mackenthun A, Pichotta P. Recovery from sevoflurane anesthesia: a comparison to isoflurane and propofol Anesthesia. *Anesthesiology* 1998; 89:1524–31.

25 Robinson B, Uhrich T, Ebert T. A review of recovery from sevoflurane anaesthesia: comparisons with isoflurane and propofol including meta-analysis. *Acta Anaesthesiol Scand* 1999; 43: 185–90.

26 Joo H, Perks W. Sevoflurane versus propofol for anesthetic induction: a meta-analysis. *Anesth Analg* 2000; 91: 213–19.

27 Burney R, Prabhu M, Greenfield M, Shanks A, O'Reilly M. Comparison of spinal vs general anaesthesia via laryngeal mask airway in inguinal hernia repair. *Archiv Surgery* 2004; 139: 183–7.

28 Korhonen A, Valanne J, Jokela R, Ravaska P, Korttila K. A comparison of selective spinal anesthesia with hyperbaric bupivocaine and general anesthesia with desflurane for outpatient knee arthroscopy. *Anesth Analg* 2004; 99: 1668–73.

29 Liu S. Effects of bispectral index monitoring on ambulatory anesthesia: a meta-analysis and a cost analysis. *Anesthesiology* 2004; 101: 311–15.

30 Chung F, Ritchie E, Su J. Postoperative pain in ambulatory surgery. *Anesth Analg* 1997; 85: 808–16.

31 McGrath B, Elgendy H, Chung F, Kamming D, Curti B, King S. Thirty percent of patients have moderate to severe pain 24 hr after ambulatory sugery: a survey of 5,703 patients. *Can J Anesth* 2004; 51; 886–91.

32 Fortier J, Chung F, Su J. Unanticipated admission after ambulatory surgery – a prospective study. *Can J Anesth* 2004; 51: 886–91.

33 Moiniche S, Kehlet H, Dahl J. A qualitative and quantitative systematic review of preemptive analgesia for postoperative pain relief. *Anesthesiology* 2002; 96: 725–41.

34 McQuay H, Moore RA. Postoperative analgesia and vomiting: with special reference to day case surgery: a systematic review. *Health Technol Assess* 1998; 2(12).

35 Moiniche S, Mikkelsen S, Wetterslev J, Dahl J. A qualitative systematic review of incisional local anaesthesia for postoperative pain relief after abdominal operations. *Br J Anaesth* 1998; 81: 377–83.

36 Moiniche S, Mikkelsen S, Wetterslev J, Dahl J. A systematic review of intra-articular local anesthesia for postoperative pain relief after arthroscopic knee surgery. *Reg Anesth Pain Med* 1999; 24: 430–7.

37 Rosseland L. No evidence for analgesic effect of intra-articular morphine after knee arthroscopy: a qualitative systematic review. *Reg Anesth Pain Med* 2005; 30: 83–98.

38 Ding Y, White P. Post-herniorrhaphy pain in outpatients after pre-incision ilioinguinal–hypogastric nerve block during monitored anaesthetia care. *Can J Anesth* 1995; 42: 12–15.

39 Klein S, Pietrobon R, Nielsen K, Steele S, Warner D, Moylan J et al. Paravertebral somatic nerve block compared with peripheral nerve blocks for outpatient inguinal herniorrhaphy. *Reg Anesth Pain Med* 2002; 27: 476–80.

40 Mulroy M, Larkin K, Batra M. Hodgson P, Owens B. Femoral nerve block with 0.25% or 0.5% bupivocaine improves postoperative analgesia following outpatient arthroscopic anterior cruciate ligament repair. *Reg Anesth Pain Med* 2001; 26: 24–9.

41 Wu C, Berenholtz S, Pronovost P, Fleisher L. Systematic review and analysis of postdischarge symptoms after outpatient surgery. *Anesthesiology* 2002; 96: 994–1003.

42 Gupta A, Wu C, Elkassabany N, Krug C, Parker S, Fleisher L. Does the routine prophylactic use of antiemetics affect the incidence of postdischarge nausea and vomiting following ambulatory surgery? A systematic review of randomized controlled trials. *Anesthesiology* 2003; 99: 488–95.

43 Tramer M. A rational approach to the control of postoperative nausea and vomiting: evidence from systematic reviews (Part I and II). *Acta Anaesthesiol Scand* 2001; 45: 4–19.

44 Aldrete J. The post-anesthesia recovery score revisited. *J Clin Anesth* 1995; 7: 89–91.

45 Chung F, Chen V, Ong D. A post-anesthetic discharge scoring system for home readiness after ambulatory surgery. *J Clin Anesth* 1995; 7: 500–6.

46 Apfelbaum J, Walawander C, Grasela T, Wise P, McLeskey C et al. Eliminating intensive postoperative care in same-day surgery patients using short-acting anesthetics. *Anesthesiology* 2002; 97: 66–74.

47 Song D, Chung F, Ronayne M, Ward B, Yogendran S, Sibbick C. Fast-tracking (by-passing the PACU) does not reduce nursing workload after ambulatory surgery. *Br J Anaesth* 2004; 93: 768–74.

48 Pavlin J, Rapp E, Polissar N, Malmgren J, Koerschgen M, Keyes H. Factors affecting discharge time in adult outpatients. *Anesth Analg* 1998; 87: 816–26.

49 Korttila K. Recovery from outpatient anaesthesia, factors affecting outcome. *Anaesthesia* 1995; 50(Suppl): 22–8.

18

Obstetrical anaesthesia

Stephen Halpern

University of Toronto, Obstetrical Anaesthesia, Sunnybrook and Women's College Health Sciences Centre, Toronto, ON, Canada

Neuraxial analgesia (epidural, and combined spinal–epidural techniques) effectively relieves labour pain. Whether or not these modalities affect progress of labour has been controversial. This chapter discusses the effect of neuraxial analgesia on caesarean section rates, instrumental delivery rates and the duration of labour. There is strong, homogeneous evidence to show that neuraxial analgesia does not increase the caesarean section rate. There is also strong, consistent evidence to show that there is an increase in the incidence of instrumental vaginal delivery in patients who have neuraxial analgesia. Further, there appears to be a dose–response relationship – parturients exposed to high concentrations of local anaesthetic are at higher risk for instrumental vaginal delivery than those exposed to low concentrations. While there appears to be a prolongation of the second stage of labour with neuraxial analgesia, these results are inconsistent and dependent on the obstetric protocol at a particular institution. In conclusion, neuraxial analgesia does not cause an increased incidence of caesarean section but may increase the incidence of instrumental vaginal delivery. This effect can be reduced by reducing the concentration of local anaesthetic. The effect on the length of first and second stage of labour is variable but is likely clinically unimportant.

Introduction

Since the introduction of anaesthesia to obstetric practice by James Young Simpson in 1847, there have been controversies concerning its use. In addition to the larger issue of the use of any medical intervention during normal childbirth, the lay public and medical community continue to struggle with the balance between the benefits and risks of analgesia and anaesthesia to the mother and fetus during labour and delivery.

During the past 20 years, there has been a major improvement in the quality of evidence that has become available to answer questions pertaining to obstetrical

Key words: Analgesia, obstetric, caesarean section, instrumental vaginal delivery, analgesia, epidural.

analgesia and anaesthesia. Practices and attitudes that were previously defended dogmatically or emotionally have been tested in well-conducted randomised controlled trials (RCTs). Of interest, some of the early work on physiological animal models in the early 1960s may prove not to be applicable to humans.

In this chapter, I will discuss the effect of neuraxial labour analgesia on the progress of labour. This question has been addressed by well-designed RCTs, high-quality trials of other designs, meta-analyses and systematic reviews.

Neuraxial analgesia (epidural, and combined spinal–epidural techniques) effectively relieves labour pain and is often chosen by parturients because of the known efficacy of the technique. However, some authors express concern about potential adverse effects of neuraxial analgesia on the progress of labour. In particular, there is concern that it may lead to an increase in the incidence of caesarean section and instrumental delivery. These questions have been addressed by numerous clinical trials and synthesised in meta-analyses and systematic reviews [1,2]. Whether or not neuraxial analgesia prolongs labour has also been discussed.

Caesarean section

Search strategy

The initial search has been reported elsewhere [1] and has been updated for this review. Of note, because of ethical considerations, there were no clinical trials that compared neuraxial analgesia to a placebo. Therefore, RCTs comparing neuraxial analgesia to parenteral opioid analgesia were sought in MEDLINE (1966 until 11 August 2005), and EMBASE (1980 until 11 August 2005) using text terms (with alternate spellings, synonyms and appropriate wild card characters) analgesia, obstetrical; analgesia, epidural; caesarean delivery; analgesics, opioid. Hand searches were performed on the abstracts from major anaesthesia meetings, and the *International Journal of Obstetric Anesthesia*. Reference lists from major textbooks, review articles and retrieved articles were searched. There was no language restriction.

Quality

Although in most cases, RCTs are the strongest study design in the sense that, when properly performed, they result in the least amount of bias, there are a number of barriers to consider when studying labour analgesia. First, it is not possible to blind the patients or the caregivers involved in these studies. Since there is some subjectivity in deciding the need for and timing of caesarean or instrumental vaginal delivery for dystocia (the main outcomes of most of the studies), knowledge of patient treatment group by the caregivers could introduce bias. A second concern is that women with a definite desire for or against epidural analgesia do not enrol in these trials. A large proportion of women make this decision before the onset of labour, eliminating many parturients from study participation. This may reduce the applicability of the results to the general obstetrical population. Finally, patients may not follow their group assignment. If patients are randomised too early, they may not require any analgesia and may refuse group assignment. Assigning the group when the patient requests analgesia can reduce this problem. Later, if the analgesia is inadequate, the patient may choose to "cross over" and receive the alternate treatment. Usually this occurs when the patient has not been assigned to the epidural group. If enough patients change groups, the randomisation may be threatened.

Retrieved studies

In spite of these difficulties, random allocation to epidural versus parenteral opioid labour analgesia was reported in 15 studies enrolling 4624 healthy patients [3–17]. In addition, 1223 patients in a single study were randomised to receive either parenteral meperidine or subarachnoid analgesia followed by a continuous epidural infusion (combined spinal–epidural, CSE) [18]. Finally, there were 854 pre-eclamptic patients in two studies [19,20]. Intention-to-treat data on one of the studies [13] has become available in a review article [21].

The study characteristics are shown in Table 18.1. All of the studies were rated for quality using the Jadad Scale [22]. Since none of the studies could be blinded, the maximum score was 3. Most of the patients were enrolled in high-quality studies. Appropriate blinding of allocation was explicitly described in seven of the studies of normal patients, and both studies that involved hypertensive patients. Nulliparous and multiparous as well as hypertensive patients are represented. In addition, there is extensive geographical diversity.

The obstetric and anaesthetic protocols are shown in Table 18.2. There was a wide diversity in the descriptions of the conduct of labour among the studies. Most of the studies used either meperidine or fentanyl for the opioid group. There was wide variation in the concentration of local anaesthetic used among the studies. Further, different methods were used for maintenance of analgesia for both groups. These included both clinician and patient-controlled techniques. It should be noted that, in some studies, there was a large number of patients who were assigned to the parenteral group that received epidural analgesia because of inadequate pain relief.

Results

The incidence of caesarean section is shown in Figure 18.1. In all cases, intent-to-treat data were used. Although there were differences in the populations studied the obstetric protocols and the analgesic protocols, there was very little heterogeneity in the data. When all the data is pooled, the caesarean section rate is 8.8%. The odds ratio (OR) for the difference in caesarean section rates is 1.03 (95% confidence

Table 18.1. Epidural analgesia versus parenteral opioid: study characteristics

Reference and year	Country of origin	Jadad quality score	Population nulliparous: multiparous	Induced labour included	Comments
Healthy parturients					
Robinson* [14]	UK	1	58:0	Unknown	
Robinson* [14]	UK	1	0:35	Unknown	
Philipsen† [11,12]	Denmark	3	104:7	Yes	
Thorp [17]	USA	3	93:0	No	The trial was stopped early for "ethical" reasons
Ramin [13]	USA	2	693:637[a] 484:385[b]	No	Parity and cervical dilatation at request for analgesia were unbalanced between groups. Intent-to-treat data available from Ref. 21
Clark [4]	USA	3[^]	318:0	No	Both intent to treat and protocol compliant data were presented
Muir [9]	Canada	Nct rated	50:0	No	Abstract
Sharma [15]	USA	3	386:329	No	
Nikkola [10]	Finland	2	20:0	Unknown	Primary outcome was the effect of analgesia on the neonate
Bofill [3]	USA	3[^]	100:0	No	The trial was stopped early because of slow recruitment
Gambling [18]	USA	3[^]	650:573	No	CSE** + continuous infusion. Analysed as intent to treat and protocol compliant
Loughnan [8]	UK	3[^]	614:0	Unknown	
Howell [6]	UK	3[^]	369:0	Yes	Primary outcome was back pain
Sharma [16]	USA	3[^]	459:0	No	
Jain [7]	India	3	123:0	No	3 groups Group 1: epidural Group 2: IM meperidine Group 3: IM tramadol
Halpern [5]	Canada	3[^]	242:0	No	Multicentered trial
Hypertensive parturients					
Lucas [20]	USA	3[^]	525:213	Yes	Admitted with the diagnosis of pre-eclampsia. Enrolled when analgesia requested
Head [19]	USA	3[^]	75:116	Yes	Admitted with the diagnosis of severe pre-eclampsia but no contraindications to epidural analgesia

* This manuscript contained data for nulliparous and multiparous patients which were analysed separately. Therefore they are presented as two studies; ** CSE: combined spinal epidural; † Data from this cohort of patients was presented in two manuscripts; [a] Total number of enrolled patients; used to calculate the caesarean delivery incidence by intent-to-treat; [b] Number of protocol-compliant patients; used for all other maternal and neonatal outcomes in this study (21); [^] blinded allocation.

Table 18.2. Epidural analgesia versus parenteral opioid: analgesic protocol

Study	Explicit protocol for conduct of labour	Criteria for operative intervention	Analgesic agents parenteral analgesia	Analgesic protocol epidural	Crossover rate
Normal parturients					
Robinson [14] (both studies)	No	No	Meperidine IM Nitrous oxide Methoxyflurane	Bupivacaine 0.5% Clinician bolus	None reported
Philipsen [11]	No	No	Meperidine IM Nitrous oxide	Lidocaine test dose Bupivacaine 0.375% clinician bolus Nitrous oxide	None reported
Thorp [17]	Yes	No	Meperidine IV	0.25% bupivacaine bolus 0.125% bupivacaine maintenance infusion	1/48 patients assigned to the epidural group did not receive an epidural 1/45 patients assigned to the parenteral opioid group also received an epidural
Ramin [13]	Yes	Criteria for low forceps, not for C/S	Meperidine IV	Bupivacaine 0.25% bolus, bupivacaine, 0.125% maintenance infusion	103/666 in the parenteral opioid group also received an epidural 232/664 randomised to receive an epidural received an epidural
Muir [9]	"Strict definitions" for diagnosis and management of labour	No	Meperidine PCA	Bupivacaine 0.125% PCEA	no medication 11/22 in the parenteral opioid group also received an epidural
Clark 1997	"Active management of labour"	"Obstetrical reasons"	Meperidine IV	Lidocaine test dose, bupivacaine 0.25% bolus Bupivacaine 0.125% maintenance infusion	84/162 in the parenteral opioid group also received an epidural 5/156 in the epidural group received IV opioids (no epidural). 4 received no medication

(Continued)

Table 18.2. (Continued)

Study	Explicit protocol for conduct of labour	Criteria for operative intervention	Analgesic agents parenteral analgesia	Analgesic protocol epidural	Crossover rate
Nikkola [10]	No	No	PCA fentanyl	Bupivacaine 0.5% clinician bolus	4/10 in the parenteral opioid group also received an epidural
Sharma 1997 [15]	Yes	Yes	PCA meperidine	Bupivacaine 0.25% bolus Bupivacaine 0.125% maintenance infusion	Of 358 women assigned to the meperidine group, 93 did not receive any medication and 5 received an epidural after receiving meperidine Of 357 women assigned to the epidural group, 115 received no medication and 8 received only parenteral opioids
Bofill [3]	Yes	Yes	Butorphanol IV	Bupivacaine 0.25% bolus Bupivacaine 0.125% maintenance infusion	2/49 in the epidural group received no medication. 12/51 in the parenteral opioid group received opioid plus an epidural
Loughnan [8]	Yes	Yes	Meperidine IM	Bupivacaine 0.25% bolus Bupivacaine 0.125% maintenance clinician bolus	Of the 304 women who were randomised to epidural, 244 received an epidural, 13 received meperidine and an epidural, 47 received either meperidine or Entonox Of the 310 women randomised to meperidine, 132 received meperidine, 89 received an epidural, 86 received an epidural and meperidine, and 3 received Entonox
Howell [6]	No	No	Meperidine IM	Bupivacaine 0.25% clinician bolus	61 of 184 women in the epidural group did not receive an epidural 52 of 185 women in the non-epidural group received an epidural
Sharma [16]	Written protocol	Written protocol	PCA Meperidine	Bupivacaine 0.25% bolus bupivacaine 0.06%	In the IV meperidine group 207/233 followed the protocol. Of the 26 violations, 14 received an

Study			Intervention	Maintenance	Comments
				maintenance PCEA	epidural. In the epidural group 214/226 followed the protocol
Jain [7]	No	No	2 groups: Meperidine IM Tramadol IM PCA fentanyl	Bupivacaine 0.15% bolus Bupivacaine 0.10% maintenance clinician bolus	None were allowed
Halpern [5]	Yes	Yes	PCA fentanyl	Bupivacaine 0.08% PCEA	51 of 118 women in the IV PCA group received an epidural. 3/124 in the PCEA group received a non-protocol epidural because of failure of analgesia
Combined spinal–epidural technique (normal parturients)					
Gambling [18]	Yes	Yes	Meperidine IV	CSE sufentanil initiation Bupivacaine 0.25% bolus Bupivacaine 0.125% maintenance infusion	In the IV meperidine group 352/607 followed the protocol. Of the 255 that did not, 102 received a CSE and 42 declined analgesia. In the CSE group, 400 of 616 followed the protocol. Of the 216 that did not, 82 received meperidine and 52 declined analgesia
Pre-eclampsia					
Lucas [20]	? Written protocol for pre-eclampsia management	No	Meperidine PCA	bupivacaine 0.25% Maintenance bupivacaine 0.125% infusion	Of the 366 women in the meperidine group, 340 followed the protocol. Of the 26 that did not, none received an epidural. Of the 372 women assigned to the epidural group, 51 did not follow the protocol. Of these none received meperidine but 7 did not receive any analgesia
Head [19]	No	No	Meperidine IV	Bupivacaine 0.25% bolus bupivacaine 0.125% with $2\,\mu g\,ml^{-1}$ infusion	One patient in the meperidine group received an epidural

CSE: combined spinal–epidural; PCA: patient controlled analgesia; IV: intravenous; IM: Intramuscular; PCEA: patient controlled epidural analgesia.

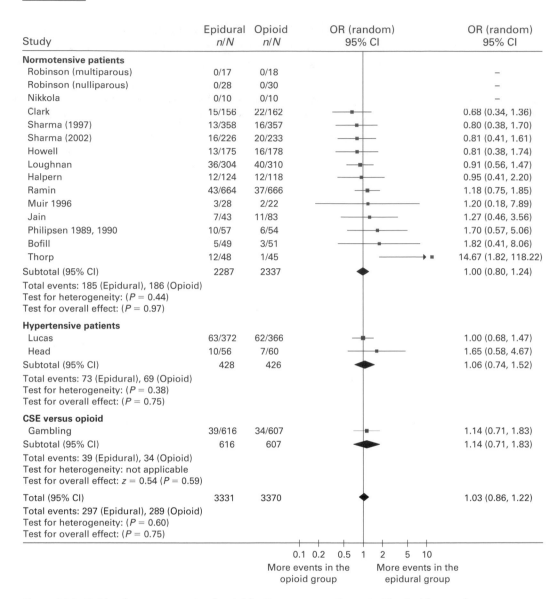

Study	Epidural n/N	Opioid n/N	OR (random) 95% CI	OR (random) 95% CI
Normotensive patients				
Robinson (multiparous)	0/17	0/18		–
Robinson (nulliparous)	0/28	0/30		–
Nikkola	0/10	0/10		–
Clark	15/156	22/162		0.68 (0.34, 1.36)
Sharma (1997)	13/358	16/357		0.80 (0.38, 1.70)
Sharma (2002)	16/226	20/233		0.81 (0.41, 1.61)
Howell	13/175	16/178		0.81 (0.38, 1.74)
Loughnan	36/304	40/310		0.91 (0.56, 1.47)
Halpern	12/124	12/118		0.95 (0.41, 2.20)
Ramin	43/664	37/666		1.18 (0.75, 1.85)
Muir 1996	3/28	2/22		1.20 (0.18, 7.89)
Jain	7/43	11/83		1.27 (0.46, 3.56)
Philipsen 1989, 1990	10/57	6/54		1.70 (0.57, 5.06)
Bofill	5/49	3/51		1.82 (0.41, 8.06)
Thorp	12/48	1/45		14.67 (1.82, 118.22)
Subtotal (95% CI)	2287	2337		1.00 (0.80, 1.24)
Total events: 185 (Epidural), 186 (Opioid)				
Test for heterogeneity: ($P = 0.44$)				
Test for overall effect: ($P = 0.97$)				
Hypertensive patients				
Lucas	63/372	62/366		1.00 (0.68, 1.47)
Head	10/56	7/60		1.65 (0.58, 4.67)
Subtotal (95% CI)	428	426		1.06 (0.74, 1.52)
Total events: 73 (Epidural), 69 (Opioid)				
Test for heterogeneity: ($P = 0.38$)				
Test for overall effect: ($P = 0.75$)				
CSE versus opioid				
Gambling	39/616	34/607		1.14 (0.71, 1.83)
Subtotal (95% CI)	616	607		1.14 (0.71, 1.83)
Total events: 39 (Epidural), 34 (Opioid)				
Test for heterogeneity: not applicable				
Test for overall effect: $z = 0.54$ ($P = 0.59$)				
Total (95% CI)	3331	3370		1.03 (0.86, 1.22)
Total events: 297 (Epidural), 289 (Opioid)				
Test for heterogeneity: ($P = 0.60$)				
Test for overall effect: ($P = 0.75$)				

0.1 0.2   0.5   1   2   5   10

More events in the   More events in the
opioid group   epidural group

Figure 18.1 Epidural versus parenteral opioids: Caesarean section rate. The incidence of caesarean section is shown for the epidural and opioid group for all studies. The OR and 95% CI are illustrated with a Forest Plot on a logarithmic scale. The squares are proportional to the effect sizes in the meta-analysis. (Modified with permission Blackwells Publishing from Figure 2.1 in Leighton BL, Halpern SH. Epidural analgesia and the progress of labor. In: Halpern SH, Douglas MJ (eds). *Evidence Based Obstetric Anesthesia*. Blackwell publishing, 2005, pp. 10–22.)

interval (CI): 0.86–1.22). The absolute risk difference is 0.3% (95% CI: −1–2%). The results are similar in all subgroups.

There have been two additional meta-analyses published on this topic [23,24]. Lui et al. studied the effect of low concentration epidural analgesia on the incidence of caesarean section [23]. They excluded all studies that used 0.375% or higher concentrations of bupivacaine [11,12,14]. They also excluded studies that did not report intent-to-treat data [13]. However, they included a large randomised trial that compared epidural analgesia to "continuous midwifery support" control rather than "opioid analgesia". In this study, the control group was encouraged to ambulate and to use parenteral pethidine or inhaled nitrous oxide for analgesia. Patients also received 1:1 nurse to patient care throughout labour. In total 2962 patients were included in this meta-analysis. Although the population of studies was different from the analysis above, the incidence of caesarean section was similar between groups (OR: 1.03; 95% CI: 0.71–1.48). Sharma et al. [24] studied data from their own institution using individual patient data. The patients were all nulliparous and were reported in previous studies [13,15,16,18,20]. Pooled analysis of patients in these studies showed that the incidence of caesarean section was very similar between groups (OR: 1.04; 95% CI: 0.81–1.34). Because this group of patients constitutes a large proportion of patients in the primary meta-analysis, some authors have questioned the generalisability to other centres. When the patients from Texas Southwest Medical Center were excluded, there were 10 studies comprised of about 2000 patients. There was still no significant difference in the incidence of caesarean section (OR: 1.09; 95% CI: 0.79–1.51). There was also no significant heterogeneity.

The greatest threat to validity of the RCTs was crossover from the opioid group to the epidural group. However, there was a subgroup of seven studies, comprised of about 2300 patients in which the crossover rate was <10% [7,11,12,16,17,19,20]. In this subgroup, there was no significant difference in the caesarean section rate. The OR was 1.15 (95% CI: 0.76–1.17; $P = 0.48$).

The conclusion that epidural analgesia does not cause an increased incidence of caesarean section is reinforced by other observations. A rapid change in availability of epidural analgesia in an institution may represent a special type of "historical control". Unlike other investigations of this type, the whole population is studied, rather than an unspecified or selected sample. This type of study may be appropriate in settings in which it is difficult to recruit to randomised trials. Further, it eliminates the "cross-over" problem because epidural analgesia was simply not an option for a portion of the study period. In order to be valid, the following criteria should be fulfilled: 1) There is a stable population. For example, the hospital continues to attract the same types of patients. 2) Treatments are stable. In this case, the criteria for obstetric intervention should not change. 3) There is stable evaluation. 4) There is stable preference. There should be no "bias" introduced by advertisement to consumers or publicised scientific reports. 5) The effect of the intervention on outcome does not change. In this case, there should be no required "learning curve". Finally, the transition should be rapid (<2 years) [25]. Segal et al. reviewed and pooled the results of nine studies, comprised of about 39 000 patients, in which there was a rapid change in the availability of epidural analgesia to a population of obstetric patients [26]. There was no change in the incidence of caesarean section between the two-study periods.

Instrumental vaginal delivery

Results from RCTs comparing neuraxial analgesia to opioid

All of the studies that reported the incidence of caesarean section also reported the incidence of instrumental vaginal deliveries. However, intent-to-treat data was not available from one of the studies and therefore those patients who were "protocol compliant" were reported [13]. There were a total of 6199 patients in the 17 studies.

There was a statistically significant increase in the instrumental delivery rate in patients who received epidural analgesia compared to those that did not (Figure 18.2). The OR was 1.92 (95% CI: 1.52–2.42). The absolute risk 16% in the epidural group and 10% in the opioid group (risk difference: 6%; 95% CI: 4–9%, $P < 0.00001$). However, there was significant heterogeneity in the data, probably because of differences in obstetric practices.

From these data it is not possible to tell whether epidural analgesia caused an excess of instrumental vaginal delivery because of a biological effect (change in muscle tone, reduction in the urge to "push" in second stage) or because of changes in physician behaviour. For example, it should be noted in one study, the authors explicitly stated that elective forceps were more common in the epidural group for the purpose of resident training [3].

In order to determine whether epidural analgesia causes an increase in forceps delivery for biological reasons the studies must, at least potentially, be blinded. As mentioned above, it is not possible to blind a "neuraxial versus no neuraxial" study. However, it is possible to study different concentrations of local anaesthetic in a blinded fashion. If a dose–response relationship is present, there is evidence for causation.

Instrumental vaginal delivery: the effect of local anaesthetic concentration

Search strategy

In order to do this, RCTs that compared a "low concentration" to a "high concentration" of local anaesthetic were sought. RCTs were sought in MEDLINE (1966

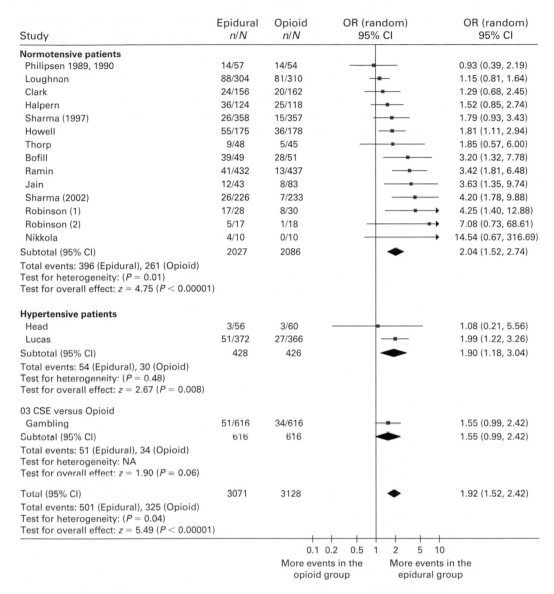

Study	Epidural n/N	Opioid n/N	OR (random) 95% CI	OR (random) 95% CI
Normotensive patients				
Philipsen 1989, 1990	14/57	14/54		0.93 (0.39, 2.19)
Loughnan	88/304	81/310		1.15 (0.81, 1.64)
Clark	24/156	20/162		1.29 (0.68, 2.45)
Halpern	36/124	25/118		1.52 (0.85, 2.74)
Sharma (1997)	26/358	15/357		1.79 (0.93, 3.43)
Howell	55/175	36/178		1.81 (1.11, 2.94)
Thorp	9/48	5/45		1.85 (0.57, 6.00)
Bofill	39/49	28/51		3.20 (1.32, 7.78)
Ramin	41/432	13/437		3.42 (1.81, 6.48)
Jain	12/43	8/83		3.63 (1.35, 9.74)
Sharma (2002)	26/226	7/233		4.20 (1.78, 9.88)
Robinson (1)	17/28	8/30		4.25 (1.40, 12.88)
Robinson (2)	5/17	1/18		7.08 (0.73, 68.61)
Nikkola	4/10	0/10		14.54 (0.67, 316.69)
Subtotal (95% CI)	2027	2086		2.04 (1.52, 2.74)

Total events: 396 (Epidural), 261 (Opioid)
Test for heterogeneity: ($P = 0.01$)
Test for overall effect: $z = 4.75$ ($P < 0.00001$)

Hypertensive patients				
Head	3/56	3/60		1.08 (0.21, 5.56)
Lucas	51/372	27/366		1.99 (1.22, 3.26)
Subtotal (95% CI)	428	426		1.90 (1.18, 3.04)

Total events: 54 (Epidural), 30 (Opioid)
Test for heterogeneity: ($P = 0.48$)
Test for overall effect: $z = 2.67$ ($P = 0.008$)

03 CSE versus Opioid				
Gambling	51/616	34/616		1.55 (0.99, 2.42)
Subtotal (95% CI)	616	616		1.55 (0.99, 2.42)

Total events: 51 (Epidural), 34 (Opioid)
Test for heterogeneity: NA
Test for overall effect: $z = 1.90$ ($P = 0.06$)

Total (95% CI)	3071	3128		1.92 (1.52, 2.42)

Total events: 501 (Epidural), 325 (Opioid)
Test for heterogeneity: ($P = 0.04$)
Test for overall effect: $z = 5.49$ ($P < 0.00001$)

```
        0.1  0.2    0.5   1    2    5   10
      More events in the      More events in the
         opioid group           epidural group
```

Figure 18.2 Epidural versus parenteral opioids: Instrumental vaginal delivery. The incidence of instrumental vaginal delivery is shown for the epidural and opioid group for all studies. The OR and 95% CI are illustrated with a Forest Plot on a logarithmic scale. The squares are proportional to the effect sizes in the meta-analysis. (Modified with permission Blackwells Publishing from Figure 2.2 in Leighton BL, Halpern SH. Epidural analgesia and the progress of labor. In: Halpern SH, Douglas MJ (eds). *Evidence Based Obstetric Anesthesia*. Blackwell publishing, 2005, pp. 10–20.)

until 30 September 2004), and EMBASE (1980 until 30 September 2004) using text terms (with alternate spellings, synonyms and appropriate wild card characters) epidural analgesia, labour analgesia, local anaesthetic concentration, forceps delivery, caesarean section. We included all RCTs that compared low concentration to a higher concentration of local anaesthetic for labour analgesia in the induction dose, maintenance or both. In order to avoid the debate concerning equipotent concentrations of local anaesthetic, only studies that compared the same local anaesthetic with (or without) the same additives were included. There was no language restriction.

Quality

In total 17 studies in 15 manuscripts, comprised of about 2200 patients, that met the inclusion criteria [27–41]. The study characteristics are shown in Table 18.3. All but four of the study had a score of 3 or more on the Jadad scale and seven explicitly mentioned blinding of allocation. Ropivacaine was used in five of the studies, bupivacaine was used in the remainder. Both nulliparous and mixed populations are represented but all patients were at term and at "low risk". Patient-controlled epidural analgesia (PCEA) was used in four studies, continuous infusion in 10 and clinician topups in three. In three of the studies, different concentrations of local anaesthetic were combined to form either the low concentration or high concentration group [30,35,37] and in one, three different regimens of the same concentration were combined for each concentration [27].

Results

These studies show a statistically significant increase in the rate of instrumental vaginal delivery in the high concentration group (OR: 1.45; 95% CI: 1.19–1.76, $P = 0.0002$). There was little heterogeneity ($P = 0.51$) among the studies in spite of significant clinical heterogeneity in the type of local anaesthetic, concentration of local anaesthetic, type of maintenance, geographical, and temporal differences. It should be noted that the incidence of caesarean section was similar between groups (OR: 0.89; 95% CI: 0.69–1.15, $P = 0.38$). In addition, there was no significant difference in maternal analgesia as measured by pain scores, clinician workload as measured by the number of unscheduled clinician topups, or neonatal outcomes [42].

These results also agree with other studies. Angle et al. reported a meta-analysis of four studies that compared patients who received bupivacaine at 0.125% or higher, compared to <0.125% [43]. This analysis was comprised of different studies because the use of different additives was not an exclusion criterion. This analysis was also different because studies were excluded if bupivacaine concentrations of >0.125% were used at any time in the low concentration group. There were four

Table 18.3. Low concentration versus high concentration local anaesthetics: study characteristics

Study	Quality score	Population	Low concentration		High concentration		Mode of maintenance and comments
			N	Local anaesthetic and concentration	N	Local anaesthetic and concentration	
Boselli [28]	5*	Mixed	63	Ropivacaine 0.1%	67	Ropivacaine 0.15%	PCEA
Brockway [29]	3	Mixed	29	Bupivacaine 0.0625%	25	Bupivacaine 0.08%	Continuous infusion
Cohen [30]	5	Mixed	15	Bupivacaire 0.625%	15	Bupivacaine 0.125%	Continuous infusion 4 group study (see study below) with and without lidocaine test dose
Cohen [30]	5	Mixed	15	Bupivacaine 0.625%	15	Bupivacaine 0.125%	Continuous infusion
Bernard [27]	4	Nulliparous induced	75	Ropivacaine 0.1%	75	Ropivacaine 0.2%	6 (N = 25) groups 3 PCEA regimens per concentration
Elliott [31]	4*	Nulliparous	27	Bupivacaire 0.125%	24	Eupivacaine 0.25%	Continuous infusion
Harms [35]	4*	Mixed	44	Bupivacaine 0.0625% and 0.125%	23	Eupivacaine 0.25%	Continuous infusion 2 low dose groups combined
Gogarten [33]	3*	Mixed	103	Ropivacaine 0.125%	100	Ropivacaine 0.175%	PCEA
Merson [36]	5*	Nulliparous	16	Bupivacaine 0.125%	17	Bupivacaine 0.25%	Continuous infusion 4 group study – 2 different concentrations of bupivacaine and 2 different concentrations of ropivacaine (see below)
Merson [36]			16	Ropivacaine 0.125%	19	Ropivacaine 0.25%	Continuous infusion
Nageotte [37]	2	Nulliparous	505	Bupivacaine 0.0625%	256	Bupivacaine 0.25%	Continuous infusion 2 low dose groups combined
Noble [38]	4	Nulliparous	35	Bupivacaine 0.0625%	21	Bupivacaine 0.125%	Continuous infusion
Stoddart [40]	3	Nulliparous	38	Bupivacaine 0.0625%	40	Bupivacaine 0.125%	Continuous infusion
Sia [39]	4*	Nulliparous	25	Ropivacaine 0.125%	25	Ropivacaine 0.2%	PCEA
Thorburn [41]	2	Mixed	183	Bupivacaine 0.25%	161	Bupivacaine 0.5%	Clinician topups
Ewen [32]	1	Mixed	25	Bupivacaine 0.08%	28	Bupivacaine 0.25%	Continuous infusion
Handley [34]	2	Mixed	20	Bupivacaine 0.125%	40	Bupivacaine 0.1875%	2 high dose groups combined clinician topups some patients eliminated from primary outcome if analgesia was not achieved with assigned solutions

* Blinded allocation, PCEA: patient controlled epidural analgesia.

studies that met these criteria [37,44–46] comprised of about 2000 patients. Only one of the studies in this meta-analysis was included in the analysis above [37]. In this meta-analysis there were more instrumental deliveries in the high concentration group compared to the low concentration group (OR: 1.31; 95% CI: 0.93–1.83, $P = 0.10$), but this was not statistically significant. In a third analysis, Reynolds et al. [47] reported the combined results of five studies [48–52] over a 3 year period in the same institution. Although there was no difference in instrumental vaginal delivery, patients were less likely to experience a spontaneous vaginal delivery if they were in the high concentration group. Logistic regression showed that there was a statistically significant incidence of obstetrical intervention as the dose (in milligrams) of local anaesthetic increased.

There was no change in the incidence of instrumental vaginal delivery in centres that rapidly acquired or lost an epidural service [26].

Duration of labour

The duration of first and second stage of labour has been compared in RCTs in patients who received neuraxial analgesia and opioid analgesia controls. These outcomes are not precise because there are no agreed criteria for the time intervals between measurements of cervical dilatation during labour. Further, the time that labour begins is sometimes difficult to determine. However nine studies (in eight manuscripts), comprised of about 2000 patients report a comparison of the duration of the first stage of labour [3,4,6–8,14,16,17]. In these studies, the mean duration of first stage of labour was between 274 and 676 min. The weighted mean difference between the groups was 25 min (95% CI: -5–54 min; $P = 0.09$). There was marked heterogeneity in the results, primarily because of the inclusion of both nulliparous and multiparous patients. The heterogeneity also reflected the difficulty in determining the beginning and end of the first stage of labour.

There were 11 studies (in 10 manuscripts), comprised of about 2400 patients, that reported the difference in duration of second stage of labour [3–8,11,14,16,17]. The mean duration was between 18 and 121 min. Of note, the study that reported a mean duration of 18 min consisted only of multiparous patients [14]. The weighted mean difference in duration of second stage was 17 min (95% CI: 10–23 min; $P = 0.003$). There was significant heterogeneity among the studies. This was likely due to the reasons outlined above concerning first stage of labour. An additional factor may have been a change in obstetric practice that allowed second stage of labour to last longer than 1 h. This change took place in many institutions between 1985 and 1995.

There were 6 studies, comprised of about 660 patients, that compared the duration of the first stage of labour in parturients who received low or high concentration of local anaesthetics [28,29,31–33,40]. There was no difference between groups (weighted mean difference 14.4 min; 95% CI: -39–10 min; $P = 0.26$). Similarly, there was no difference in duration of second stage in the 4 studies that reported this outcome (weighted mean difference 5 min; 95% CI: -18–8 min; $P = 0.44$) [28,31,33,40].

Practice points

- Neuraxial analgesia is the most effective means of alleviating labour pain.
- Whether or not neuraxial analgesia is detrimental to the progress of labour has been controversial.
- Recent evidence shows that neuraxial analgesia does not increase the incidence of caesarean sections.
- The incidence of instrumental vaginal delivery may be increased by neuraxial analgesia. This appears to be a dose related phenomenon and may be decreased by decreasing the concentration of local anaesthetic.
- Currently, it is recommended that the lowest concentration of local anaesthetic be used to achieve analgesia.

Research agenda

Current research is directed at:

- Determining the appropriate dose of local anaesthetic.
- Determining the role for adjuvants such as opioids
- Determining the role of spinal opioids for initiation of analgesia.

Conclusions

Over the past 25 years, the effects of neuraxial analgesia on the progress of labour have become better defined. There is clear evidence that there is no effect on the incidence of caesarean section. This has been established by examining numerous RCTs as well as well-designed historical cohort studies. Further, in studies that compared low concentration to high concentration local anaesthetics, there was no difference in the caesarean section rate.

Conversely, neuraxial analgesia may cause an increase in the incidence of instrumental vaginal delivery. This is particularly true if high concentrations of local anaesthetics are used. Neuraxial analgesia does not prolong the first stage of labour. The second stage of labour may be prolonged by approximately 17 min, although this difference is unlikely to be clinically significant.

When deciding which type of analgesia to offer a parturient, the benefits and risks must be assessed. Neuraxial analgesia provides the most complete analgesia when compared to any other mode of treatment. Using the lowest concentration of local anaesthetic compatible with patient comfort can reduce its impact on progress of labour.

REFERENCES

1 Halpern SH, Leighton BL, Ohlsson A, Barrett JF, Rice A. Effect of epidural vs parenteral opioid analgesia on the progress of labor: a meta-analysis. *JAMA* 1998; 280: 2105–10.

2 Lieberman E. Epidemiology of epidural analgesia and cesarean delivery. *Clin Obstet Gynecol* 2004; 47: 317–31.

3 Bofill JA, Vincent RD, Ross EL. Nulliparous active labor, epidural analgesia, and cesarean delivery for dystocia. *Am J Obstet Gynecol* 1997; 177: 1465–70.

4 Clark A, Carr D, Loyd G, Cook V, Spinnato J. The influence of epidural analgesia on cesarean delivery rates: a randomized, prospective clinical trial. *Am J Obstet Gynecol* 1998; 179: 1527–33.

5 Halpern SH, Muir H, Breen TW et al. A multicenter randomized controlled trial comparing patient-controlled epidural with intravenous analgesia for pain relief in labor. *Anesth Analg* 2004; 99: 1532–8.

6 Howell C, Kidd C, Roberts W et al. A randomized controlled trial of epidural compared with non-epidural analgesia in labour. *Br J Obstet Gynaecol* 2001; 108: 27–33.

7 Jain S, Arya VK, Gopalan S, Jain V. Analgesic efficacy of intramuscular opioids versus epidural analgesia in labor. *Int J Gynaecol Obstet* 2003; 83: 19–27.

8 Loughnan BA, Carli F, Romney M, Dorè CJ, Gordon H. Randomized controlled comparison of epidural bupivacaine versus pethidine for analgesia in labour. *Br J Anaesth* 2000; 84: 715–9.

9 Muir HA, Shukla R, Liston R, Writer D. Randomized trial of labour analgesia: A pilot study to compare patient-controlled intravenous analgesia with patient-controlled epidural analgesia to determine if analgesic method affects delivery outcome. *Can J Anaesth* 1996; 43: A60.

10 Nikkola EM, Ekblad UU, Kero PO, Alihanka JM, Salonen MAO. Intravenous PCA in labor. *Can J Anaesth* 1997; 44: 1248–55.

11 Philipsen T, Jensen N-H. Epidural block or parenteral pethidine as analgesic in labour; a randomized study conerning progress in labour and instrumental deliveries. *Eur J Obstet Gynecol Reproduct Biol* 1989; 30: 27–33.

12 Philipsen T, Jensen N-H. Maternal opinion about analgesia in labour and delivery. A comparison of epidural blockade and intramuscular pethidine. *Eur J Obstet Gynecol Reproduct Biol* 1990; 34: 205–10.

13 Ramin S.M, Gambling DR, Lucas MJ, Sharma SK, Sidawi JE, Leveno KJ. Randomized trial of epidural versus intravenous analgesia during labor. *Obstet Gynecol* 1995; 86: 783–9.

14 Robinson JO, Rosen M, Evans JM, Revill SI, David H, Rees GA. Maternal opinion about analgesia for labour: A controlled trial between epidural block and intramuscular pethidine. *Anaesthesia* 1980; 35: 1173–81.

15 Sharma SK, Sidawi JE, Ramin SM, Lucas MJ, Leveno KJ, Cunningham FG. Cesarean delivery: a randomized trial of epidural versus patient-controlled meperidine analgesia during labor. *Anesthesiology* 1997; 87: 487–94.

16 Sharma SK, Alexander JM, Messick G et al. Cesarean delivery: a randomized trial of epidural analgesia versus intravenous meperidine analgesia during labor in nulliparous women. *Anesthesiology* 2002; 96: 546–51.

17 Thorp JA, Hu DH, Albin RM et al. The effect of intrapartum epidural analgesia on nulliparous labor: a randomized, controlled, prospective trial. *Am J Obstet Gynecol* 1993; 169: 851–8.

18 Gambling DR, Sharma SK, Ramin SM et al. A randomized study of combined spinal–epidural analgesia versus intravenous meperidine during labor: impact on cesarean delivery rate. *Anesthesiology* 1998; 89: 1336–44.

19 Head BB, Owen J, Vincent Jr RD, Shih G, Chestnut DH, Hauth JC. A randomized trial of intrapartum analgesia in women with severe preeclampsia. *Obstet Gynecol* 2002; 99: 452–7.

20 Lucas MJ, Sharma SK, McIntire DD et al. A randomized trial of labor analgesia in women with pregnancy-induced hypertension. *Am J Obstet Gynecol* 2001; 185: 970–5.

21 Sharma SK, Leveno KJ. Update: epidural analgesia does not increase cesarean births. *Curr Anesthesiol Rep* 2000; 2: 18–24.

22 Jadad AR, Moore RA, Carroll D et al. Assessing the quality of reports of randomized clinical trials: is blinding necessary? *Control Clin Trials* 1996; 17: 1–12.

23 Liu EH, Sia AT. Rates of caesarean section and instrumental vaginal delivery in nulliparous women after low concentration epidural infusions or opioid analgesia: systematic review. *BMJ* 2004; 328: 1410–5.

24 Sharma SK, McIntire DD, Wiley J, Leveno KJ. Labor analgesia and cesarean delivery: an individual patient meta-analysis of nulliparous women. *Anesthesiology* 2004; 100: 142–8.

25 Baker SG, Lindeman KS, Kramer BS. The paired availability design for historical controls. *BMC Med Res Methodol* 2001; 1: 9.

26 Segal S, Su M, Gilbert P. The effect of a rapid change in availability of epidural analgesia on the cesarean delivery rate: a meta-analysis. *Am J Obstet Gynecol* 2000; 183: 974–8.

27 Bernard JM, Le RD, Frouin J. Ropivacaine and fentanyl concentrations in patient-controlled epidural analgesia during labor: a volume-range study. *Anesth Analg* 2003; 97: 1800–7.

28 Boselli E, Debon R, Duflo F, Bryssine B, Allaouchiche B, Chassard D. Ropivacaine 0.15% plus sufentanil 0.5 microg/mL and ropivacaine 0.10% plus sufentanil 0.5 microg/mL are equivalent for patient-controlled epidural analgesia during labor. *Anesth Analg* 2003; 96: 1173–7.

29 Brockway MS, Noble D, Tunstall ME. A comparison of 0.08% and 0.0625% bupivacaine for continuous epidural analgesia in labour. *Eur J Anaesthesiol* 1990; 7: 227–34.

30 Cohen SE, Yeh JY, Riley ET, Vogel TM. Walking with labor epidural analgesia: the impact of bupivacaine concentration and a lidocaine-epinephrine test dose. *Anesthesiology* 2000; 92: 387–92.

31 Elliott RD. Continuous infusion epidural analgesia for obstetrics: bupivacaine versus bupivacaine-fentanyl mixture. *Can J Anaesth* 1991; 38: 303–10.

32 Ewen A, McLeod DD, MacLeod DM, Campbell A, Tunstall ME. Continuous infusion epidural analgesia in obstetrics. A comparison of 0.08% and 0.25% bupivacaine. *Anaesthesia* 1986; 41: 143–7.

33 Gogarten W, Van de Velde M, Soetens F et al. A multicentre trial comparing different concentrations of ropivacaine plus sufentanil with bupivacaine plus sufentanil for patient-controlled epidural analgesia in labour. *Eur J Anaesthesiol* 2004; 21: 38–45.

34 Handley G, Perkins G. The addition of pethidine to epidural bupivacaine in labour – effect of changing bupivacaine strength. *Anaesth Intens Care* 1992; 20: 151–5.

35 Harms C, Siegemund M, Marsch SC, Surbek DV, Hosli I, Schneider MC. Initiating extradural analgesia during labour: comparison of three different bupivacaine concentrations used as the loading dose. *Fetal Diag Ther* 1999; 14: 368–74.

36 Merson N. A comparison of motor block between ropivacaine and bupivacaine for continuous labor epidural analgesia. *AANA* 2001; 69: 54–8.

37 Nageotte MP, Larson D, Rumney PJ, Sidhu M, Hollenbach K. Epidural analgesia compared with combined spinal–epidural analgesia during labor in nulliparous women. *New Engl J Med* 1997; 337: 1715–9.

38 Noble HA, Enever GR, Thomas TA. Epidural bupivacaine dilution for labour – A comparison of three concentrations infused with a fixed dose of fentanyl. *Anaesthesia* 1991; 46: 549–52.

39 Sia AT, Ruban P, Chong JL, Wong K. Motor blockade is reduced with ropivacaine 0.125% for parturient-controlled epidural analgesia during labour. *Can J Anaesth* 1999; 46: 1019–23.

40 Stoddart AP, Nicholson KE, Popham PA. Low dose bupivacaine/fentanyl epidural infusions in labour and mode of delivery. *Anaesthesia* 1994; 49: 1087–90.

41 Thorburn J, Moir DD. Extradural analgesia: the influence of volume and concentration of bupivacaine on the mode of delivery, analgesic efficacy and motor block. *Br J Anaesth* 1981; 53: 933–9.

42 Halpern SH, Davallou M, Yee J, Angle PA, Tang S. Is obstetric outcome related to epidural analgesia local anesthetic concentration? *Anesthesiology* 2005; 102: A10.

43 Angle P, Halpern S, Morgan A. Effect of low dose mobile versus high dose epidural techniques on the progress of labor: A meta-analysis. *Anesthesiology* 2002; 96: P52.

44 Collis RE, Davies DWL, Aveling W. Randomised comparison of combined spinal-epidural and standard epidural analgesia in labour. *Lancet* 1995; 345: 1413–6.

45 Comparative obstetric mobile epidural trial (COMET) study group UK. Effect of low-dose mobile versus traditional epidural techniques on mode of delivery: a randomized trial. *Lancet* 2001; 358: 19–23.

46 James KS, McGrady E, Quasim I, Patrick A. Comparison of epidural bolus administration of 0.25% bupivacaine and 0.1% bupivacaine with 0.0002% fentanyl for analgesia during labour. *Br J Anaesth* 1998; 81: 507–10.

47 Reynolds F, Russell R, Porter J, Smeeton N. Does the use of low dose bupivacaine/opioid epidural infusion increase the normal delivery rate? *Int J Obstet Anesth* 2003; 12: 156–63.

48 Russell R, Quinlan J, Reynolds F. Motor block during epidural infusions for nulliparous women in labour. A randomized double blind comparison of 0.125% bupivacaine and 0.0625% bupivacaine with 2.5 μg/mL fentanyl. *Int J Obstet Anesth* 1994; 3(3): 174–5.

49 Russell R, Dundas R, Reynolds F. Long term backache after childbirth: prospective search for causative factors. *BMJ* 1996; 312: 1384–8.

50 Porter JS, Bonello E, Reynolds F. The effect of epidural opioids on maternal oxygenation during labour and delivery. *Anaesthesia* 1996; 51: 899–903.

51 Porter JS, Bonello E, Reynolds F. The influence of epidural administration of fentanyl infusion on gastric emptying in labour. *Anaesthesia* 1997; 52: 1151–6.

52 Porter J, Bonello E, Reynolds F. Effect of epidural fentanyl on neonatal respiration. *Anesthesiology* 1998; 89: 79–85.

19

Anaesthesia for major abdominal and urological surgery

Paul Myles[1] and Kate Leslie[2]

[1]Department of Anaesthesia and Perioperative Medicine, Alfred Hospital and Monash University, Melbourne, Australia

[2]Department of Anaesthesia and Pain Management, Royal Melbourne Hospital and Department of Pharmacology, University of Melbourne, Melbourne, Australia

Abstract

There is good evidence that epidural analgesia provides slightly better analgesia when compared with intravenous (IV) opioid regimens; incisional local anaesthetic infiltration has minimal analgesic effectiveness; supplemental IV fluids improve patient comfort, but a restrictive fluid regimen promotes return of gastrointestinal (GI) function; normothermia prevents shivering and wound infection, prophylactic antibiotics prevent infections; heparin and graduated compression stockings reduce thromboembolism; nasogastric drainage has no benefit, but early enteral feeding reduces postoperative infection and hospital stay, and may have other benefits after abdominal surgery. There is inconclusive evidence that supplemental IV fluids improve postoperative nausea and vomiting (PONV), headache and pain; a restrictive fluid regimen reduces postoperative complications and hospital stay; choice of IV fluid has any clinically important effects; optimisation of tissue oxygen delivery with inotrope therapy improves outcome; supplemental oxygen reduces serious complications; nitrous oxide reduces wound infection and pneumonia; and whether or not beta-blockers reduce cardiac mortality.

Major abdominal surgery includes many types of GI, as well as hepatobiliary, aortic, renal, and prostatic surgery. Naturally there are specific anaesthetic considerations inherent in each of these procedures, and some institutions will have unique issues for the anaesthetist to consider, such as innovative surgical techniques or the extent of hospital resources available for the perioperative care of the patient. However, despite these understandable modifiers of anaesthetic technique, there is

Key words: Morbidity, mortality, surgery, epidural analgesia, local anaesthesia, fluid therapy, colloid, oxygen delivery, transfusion, supplemental oxygen, nitrous oxide, normothermia, beta-blockade, alpha$_2$-agonists, thromboembolism, nasogastric drainage.

good evidence that variations in surgical and anaesthetic practice occur [1], and these could have a substantial impact on patient outcome [2].

The major issues confronting anaesthetists caring for patients undergoing major abdominal surgery include effective pain relief, optimisation of respiratory function, and avoidance of serious complications and death. Choice of general anaesthetic agent appears to have little effect on outcome [3–5], although overall rates of death and serious complications are very low and so the ability for trials to identify clinically useful treatments is limited [6]. In this chapter we describe many evidence-based interventions relevant to anaesthesia for abdominal surgery.

Pain relief

Observational studies suggest that an integrated approach to perioperative care of abdominal surgical patients that includes minimally invasive surgery, optimal pain relief (with or without epidural analgesia), early oral nutrition, and active mobilisation, leads to shorter hospital stays and, possibly, reduced postoperative complications. However, this has yet to be confirmed with large randomised trials, although a small trial has found some benefits of epidural analgesia in enhancing quality of life after colorectal surgery [7]. Analgesic studies typically use a visual analogue scale (VAS) to measure pain intensity; a clinically useful reduction in pain is a reduction in VAS score of at least 15–20 mm [8].

The two most common analgesic therapies after abdominal surgery are patient controlled analgesia (PCA) and epidural analgesia. These techniques have been compared after abdominal surgery in a systematic review (SR) that included nine randomised trials with 711 patients [9]. Epidural analgesia provided better pain relief as assessed by VAS pain scores at 6, 24, and 72 h after surgery: weighted mean difference (WMD) 1.74 (95% confidence interval, CI: 1.30–2.19), 0.99 (95% CI: 0.65–1.33), and 0.63 (95% CI: 0.24–1.01), respectively. The incidence of pruritus was lower in the PCA group (odds ratio,OR: 0.27, 95% CI: 0.11–0.64), but there was insufficient evidence of other possible benefits or risks of these two techniques in this setting. An earlier SR which focused on serious complications and mortality found no significant effect of neuraxial blockade in the abdominal surgery sub-group [10], but the pooled estimates had wide CIs and so further trials are required before definitive conclusions can be made. A large randomised trial in abdominal surgical patients found that postoperative epidural analgesia was associated with lower pain scores during the first three postoperative days, as assessed by VAS scores [11]. However, the magnitude of the effect lost clinical significance (VAS score difference <15 mm) after the first 24 h.

An SR comparing epidural local anaesthesia with opioid-based regimens to assess postoperative GI function, PONV, pain and complications found that most

Review: Patient controlled intravenous opioid analgesia (PCA) versus continuous epidural analgesia (CEA)
        for pain after intra-abdominal surgery
Comparison: 01 Efficacy (continuous)
Outcome: 01 Pain VAS: Early phase

Study	PCA N	Mean (SD)	CEA N	Mean (SD)	WMD (fixed) (95% CI)	Weight (%)	WMD (fixed) (95% CI)
01 Resting pain: Early phase (cm)							
Allaire 1992	29	3.30 (1.70)	39	2.00 (1.90)		23.8	1.30 (0.38, 2.22)
Bois 1997	59	3.30 (2.80)	55	1.40 (1.90)		26.3	1.90 (1.03, 2.77)
Boylan 1998	21	2.10 (3.70)	19	1.30 (2.10)		5.9	0.80 (−1.04, 2.64)
Kowalski 1992	9	5.40 (2.20)	9	4.90 (3.10)		3.3	0.50 (−1.98, 2.98)
Tsui 1997	54	4.47 (2.19)	57	2.33 (1.50)		40.7	2.14 (1.44, 2.84)
Subtotal (95% CI)	172		170			100.0	1.74 (1.30, 2.19)

Test for heterogeneity: $\chi^2 = 4.21$, df = 4, $P = 0.38$, $I^2 = 5.1\%$
Test for overall effect: $z = 7.63$, $P < 0.00001$

02 Dynamic pain: Early phase (cm)							
Boylan 1998	21	4.00 (6.00)	19	3.00 (4.00)		6.1	1.00 (−2.13, 4.13)
Tsui 1997	54	5.86 (2.17)	57	4.11 (2.12)		93.9	1.75 (0.95, 2.55)
Subtotal (95% CI)	75		76			100.0	1.70 (0.93, 2.48)

Test for heterogeneity: $\chi^2 = 0.21$, df = 1, $P = 0.65$, $I^2 = 0.0\%$
Test for overall effect: $z = 4.32$, $P < 0.00002$

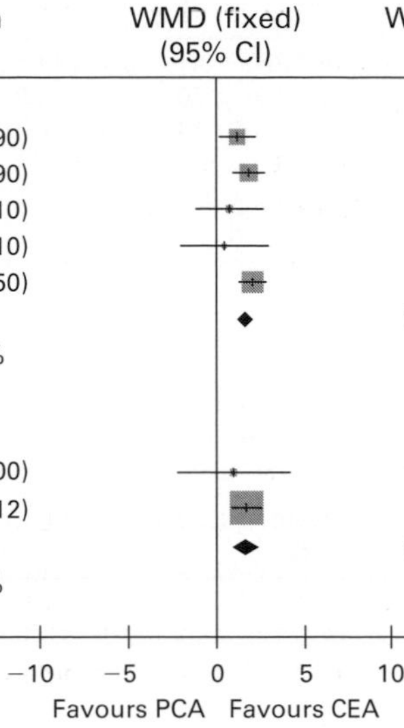

```
      −10    −5     0     5    10
         Favours PCA  Favours CEA
```

Figure 19.1 PCA versus epidural analgesia for pain relief after abdominal surgery. The forest plot
illustrates differences in pain score at about 6 h after surgery (see Werawatganon and
Charuluxanun [10], Copyright Cochrane Library, reproduced with permission from Elsevier.
© 2005 Elsevier Ltd)

trials involved a small number of patients, had poor methodology, and the subsequent meta-analyses had marked heterogeneity [12]. However, one consistent
result was earlier return of GI function in the epidural local anaesthetic group
compared with groups receiving systemic or epidural opioid, 37 h versus 24 h,
respectively. Postoperative pain was comparable (Figure 19.1).

> Epidural analgesia is superior to opioid PCA in relieving postoperative pain in patients
> after abdominal surgery, but is associated with a higher incidence of pruritus. The
> analgesic benefit is small and transitory (<24 h). Administration of epidural local
> anaesthetics to patients undergoing abdominal surgery assists return of GI function
> compared with systemic or epidural opioid regimens. There is no evidence of other
> benefits of epidural analgesia in abdominal surgery patients.
>   Further research is needed, with studies focusing on major complications such as
> respiratory failure, pneumonia, and mortality.

An SR of 26 trials with 1211 patients evaluated the analgesic efficacy of incisional
infiltration with local anaesthetic after abdominal surgery [13]. The study populations included inguinal hernia repair, hysterectomy, and cholecystectomy. There

Comparison: 01 Postop pain (0–24 h)
Outcome: 08 Abdominal pain (0–2 h)

Study	Local anaesthetic n	Mean (SD)	Placebo n	Mean (SD)	WMD (95% CI random)	Weight (%)	WMD (95% CI random)
Jiranantarat et al.	39	3.18 (2.64)	41	3.40 (2.70)		33.9	−0.22 (−1.39, 0.95)
Lepner et al.	20	2.11 (1.83)	20	2.68 (2.00)		33.5	−0.57 (−1.76, 0.62)
Pasqualucci et al.	14	0.08 (0.28)	14	2.31 (2.35)		32.6	−2.23 (−3.47, −0.99)
Total (95% CI)	73		75			100.0	−0.99 (−2.19, 0.20)

Test for heterogeneity: $\chi^2 = 5.98$, df $= 2$, $P = 0.05$
Test for overall effect: $z = 1.62$, $P = 0.10$

−10   −5   0   5   10
Favours treatment   Favours control

Comparison: 01 Postop pain (0–24 h)
Outcome: 09 Abdominal pain (2–6 h)

Study	Local anaesthetic n	Mean (SD)	Placebo n	Mean (SD)	WMD (95% CI random)	Weight (%)	WMD (95% CI random)
Jiranantarat et al.	39	3.00 (2.02)	41	3.68 (2.85)		34.1	−0.65 (−1.73, 0.43)
Lepner et al.	20	2.62 (1.70)	20	2.05 (2.26)		32.6	0.57 (−0.67, 1.81)
Pasqualucci et al.	14	0.99 (1.04)	14	3.36 (1.96)		33.3	−2.37 (−3.53, −1.21)
Total (95% CI)	73		75			100.0	−0.83 (−2.45, 0.79)

Test for heterogeneity: $\chi^2 = 11.74$, df $= 2$, $P = 0.0028$
Test for overall effect: $z = 1.00$, $P = 0.3$

−10   −5   0   5   10
Favours treatment   Favours control

Figure 19.2   The early analgesic efficacy of local anaesthetic infiltration after laparoscopic cholecystectomy (reprinted from *Practice and Research Clinical Anaesthesiology*, Ref. [14] With permission from Elsevier. © *2005 Elesevier Ltd*)

was marginal evidence of benefit in some of these settings, but the authors concluded that further clinical trials were needed before recommendations could be made. A subsequent meta-analysis, restricted to laparoscopic cholecystectomy, was completed recently [14]. A total of 31 trials with 2116 patients were identified, and once again only small differences were found. The authors noted that postoperative pain was generally mild to moderate after this type of surgery, suggesting that additional analgesic interventions had limited capacity to improve analgesic effectiveness. Importantly, they reported toxic plasma concentrations of local anaesthetics in some patients, and recommended that if local infiltration is to be used, the dose should be monitored closely to avoid toxicity (Figure 19.2).

Incisional infiltration with local anaesthetic has marginal analgesic effectiveness after abdominal surgery.

Fluid therapy

Traditional anaesthetic teaching has encouraged liberal IV fluid administration in the perioperative setting, in a belief that this will restore hydration status and tissue perfusion. Yet there are conflicting reports in the literature regarding the effect of various IV fluids and the optimal volume of administration during and after surgery.

Preoperative fasting leads to a fluid deficit of about 1 L and is likely to contribute to preoperative thirst, perioperative discomfort, patient dissatisfaction, and, possibly, morbidity. Holte and Kehlet [15] did an SR of 17 trials in 2002 comparing no fluids with correction of the preoperative fluid deficit. Low-volume fluid therapies reduced preoperative thirst, and larger volumes (at least 1 L) reduced postoperative drowsiness and dizziness, but there was insufficient data to draw conclusions on outcomes such as PONV, headache and pain.

Several small trials have found that balanced electrolyte solutions result in better clinical outcomes when compared with saline-based fluids [16–18]. This is most apparent in patients undergoing minor surgery, mostly in the ambulatory setting, where higher-volume fluid regimens improve early recovery measures such as dizziness, nausea, and thirst [16–19], and may improve pulmonary function, exercise capacity, and shorten hospital stay [17,18].

> In patients undergoing minor surgery the routine administration of about 1 L of IV fluid improves patient comfort before and after surgery. There is insufficient evidence to draw conclusions for an effect on PONV, headache and pain.

However, the results of such trials may not be applicable to patients undergoing major abdominal surgery in which substantially larger fluid shifts, and a complex inflammatory response occurs [20]. Recently, the effects of different fluid regimens on outcome were evaluated in this setting, where three trials in abdominal surgical patients concluded that a restrictive fluid regimen improves outcome [21–23]. However, a more recent trial was not able to replicate these findings [24].

Lobo et al. [21] did a randomised trial of salt and water restriction on recovery of GI function after elective colorectal surgery. They randomised 20 patients to either a standard postoperative fluid regimen (about 3 L and 154 mmol sodium per day) or a restrictive fluid regimen of about 2 L and 77 mmol sodium per day. They found that GI function (gastric emptying, passage of flatus) was improved in the restrictive group. Patients in the restrictive fluid group had fewer complications ($P = 0.01$), and their median hospital stay was shorter (6 days versus 9 days; $P = 0.001$). Brandstrup et al. [22] did a randomised trial comparing similar fluid regimens in 172 colorectal surgical patients. The restrictive fluid group had fewer postoperative complications (33% versus 51%; $P = 0.013$), and there were no deaths in the restrictive group compared with four deaths in the standard group ($P = 0.12$). Nisanevich et al. [23] did a randomised trial comparing restrictive and liberal fluid regimens in 152 patients undergoing a broader range of abdominal surgical procedures (gastric, small bowel, pancreatic, colorectal). Once again, the restrictive group had fewer complications ($P = 0.046$), shorter durations of ileus ($P < 0.001$), and shorter hospital stay, 8 days versus 9 days ($P = 0.01$). The latter trial is notable in that the study population included a broad range of patients, many of whom were judged to be at increased risk of postoperative complications. However, Kabon et al. [24] did a randomised trial comparing similar fluid regimens in 253 colorectal surgical patients, with the primary outcome being wound infection. There was no difference in the rates of wound infection, restrictive fluid group 14% versus liberal fluid group 11% ($P = 0.46$).

We did a meta-analysis of relevant trials to evaluate the effect of fluid restriction on hospital stay, major morbidity and mortality (Figure 19.3). This suggests there may be some benefit of fluid restriction, though a large definitive trial is warranted to confirm any beneficial effect on major morbidity or mortality.

> In patients undergoing major abdominal surgery, a restrictive fluid regimen promotes return of GI function, and may reduce postoperative complications and hospital stay. In addition, there may be reduced mortality. Further studies are warranted.

Although a large trial in a critical care setting found no difference in outcome between colloids and crystalloids [25], choice of IV fluid therapy in abdominal surgery has been investigated in small trials only. One of the best compared three solutions, 6% hetastarch in saline, 6% hetastarch in balanced salt, or Ringer's lactate, in a randomised trial in 90 patients undergoing major abdominal, gynaecological, or urological surgery [26]. Fluid administration was directed at maintaining standard haemodynamic goals. Both colloid groups had a significantly lower incidence of tissue oedema, PONV, and severe pain [26]. An SR of nine trials with 412 patients compared different IV fluids in abdominal aortic surgery [27]. Endpoints of interest included various surrogate markers of cardiac, respiratory, haematological, and nutritional status. Ten fluids were studied, but no single fluid was found to be superior to any other. However, each trial compared different fluids and so there was limited ability to identify any clinically important effects. The authors of this review concluded that further trials with sufficient sample size and power are required, and that the effect of fluid choice in aortic and other abdominal surgery is currently unclear.

> There is insufficient evidence to draw conclusions as to whether choice of fluid – crystalloid or colloid, balanced salt or normal saline – has any clinically important effects in abdominal surgery.

Review: Fluid restriction
Comparision: 03 Mortality
Outcome: 01 Mortality

Study or sub-category	Restrictive group (n/N)	Control n/N	OR (fixed) (95% CI)	Weight (%)	OR (fixed) (95% CI)
Lobo	0/10	1/10		24.66	0.30 (0.01, 8.33)
Brandstrup	0/69	4/72		75.34	0.11 (0.01, 2.07)
Kabon	0/124	0/129			Not estimable
Nisanevich	0/77	0/75			Not estimable
Total (95% CI)	280	286		100.00	0.16 (0.02, 1.37)

Total events: 0(Restrictive group), 5(Control)
Test for heterogeneity: $\chi^2 = 0.21$, df $= 1$ ($P = 0.65$), $I^2 = 0\%$
Test for overall effect: $z = 1.68$ ($P = 0.97$)

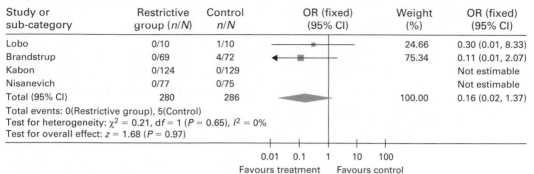

```
         0.01   0.1    1    10   100
        Favours treatment   Favours control
```

Review: Fluid restriction
Comparision: 02 Complications
Outcome: 01 Complications

Study or sub-category	Restrictive group (n/N)	Control n/N	OR (fixed) (95% CI)	Weight (%)	OR (fixed) (95% CI)
Lobo	1/10	7/10		10.17	0.05 (0.00, 0.56)
Brandstrup	21/69	40/72		43.95	0.35 (0.18, 0.70)
Kabon	14/124	11/129		15.43	1.37 (0.59, 3.14)
Nisanevich	13/77	23/79		30.45	0.49 (0.23, 1.07)
Total (95% CI)	280	290		100.00	0.52 (0.34, 0.79)

Total events: 49(Restrictive group), 81(Control)
Test for heterogeneity: $\chi^2 = 10.05$, df $= 3$ ($P = 0.02$), $I^2 = 70.2\%$
Test for overall effect: $z = 3.08$ ($P = 0.002$)

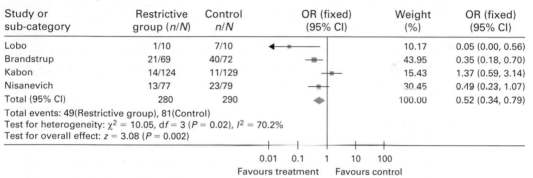

```
         0.01   0.1    1    10   100
        Favours treatment   Favours control
```

Review: Fluid restriction
Comparision: 01 LOS
Outcome: 01 Hospital length of stay (days)

Study or sub-category	N	Restrictive group mean (SD)	N	Control mean (SD)	WMD (fixed) (95% CI)	Weight (%)	WMD (fixed) (95% CI)
Lobo	10	6.00 (2.00)	10	9.00 (2.00)		18.71	−3.00 (−4.75, −1.25)
Brandstrup	69	8.00 (8.00)	72	9.00 (18.00)		2.76	−1.00 (−5.57, 3.57)
Kabon	124	7.30 (4.00)	129	7.00 (5.30)		43.17	0.30 (−0.85, 1.45)
Nisanevich	77	8.00 (3.75)	75	9.00 (4.25)		35.35	−1.00 (−2.28, 0.28)
Total (95% CI)	280		286			100.00	−0.81 (−1.57, −0.05)

Test for heterogeneity: $\chi^2 = 9.84$, df $= 3$ ($P = 0.02$), $I^2 = 68.9\%$
Test for overall effect: $z = 2.10$ ($P = 0.04$)

```
        −10   −5    0    5    10
        Favours treatment   Favours control
```

Figure 19.3 The effects of restrictive fluid therapy on mortality, complications and hospital stay after major abdominal surgery (for the Kabon study, wound infection only and this does not account for variations in hospital discharge practices)

Goal-directed therapies

It has been suggested that a strategy of targeting tissue oxygen delivery, so-called "optimisation" or "goal-directed" therapy, can improve postoperative outcome. One of the most compelling sources of evidence is a trial by Wilson et al. [28], who did a randomised trial to test the effect of inotropic therapy to enhance oxygen delivery in 138 patients undergoing major elective surgery. Two groups received invasive haemodynamic monitoring, fluid, and either adrenaline or dopexamine to increase oxygen delivery. Inotropic support was continued during surgery and for at least 12 h afterwards. The third group (control) received routine perioperative care. Mortality was reduced in the groups receiving inotropic support, 3% versus 17% ($P = 0.007$). There were no differences in mortality between the two inotropic therapy groups, but 30% of patients in the dopexamine group developed complications compared with 52% of patients in the adrenaline group (difference 22%, 95% CI: 2–41%) and 28 patients (61%) in the control group (31%, 95% CI: 11–50%). The use of dopexamine was associated with a decreased hospital stay. These beneficial findings may be due to the inotropic treatment, or may have resulted from the improved postoperative care in a high-dependency environment. Interestingly, support for positive inotropic therapy seems to contradict the supposed beneficial effect of perioperative beta-blockade [29–31].

Boyd et al. [32] randomly allocated 107 surgical patients to a dopexamine infusion or a standard care group, with the dopexamine infusion titrated to increase oxygen delivery index to $>600 \, \text{mL min}^{-1} \text{m}^{-2}$. The dopexamine group had a 75% reduction in mortality, 5.7% versus 22.2% ($P = 0.015$), and a 50% reduction in postoperative complications ($P = 0.008$). However, an SR of goal-directed therapies in the critical care population found equivocal results [33].

> There is some evidence that optimisation of tissue oxygen delivery with inotrope therapy may improve outcome after abdominal surgery, but further confirmatory trials are required before definitive recommendations can be made.

Some small trials have found some benefits of oesophageal Doppler-guided fluid optimisation in patients undergoing elective major surgery [34,35]. This and other technologies designed to optimise tissue oxygen delivery may be beneficial, but given they may lead to increase fluid administration and possibly more complications (Figure 19.3), definitive large multicentre randomised trials are required before they are adopted into routine practice.

McAlister et al. [36] did an SR to investigate the effect of red cell transfusion in patients undergoing cancer surgery. A meta-analysis of 17 studies, only six of which were randomised trials, found no evidence of increased mortality (risk ratio, RR: 0.95, 9% CI: 0.79–1.15), cancer recurrence (RR: 1.06, 95% CI: 0.88–1.28), or infection (RR: 1.00, 95% CI: 0.76–1.32). However, this meta-analysis was limited by heterogeneity, and dependence on small trials and other uncontrolled studies.

> To date there is no evidence that blood transfusion increases the risk of serious complications or death in patients undergoing cancer surgery.

Respiratory therapies

Overend et al. [37] did an SR comparing incentive spirometry with a variety of less complex interventions (including early mobilisation) to reduce postoperative pulmonary complications. Most studies were of poor methodological quality, with only 10 of 85 being suitable for inclusion, and they found no beneficial effects in abdominal surgery. One of the best trials comparing incentive spirometry, deep breathing, and intermittent positive-pressure breathing found they were equally more effective than no treatment in preventing pulmonary complications after abdominal surgery [38].

Supplemental oxygen therapy

Wound infection is a common complication of surgery and has significant cost implications because of greater resource utilisation and increased hospital stay [39]. The use of high-inspired oxygen concentration during the perioperative period has theoretical benefits because of improved tissue oxygenation and bacteriocidal activity. Two trials with conflicting results have been published.

Greif et al. [40] enrolled 500 patients undergoing colorectal surgery, and randomly allocated them to receive 30% or 80% oxygen during surgery and for 2 h afterward. The supplemental oxygen group had a 50% reduction in the incidence of wound infection, 5.2% versus 11.2% ($P = 0.01$). Pryor et al. [39] did a similar study, but this time in a broader range of abdominal surgical procedures and with less specified perioperative care, aiming to reflect routine practice. It thus can be considered an effectiveness trial. They randomly allocated 165 patients to receive either 80% or 35% oxygen during surgery and for the first 2 h after surgery. Unlike the earlier trial [40] in which nitrogen made up the remainder of the inspired gas mixture, in this study both groups were administered nitrous oxide, 20% or 65%, respectively. The incidence of infection was significantly higher in the supplemental oxygen group, 25% versus 11%, $P = 0.02$. Given the conflicting results, further large trials are required to determine whether some surgical groups may benefit from supplemental oxygen therapy.

Another purported benefit of supplemental oxygen is a reduction in PONV [41]. In an analysis of 231 patients from the study of Grief et al. [40], use of 80% oxygen was associated with a reduction in early PONV, 30% versus 17% ($P = 0.02$). A more recent study enrolled 240 patients undergoing gynaecological laparoscopy, and randomly allocated them to one of three groups: 30% oxygen, 80% oxygen, and 30% oxygen plus ondansetron 8 mg [42]. The overall incidence of PONV within 24 h was 44%, 22%, and 30%, respectively. The difference between 30% and 80% oxygen groups was statistically significant, but not between other groups. However, another trial has failed to replicate these findings in 100 patients undergoing gynaecologic laparoscopy [43].

> There is insufficient evidence to draw conclusions as to whether supplemental oxygen reduces serious complications after abdominal surgery. Supplemental oxygen may reduce early PONV.

Induction of anaesthesia in obese patients

Obese patients have reduced functional residual capacity and so oxygen stores are quickly depleted with apnoeic episodes during induction of anaesthesia. The effect of preoxygenation with the patient in the 25° head-up position was tested with a randomised trial in 42 morbidly obese patients undergoing laparoscopic gastric banding [44]. The head-up position group took 45 s longer to desaturate to 92% ($P = 0.023$), and so this simple technique provides a greater safety margin during induction of anaesthesia in obese subjects.

Avoidance of nitrous oxide

An SR of 24 trials with 2478 patients completed in 1997 found that avoidance of nitrous oxide with anaesthesia reduced the risk of PONV [45], and a practice guideline has been produced [46]. Whether or not nitrous oxide has other major adverse effects has been unclear [47]. Fleischmann et al. [48] evaluated the effect of nitrous oxide in a randomised trial in 418 colorectal surgical patients. Patients were randomly assigned 65% nitrous oxide or nitrogen (both groups FiO$_2$ 0.35) with a remifentanil–isoflurane anaesthetic. The incidence of wound infection was similar in both groups, nitrous oxide 15% versus nitrogen 20% ($P = 0.21$). In contrast, we have recently completed a large, multicentre randomised trial, comparing 70% nitrous oxide in oxygen (FiO$_2$ 0.3) with a nitrous-free anaesthetic (FiO$_2$ 0.8–1.0), in

2050 patients, of which two-thirds underwent abdominal surgery [49]. We found that patients receiving nitrous oxide had a significant increased hospital stay and intensive care unit (ICU) stay, and increased risk of postoperative wound infection, severe vomiting, atelectasis, and pneumonia (all $P < 0.05$). There was no evidence of a confounding effect of FiO_2 in this study. Thus nitrous oxide could be associated with a number of serious complications after surgery and its routine use should be questioned.

> Nitrous oxide is associated with increased risk of postoperative complications, including severe vomiting, and possibly wound infection and pneumonia. The routine use of nitrous oxide in patients undergoing major abdominal surgery should be questioned.

Maintenance of normothermia

Both general and major regional anaesthesia impair central thermoregulation and will result in core hypothermia ($<34°C$) unless preventative measures are implemented [50]. Patients undergoing major abdominal surgery are particularly at risk of hypothermia, because of the potential for significant heat loss. There is substantial evidence in the literature that maintenance of normothermia during major abdominal surgery may lead to improved outcomes.

Wound infection and wound healing

Kurz et al. [51] studied 200 patients undergoing colorectal surgery, randomly allocating them to routine care or active forced-air warming. The incidence of postoperative wound infection was significantly higher in hypothermic patients, 19% versus 6% ($P = 0.009$). Hypothermia also affected several measures of wound healing, and the duration of hospitalisation was prolonged, 15 ± 6.5 days versus 12 ± 4.4 days ($P < 0.001$).

Blood loss and blood transfusion

Coagulation and platelet function are both temperature-dependent physiological functions [52] with important implications for surgical outcome. Bock et al. [53] did a randomised trial of active warming in 40 patients undergoing major abdominal surgery. Intraoperative blood loss was greater in hypothermic patients, 1.1 ± 0.8 versus 0.6 ± 0.5 L, and they received more blood products, 0.5 ± 0.8 versus 0.1 ± 0.3 L (both $P < 0.05$). These data confirm two previous reports in patients undergoing major joint replacement surgery [54,55]. However, increased blood loss and transfusion requirement have not been linked to any longer-term adverse outcomes.

Myocardial ischaemia and infarction

Mild hypothermia is associated with activation of the sympathetic nervous system, inducing vasoconstriction, shivering and the release of stress hormones [56], all of which have been postulated to increase the likelihood of myocardial ischaemia and infarction in at-risk patients undergoing surgery. Frank et al. [57] randomly allocated 300 patients undergoing abdominal (46%), thoracic (13%), or peripheral vascular (41%) surgery, to passive or active warming and reported hypothermia was an independent risk factor for morbid cardiac events (unstable angina/ischaemia, cardiac arrest, and myocardial infarction) in multivariate analyses (RR: 2.2, 95% CI: 1.1–4.1), $P = 0.04$. Length of ICU stay was significantly longer in patients suffering a myocardial event, but hospital stay and mortality were not affected.

Recovery from anaesthesia

Recovery room stay potentially may be prolonged in hypothermic patients, by mechanisms including prolonged anaesthetic drug effects, cardiovascular instability, the need to treat shivering and the need to meet discharge requirements that include core temperature [52]. Two randomised trials have demonstrated prolonged recovery room stays in hypothermic patients following major abdominal surgery [53,58].

Shivering

Postoperative shivering is a troublesome complication of hypothermia, that can impair quality of patient recovery [59]. Skin warming [60] and a wide variety of drugs [59] effectively abolish shivering. Kranke et al. [61] did an SR of 20 randomised trials comparing drug therapies with placebo. The short-term efficacies of pethidine 25 mg, clonidine 0.15 mg, ketanserin 10 mg, and doxapram 100 mg were reported in at least three trials and all were more effective than placebo, with NNT (number needed to treat) 2. Long-term outcomes were not reported and adverse event reporting was infrequent. Ten of these studies included patients having major and minor intra-abdominal surgery. The applicability of these data to major abdominal surgery patients, who are more prone to hypothermia, therefore may be limited.

> Evidence supports maintenance of normothermia, and drug treatment of shivering to prevent adverse outcomes, following major abdominal surgery.

Benefits of beta-blockers and alpha$_2$-agonists

Perioperative cardiac events, such as myocardial infarction, cardiac arrest, and cardiac death, represent a great burden on health care resources in developed nations.

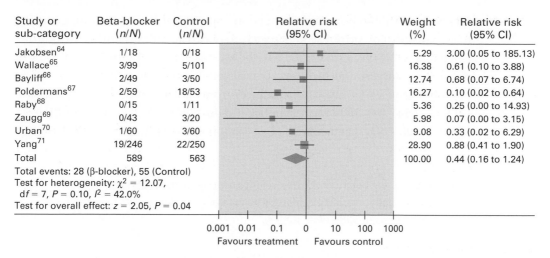

Study or sub-category	Beta-blocker (n/N)	Control (n/N)	Relative risk (95% CI)	Weight (%)	Relative risk (95% CI)
Jakobsen[64]	1/18	0/18		5.29	3.00 (0.05 to 185.13)
Wallace[65]	3/99	5/101		16.38	0.61 (0.10 to 3.88)
Bayliff[66]	2/49	3/50		12.74	0.68 (0.07 to 6.74)
Poldermans[67]	2/59	18/53		16.27	0.10 (0.02 to 0.64)
Raby[68]	0/15	1/11		5.36	0.25 (0.00 to 14.93)
Zaugg[69]	0/43	3/20		5.98	0.07 (0.00 to 3.15)
Urban[70]	1/60	3/60		9.08	0.33 (0.02 to 6.29)
Yang[71]	19/246	22/250		28.90	0.88 (0.41 to 1.90)
Total	589	563		100.00	0.44 (0.16 to 1.24)

Total events: 28 (β-blocker), 55 (Control)
Test for heterogeneity: $\chi^2 = 12.07$,
  df = 7, $P = 0.10$, $I^2 = 42.0\%$
Test for overall effect: $z = 2.05$, $P = 0.04$

0.001 0.01 0.1 0 10 100 1000
Favours treatment   Favours control

Figure 19.4 Relative risks for major perioperative cardiovascular events (cardiovascular death, non-fatal myocardial infarction, or non-fatal cardiac arrest) in non-cardiac surgery (provided by PJ Devereaux)

Perioperative beta-blockade has been the subject of many randomised trials, several SRs (29–31), and an influential clinical practice guideline [62]. This guideline, revised in 2002, made a Class I recommendation for perioperative beta-blockade in patients with documented ischaemia having vascular surgery and a Class IIa recommendation for patients with, or at risk of, ischaemic heart disease having non-cardiac surgery, despite acknowledging that the trials "do not provide enough data from which to draw firm conclusions" [62].

Earlier SRs [29,30] included only 5 and 11 trials, respectively. These reviews have been supplanted by the recent review of Devereaux et al. [31] that included 22 trials with 2437 patients. Eleven of the trials included patients having major abdominal surgery. The recently completed DIPOM study of beta-blockade in diabetic patients having non-cardiac surgery, which had a negative result, was not included [63].

Perioperative beta-blockers did not affect any individual outcome and had a marginal statistically significant beneficial effect on cardiovascular mortality, non-fatal myocardial infarction, and non-fatal cardiac arrest combined (RR: 0.44, 95% CI: 0.20–0.97). The authors argued that because the cumulative Z value did not reach the Lan-deMets sequential monitoring boundary, the current evidence is inconclusive [31]. The relative risks for bradycardia (2.27; 95% CI: 1.53–3.36) and hypotension (1.27; 95% CI: 1.04–1.56) needing treatment reached statistical significance. A randomised trial in 10 000 at-risk patients having non-cardiac surgery (the POISE study) is underway (Figure 19.4).

Fewer randomised trials have evaluated the effects of alpha$_2$-agonists. Nishana et al. [72] included seven trials of clonidine to prevent perioperative myocardial events in an SR, but none included abdominal surgical patients (cardiac surgery, $n = 5$, vascular or orthopaedic surgery, $n = 2$). Clonidine reduced myocardial ischaemia (OR: 0.49, 95% CI: 0.34–0.71). Stevens et al. [30] restricted their SR to non-cardiac surgery and included six trials of clonidine or mivazerol. The effect of alpha$_2$-agonists on myocardial infarction was not significant (OR: 0.85, 95% CI: 0.62–1.14), but there was a significant reduction in cardiac deaths (OR: 0.50, 95% CI: 0.28–0.91). Further large-scale randomised trials were advocated [30,72].

> There is promising but inconclusive evidence supporting the routine use of beta-blockers and alpha$_2$-agonists to prevent perioperative cardiac events in at-risk patients presenting for major abdominal surgery.

Antibiotic prophylaxis

The Centers of Disease Control (CDC) Hospital Infections Programme produced a comprehensive evidence-based guideline for prevention of surgical site infection in 1999 [73]. Most major elective abdominal operations may be considered as clean/contaminated, where cefazolin provides an adequate spectrum of activity. Cefoxitin and metronidazole are recommended for colorectal surgery. Antibiotic prophylaxis should be given before the first skin incision is made and bactericidal concentrations should be maintained until closure of the wound (but not beyond). There is also evidence presented in the guideline supporting the use of mechanical bowel preparation to prevent wound infection in colorectal surgery.

Two subsequent SRs on antibiotic prophylaxis during abdominal surgery are reported in the Cochrane database, although neither involved "major" surgery. Catarci et al. [74] examined six trials with 974 patients undergoing laparoscopic cholecystectomy, and did not demonstrate a significant effect of antibiotic prophylaxis on wound infection (OR: 0.82, 95% CI: 0.36–1.86), $P = 0.63$. However the authors believed that the number of patients enrolled to date was insufficient to rule out a type II error and that a large trial was required. A more recent SR [75] evaluated the effectiveness of antibiotic prophylaxis with appendicectomy. Nineteen studies with 2191 patients found single-dose antibiotic prophylaxis had beneficial effects (OR: 0.34, 95% CI: 0.25–0.45).

An SR and meta-analysis of 28 trials with 4694 patients evaluated whether antibiotic prophylaxis can reduce the risk of postoperative infective complications after transurethral resection of the prostate (TURP) [76]. Prophylactic antibiotics decrease the incidence of post-TURP bacteriuria, fever, bacteraemia, and additional antibiotic treatment.

Appropriately chosen and administered antibiotics should be prescribed prophylactically for all patients undergoing major abdominal surgery. If possible, these should be given before the first skin incision.

Venous thromboembolism prophylaxis

Major abdominal surgery patients, in particular cancer patients, are at relatively high risk of deep venous thrombosis (DVT) and pulmonary embolism [77]. Numerous randomised trials and several SRs have compared various pharmacological and mechanical preventative measures, alone or in combination, with placebo or each other in general surgical patients.

Mismetti et al. [78] evaluated 51 studies (32 in abdominal surgery) comparing low-molecular-weight heparin (LMWH) with unfractionated heparin (UFH) and 8 studies (5 in abdominal surgery) comparing LMWH with placebo. LMWH significantly decreased the risk of DVT compared with placebo (RR: 0.28, 95% CI: 0.14–0.54), $P < 0.001$, but not compared with UFH (RR: 0.90, 95% CI: 0.79–1.02), $P = 0.1$. The authors concluded that the optimal-dose regimen of LMWH for this indication requires further investigation. Wille-Jorgensen et al. [79] did a meta-analysis of 19 randomised trials in colorectal surgery patients. They concluded that any type of heparin was better than no treatment or placebo (OR: 0.32, 95% CI: 0.20–0.53). UFH and LMWH were equally effective (OR: 1.01, 95% CI: 0.67–1.52). The combination of graduated compression stockings and LMWH was better than LMWH alone (OR: 4.17, 95% CI: 1.37–12.70). The data were insufficient to evaluate the effectiveness of intermittent pneumatic compression against heparin or no treatment. Another SR that included eight trials in patients having major gynaecological surgery [80] found that heparin (OR: 0.30, 95% CI: 0.12–0.76) and warfarin (OR: 0.22, 95% CI: 0.06–0.86) decreased the risk of DVT compared with placebo, including in patients with malignancy. There was no difference between UFH and LMWH (Figure 19.5).

Prophylaxis against thromboembolism should be instituted in all patients undergoing major abdominal surgery, with a combination of heparin and graduated compression stockings.

Nasogastric tubes

Routine nasogastric drainage after abdominal surgery is intended to reduce gastric distension, hasten the return of bowel function, and hopefully reduce the risk of

Review: Heparins and mechanical methods for thromboprophylaxis in colorectal surgery
Comparison: 03 Thromboembolic events (TE). LDH versus no treatment or placebo
Outcome: 03 DVT and/or PE.

Study	LDH n/N	No treatment/ placebo n/N	Peto OR (95% CI)	Weight (%)	Peto OR (95% CI)
Covey 1975	3/9	1/11		6.8	4.22 (0.49, 36.09)
Gallus 1976	5/44	13/46		29.8	0.35 (0.13, 0.98)
Joffe 1976	2/8	3/6		7.0	0.36 (0.04, 3.06)
✕ Kosir 1996	0/3	0/7		0.0	Not estimable
Lahnborg 1974	0/11	2/8		3.8	0.08 (0.00, 1.45)
Negus 1980	0/14	6/19		10.1	0.13 (0.02, 0.74)
Rem 1975	4/19	7/12		14.3	0.21 (0.05, 0.91)
Tomgren 1978	7/41	11/34		28.2	0.44 (0.15, 1.26)
Total (95% CI)	149	143		100.0	0.35 (0.20, 0.62)

Total events: 21 (LDH), 43 (No treatment/placebo)
Test for heterogeneity: $\chi^2 = 8.07$, df $= 6$, $P = 0.23$, $I^2 = 25.6\%$
Test for overall effect: $z = 3.65$, $P = 0.0003$

0.1 0.2   0.5   1   2   5   10
Favours treatment   Favours control

Figure 19.5 The effect of low-dose heparin (LDH) on venous thromboembolism (deep vein thrombosis or pulmonary embolism); see Wille-Jorgensen et al. [79], Copyright Cochrane Library, reproduced with permission

anastomotic leakage and shorten hospital stay. An earlier meta-analysis found no evidence that routine nasogastric decompression is efficacious [81]. A recent Cochrane review has been published [82]. The authors included patients having any type of emergency or elective abdominal surgery. They identified 28 trials with 4194 patients. Patients not having routine nasogastric drainage had an earlier return of bowel function ($P < 0.001$), and possibly decreased pulmonary complications ($P = 0.07$); however, there could be an increased risk of wound infection ($P = 0.08$). Anastomotic leak was no different between groups ($P = 0.70$). There were also possible beneficial effects on patient comfort, PONV, and hospital stay, but the heterogeneity of these data limited definitive conclusions (Figures 19.6–19.8).

Routine postoperative nasogastric drainage has no demonstrable beneficial effects in abdominal surgery.

Nutrition

Although nutritional status is considered to be a marker of health and is likely to impact on perioperative risk, the clinical benefits of early postoperative nutrition in patients undergoing elective abdominal surgery are unclear. Traditional surgical

Review: Prophylactic nasogastric decompression after abdominal surgery
Comparison: 01 Time to flatus
Outcome: 01 Does postoperative nasogastric decompression hasten recovery
        of gastrointestinal function?

Study	Tube N	Mean (SD)	No tube N	Mean (SD)	WMD (fixed) (95% CI)	Weight (%)	WMD (fixed) (95% CI)
Cheadle 1985	100	3.10 (1.84)	100	2.50 (2.26)		2.1	0.60 (0.03, 1.17)
Colvin 1986	44	5.10 (2.10)	46	4.03 (1.40)		1.2	1.07 (0.33, 1.81)
Cunningham 1992	50	4.17 (2.60)	52	3.08 (2.60)		0.7	1.09 (0.08, 2.10)
Friedman 1996	40	4.90 (1.65)	40	4.10 (1.39)		1.5	0.80 (0.13, 1.47)
Koukouras 2001	50	4.10 (1.40)	50	3.40 (1.40)		2.2	0.70 (0.15, 1.25)
Lee 2002	70	3.80 (0.90)	66	3.50 (0.90)		7.4	0.30 (0.00, 0.60)
Montgomery 1996	37	4.33 (2.23)	39	4.51 (0.25)		1.3	−0.18 (−0.90, 0.54)
Nathan 1991	97	3.40 (0.69)	100	3.34 (0.75)		16.6	0.06 (−0.14, 0.26)
Olesen 1983	46	3.20 (0.98)	51	2.70 (0.95)		4.5	0.50 (0.12, 0.88)
Ortiz 1996	95	4.30 (2.07)	95	4.70 (2.07)		1.9	−0.40 (−0.99, 0.19)
Pearl 1996	55	4.30 (1.70)	54	3.60 (1.30)		2.1	0.70 (0.13, 1.27)
Racette 1987	28	4.00 (0.36)	28	3.90 (0.36)		18.9	0.10 (−0.09, 0.29)
Sakadamis 1999	500	3.25 (1.11)	500	2.72 (1.11)		35.6	0.53 (0.39, 0.67)
Savassi-Rocha 1992	57	3.40 (1.50)	52	3.70 (1.50)		2.1	−0.30 (−0.86, 0.26)
Sitges-Serra 1984	22	3.40 (1.34)	22	4.50 (1.34)		1.1	−1.10 (−1.89, −0.31)
✕ Wolff 1989	274	3.92 (0.00)	261	3.92 (0.00)		0.0	Not estimable
Wu 1994	37	4.30 (2.30)	37	4.20 (1.90)		0.7	0.10 (−0.86, 1.06)
Total (95% CI)	1602		1593			100.0	0.31 (0.23, 0.39)

Test for heterogeneity: $\chi^2 = 58.82$, df = 15, $P \leq 0.0001$, $I^2 = 74.5\%$
Test for overall effect: $z = 7.40$, $P < 0.00001$

       −4.0   −2.0   0   2.0   4.0
      Favours NG tube   Favours no tube

Figure 19.6 The effect of postoperative nasogastric drainage on recovery of GI function (days), as assessed by time to flatus after abdominal surgery (see Nelson et al. [82], Copyright Cochrane Library, reproduced with permission)

practice has been to "drip and suck" after major abdominal surgery, but recent observational studies and some randomised trials have questioned this practice. Early enteral feeding may improve tissue healing and reduce complications after GI surgery.

Lewis et al. [83] did an SR and identified 11 trials with 837 patients comparing enteral feeding started within 24 h after surgery with nil by mouth management in elective GI surgery. Early feeding reduced the risk of any type of infection (RR: 0.72, 95% CI: 0.54–0.98), $P = 0.036$, and hospital stay, 0.84 days (95% CI: 0.36–1.33 days), $P = 0.001$. There were non-significant reductions in anastomotic dehiscence, wound infection, pneumonia, intra-abdominal abscess, and mortality. The SR did not include trials using parenteral nutrition, and when later trial data [84] are considered, it provides additional support for early enteral nutrition.

A subsequent randomised trial [84] compared enteral nutrition with parenteral nutrition in 317 patients with GI cancer who were malnourished, and measured postoperative complications and hospital stay. Postoperative complications were

Review: Prophylactic nasogastric decompression after abdominal surgery
Comparison: 02 Pulmonary complications
Outcome: 01 Does postoperative nasogastric decompression diminish the risk
    of pulmonary complications?

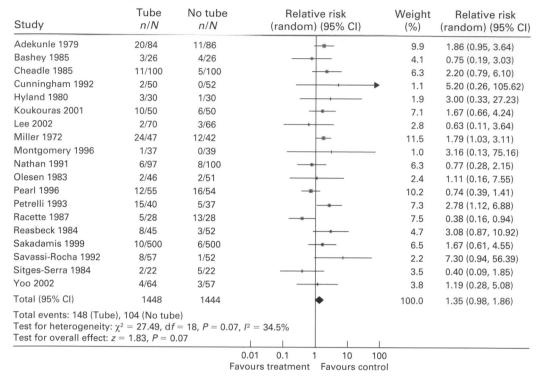

Study	Tube n/N	No tube n/N	Relative risk (random) (95% CI)	Weight (%)	Relative risk (random) (95% CI)
Adekunle 1979	20/84	11/86		9.9	1.86 (0.95, 3.64)
Bashey 1985	3/26	4/26		4.1	0.75 (0.19, 3.03)
Cheadle 1985	11/100	5/100		6.3	2.20 (0.79, 6.10)
Cunningham 1992	2/50	0/52		1.1	5.20 (0.26, 105.62)
Hyland 1980	3/30	1/30		1.9	3.00 (0.33, 27.23)
Koukouras 2001	10/50	6/50		7.1	1.67 (0.66, 4.24)
Lee 2002	2/70	3/66		2.8	0.63 (0.11, 3.64)
Miller 1972	24/47	12/42		11.5	1.79 (1.03, 3.11)
Montgomery 1996	1/37	0/39		1.0	3.16 (0.13, 75.16)
Nathan 1991	6/97	8/100		6.3	0.77 (0.28, 2.15)
Olesen 1983	2/46	2/51		2.4	1.11 (0.16, 7.55)
Pearl 1996	12/55	16/54		10.2	0.74 (0.39, 1.41)
Petrelli 1993	15/40	5/37		7.3	2.78 (1.12, 6.88)
Racette 1987	5/28	13/28		7.5	0.38 (0.16, 0.94)
Reasbeck 1984	8/45	3/52		4.7	3.08 (0.87, 10.92)
Sakadamis 1999	10/500	6/500		6.5	1.67 (0.61, 4.55)
Savassi-Rocha 1992	8/57	1/52		2.2	7.30 (0.94, 56.39)
Sitges-Serra 1984	2/22	5/22		3.5	0.40 (0.09, 1.85)
Yoo 2002	4/64	3/57		3.8	1.19 (0.28, 5.08)
Total (95% CI)	1448	1444		100.0	1.35 (0.98, 1.86)

Total events: 148 (Tube), 104 (No tube)
Test for heterogeneity: $\chi^2 = 27.49$, d$f = 18$, $P = 0.07$, $I^2 = 34.5\%$
Test for overall effect: $z = 1.83$, $P = 0.07$

0.01   0.1   1   10   100
Favours treatment   Favours control

Figure 19.7   The risk of pulmonary complications with postoperative nasogastric drainage after abdominal
surgery (see Nelson et al. [82], Copyright Cochrane Library, reproduced with permission)

reduced in the enterally fed group, 34% versus 49% (RR: 0.69, 95% CI: 0.53–0.90),
$P = 0.005$. Length of stay was also reduced, 13 days versus 15 days ($P = 0.009$).
Adverse effects, which consisted mainly of abdominal distension and cramps, were
more common in the enteral group, 35% versus 14% (RR: 2.50, 95% CI: 1.61–3.86),
$P < 0.001$. Another study was published by this group [85], which focused on
metabolic and economic advantages of enteral nutrition, but it is unclear how much
of the data had been included in previous publications. They found no significant
differences in surrogate nutritional and inflammatory markers between the two
groups, nor in complications or hospital stay [85].

> Early enteral feeding reduces postoperative infection and hospital stay, and may have
> other benefits after abdominal surgery.

Review: Prophylactic nasogastric decompression after abdominal surgery
Comparison: 03 Wound infection
Outcome: 01 Does postoperative nasogastric decompression diminish the risk if wound infection?

Study	Tube n/N	No tube n/N	OR (fixed) (95% CI)	Weight (%)	OR (fixed) (95% CI)
Adekunle 1979	0/84	4/86		6.7	0.11 (0.01, 2.05)
Bashey 1985	1/26	2/26		2.9	0.48 (0.04, 5.65)
Cheadle 1985	10/100	11/100		15.0	0.90 (0.36, 2.22)
Cunningham 1992	2/50	3/52		4.3	0.68 (0.11, 4.25)
X Hyland 1980	0/1	0/1		0.0	Not estimable
Koukouras 2001	1/50	1/50		1.5	1.00 (0.06, 16.44)
Lee 2002	0/70	2/66		3.9	0.18 (0.01, 3.88)
Miller 1972	6/47	2/42		2.8	2.93 (0.56, 15.37)
Montgomery 1996	2/37	1/39		1.4	2.17 (0.19, 25.01)
Nathan 1991	8/97	9/100		12.3	0.91 (0.34, 2.46)
Pearl 1996	17/55	27/54		28.4	0.45 (0.20, 0.98)
Reasbeck 1984	3/45	11/52		14.4	0.27 (0.07, 1.02)
Sakadamis 1999	1/500	2/500		3.0	0.50 (0.05, 5.52)
Savassi-rocha 1992	4/57	0/52		0.7	8.83 (0.46, 168.14)
Yoo 2002	3/64	2/67		2.8	1.60 (0.26, 9.89)
Total (95% CI)	1283	1287		100.0	0.72 (0.50, 1.04)

Total events: 58 (Tube), 77 (No tube)
Test for heterogeneity: $\chi^2 = 13.62$, d$f = 13$, $P = 0.40$, $I^2 = 4.6\%$
Test for overall effect: $z = 1.74$, $P = 0.08$

0.1 0.2   0.5 1   2   5   10
Favours treatment   Favours control

Figure 19.8 The risk of wound infection with postoperative nasogastric drainage after abdominal surgery (see Nelson et al. [82], Copyright Cochrane Library, reproduced with permission)

TURP

Spinal anaesthesia is commonly used for TURP, but there is no evidence that it improves outcomes [11,86]. An earlier SR which included 952 urological surgical patients found no significant effect of neuraxial blockade on mortality [11]. A matched cohort study compared spinal with general anaesthetic in 261 patients after TURP [87], and although there was a higher incidence of some minor adverse events in the general anaesthesia group, back pain was more common after spinal anaesthesia. Major complications were comparable.

Conclusions

There is a large amount of evidence derived from randomised trials and meta-analyses of trials in abdominal surgical practice to guide anaesthetic practice. In many cases however there is a need for definitive large trials investigating major morbidity and mortality as primary endpoints.

REFERENCES

1 Lassen K, Hannemann P, Ljungqvist O et al. Patterns in current perioperative practice: survey of colorectal surgeons in five northern European countries. *BMJ* 2005; 330: 1420–1.

2 Birkmeyer JD, Siewers AE, Finlayson EV et al. Hospital volume and surgical mortality in the United States. *New Engl J Med* 2002; 346: 1128–37.

3 Cohen MM, Duncan DG, Pope WDB et al. A survey of 112,000 anaesthetics at one teaching hospital (1975–1983). *Can J Anaesth* 1987; 33: 22–31.

4 Forrest JB, Cahalan MK, Rehder K et al. Multicenter study of general anesthesia. 11. Results. *Anesthesiology* 1990; 72: 262–8.

5 Myles PS, Williams DL, Hendrata M, Anderson H, Weeks AM. Patient satisfaction after anaesthesia and surgery: results of a prospective survey of 10,811 patients. *Br J Anaesth* 2000; 84: 6–10.

6 Rigg JR, Jamrozik K, Clarke M. How can we demonstrate that new developments in anesthesia are of real clinical importance? *Anesthesiology* 1997; 86: 1008–11.

7 Carli F, Mayo N, Klubien K et al. Epidural analgesia enhances functional exercise capacity and health-related quality of life after colonic surgery: results of a randomized trial. *Anesthesiology* 2002; 97: 540–9.

8 Campbell WI, Patterson CC. Quantifying meaningful changes in pain. *Anaesthesia* 1998; 53: 121–5.

9 Werawatganon T, Charuluxanun S. Patient controlled intravenous opioid analgesia versus continuous epidural analgesia for pain after intra-abdominal surgery. *The Cochrane Database Syst Rev* 2005, Issue 1. Art. No.: CD004088. DOI: 10.1002/14651858.

10 Rodgers A, Walker N, Schug S et al. Reduction of postoperative mortality and morbidity with epidural or spinal anaesthesia: results from overview of randomised trials. *BMJ* 2000; 321: 1493–7.

11 Rigg JRA, Jamrozik K, Myles PS et al. Epidural anaesthesia and analgesia and outcome of major surgery: a randomised trial. *Lancet* 2002; 359: 1276–82.

12 Jørgensen H, Wetterslev J, Møiniche S, Dahl JB. Epidural local anaesthetics versus opioid-based analgesic regimens on postoperative gastrointestinal paralysis, PONV and pain after abdominal surgery. *The Cochrane Database Syst Rev* 2000, Issue 1. Art. No.: CD001893. DOI: 10.1002/14651858.

13 Moiniche S, Mikkelsen S, Wetterslev J, Dahl JB. A qualitative systematic review of incisional local anaesthesia for postoperative pain relief after abdominal operations. *Br J Anaesth* 1998; 81: 377–83.

14 Gupta A. Local anaesthesia for pain relief after laparoscopic cholecystectomy – a systematic review. *Best Pract Res Clin Anaesthesiol* 2005; 19: 275–92.

15 Holte K, Kehlet H. Compensatory fluid administration for preoperative dehydration – does it improve outcome? *Acta Anaesthesiol Scand* 2002; 46: 1089–93.

16 Grocott MP, Mythen MG, Gan TJ. Perioperative fluid management and clinical outcomes in adults. *Anesth Analg* 2005; 100: 1093–106.

17 Holte K, Klarskov B, Christensen DS et al. Liberal versus restrictive fluid administration to improve recovery after laparoscopic cholecystectomy: a randomized, double-blind study. *Ann Surg* 2004; 240: 892–9.

18 Carton E, Gardiner J, Buggy D. Effect of intraoperative intravenous crystalloid infusion on postoperative nausea and vomiting after gynaecological laparoscopy: comparison of 30 and $10 \, ml \, kg^{-1}$. *Br J Anaesth* 2004; 93: 381–5.

19 Yogendran S, Asokumar B, Cheng DC, Chung F. A prospective randomized double-blinded study of the effect of intravenous fluid therapy on adverse outcomes on outpatient surgery. *Anesth Analg* 1995; 80: 682–6.

20 Mythen MG. Postoperative gastrointestinal tract dysfunction. *Anesth Analg* 2005; 100: 196–204.

21 Lobo DN, Bostock KA, Neal KR et al. Effect of salt and water balance on recovery of gastrointestinal function after elective colonic resection: a randomised controlled trial. *Lancet* 2002; 359: 1812–8.

22 Brandstrup B, Tonnesen H, Beier-Holgersen R et al. Effects of intravenous fluid restriction on postoperative complications: comparison of two perioperative fluid regimens: a randomized assessor-blinded multicenter trial. *Ann Surg* 2003; 238: 641–8.

23 Nisanevich V, Felsenstein I, Almogy G et al. Effect of intraoperative fluid management on outcome after intraabdominal surgery. *Anesthesiology* 2005; 103: 25–32.

24 Kabon B, Akça O, Taguchi A et al. Supplemental fluid administration does not reduce the risk of surgical wound infection. *Anesth Analg* 2005; 101(5): 1546–53.

25 Finfer S, Bellomo R, Boyce N et al. A comparison of albumin and saline for fluid resuscitation in the intensive care unit. *New Engl J Med* 2004; 350: 2247–56.

26 Moretti EW, Robertson KM, El Moalem H, Gan TJ. Intraoperative colloid administration reduces postoperative nausea and vomiting and improves postoperative outcomes compared with crystalloid administration. *Anesth Analg* 2003; 96: 611–7.

27 Zavrakidis N. Intravenous fluids for abdominal aortic surgery. *The Cochrane Database Syst Rev* 2000, Issue 3: Art. No.: CD000991. DOI: 10.1002/14651858.

28 Wilson J, Woods I, Fawcett J et al. Reducing the risk of major elective surgery: randomised controlled trial of preoperative optimisation of oxygen delivery. *BMJ* 1999; 318: 1099–103.

29 Auerbach A, Goldman L. Beta-blockers and reduction of cardiac events in non-cardiac surgery. *JAMA* 2002; 287: 1435–44.

30 Stevens R, Burri H, Tramer M. Pharmacologic myocardial protection in patients undergoing noncardiac surgery: a quantitative systematic review. *Anesth Analg* 2003; 97: 623–33.

31 Devereaux P, Beattie W, Choi P et al. How strong is the evidence for the use of perioperative beta-blockers in non-cardiac surgery? Systematic review and meta-analysis of randomised controlled trials. *BMJ* 2005; 331: 313–21.

32 Boyd O, Grounds RM, Bennett ED. A randomized clinical trial of the effect of deliberate perioperative increase of oxygen delivery on mortality in high-risk surgical patients. *JAMA* 1993; 270: 2699–707.

33 Kern JW, Shoemaker WC. Meta-analysis of hemodynamic optimization in high-risk patients. *Crit Care Med* 2002; 30: 1686–92.

34 Gan TJ, Soppitt A, Maroof M et al. Goal-directed intraoperative fluid administration reduces length of hospital stay after major surgery. *Anesthesiology* 2002; 97: 820–6.

35 Conway DH, Mayall R, Abdul-Latif MS et al. Randomised controlled trial investigating the influence of intravenous fluid titration using oesophageal Doppler monitoring during bowel surgery. *Anaesthesia* 2002; 57: 845–9.

36 McAlister FA, Clark HD, Wells PS, Laupacis A. Perioperative allogeneic blood transfusion does not cause adverse sequelae in patients with cancer: a meta-analysis of unconfounded studies. *Br J Surg* 1998; 85: 171–8.

37 Overend TJ, Anderson CM, Lucy SD et al. The effect of incentive spirometry on postoperative pulmonary complications: a systematic review. *Chest* 2001; 120: 971–8.

38 Hall JC, Tarala RA, Tapper J, Hall JL. Prevention of respiratory complications after abdominal surgery: a randomised clinical trial. *BMJ* 1996; 312: 148–52.

39 Pryor KO, Fahey III TJ, Lien CA, Goldstein PA. Surgical site infection and the routine use of perioperative hyperoxia in a general surgical population: a randomized controlled trial. *JAMA* 2004; 291: 79–87.

40 Greif R, Akça O, Horn EP, Kurz A, Sessler DI. Supplemental perioperative oxygen to reduce the incidence of surgical-wound infection. *New Engl J Med* 2000; 342: 161–7.

41 Greif R, Laciny S, Rapf B, Hickle RS, Sessler DI. Supplemental oxygen reduces the incidence of postoperative nausea and vomiting. *Anesthesiology* 1999; 91: 1246–52.

42 Goll V, Akca O, Greif R et al. Ondansetron is no more effective than supplemental intraoperative oxygen for prevention of postoperative nausea and vomiting. *Anesth Analg* 2001; 92: 112–7.

43 Purhonen S, Turunen M, Ruohoaho UM, Niskanen M, Hynynen M. Supplemental oxygen does not reduce the incidence of postoperative nausea and vomiting after ambulatory gynecologic laparoscopy. *Anesth Analg* 2003; 96: 91–6.

44 Dixon BJ, Dixon JB, Carden JR et al. Preoxygenation is more effective in the 25 degrees head-up position than in the supine position in severely obese patients: a randomized controlled study. *Anesthesiology* 2005; 102: 1110–5.

45 Tramer M, Moore A, McQuay H. Omitting nitrous oxide in general anaesthesia: meta-analysis of intraoperative awareness and postoperative emesis in randomized controlled trials. *Br J Anaesth* 1996; 76: 186–93.

46 Gan TJ, Meyer T, Apfel CC et al. Consensus guidelines for managing postoperative nausea and vomiting. *Anesth Analg* 2003; 97: 62–71.

47 Myles PS, Leslie K, Silbert B, Paech M, Peyton P. A review of the risks and benefits of nitrous oxide in current anaesthetic practice. *Anaesth Intens Care* 2004; 32: 165–72.

48 Fleischmann E, Lenhardt R, Kurz A et al. Nitrous oxide and risk of surgical wound infection: a randomised trial. *Lancet* 2005; 366: 1101–7.

49 Myles PS, Leslie K, Chan MTV et al. A randomised controlled trial of nitrous oxide in patients undergoing major surgery: the ENIGMA trial (in press).

50 Sessler D. Perioperative heat balance. *Anesthesiology* 2000; 92: 578–96.

51 Kurz A, Sessler DI, Lenhardt R. Perioperative normothermia to reduce the incidence of surgical wound infection and shorten hospitalization. *New Engl J Med* 1996; 334: 1209–15.

52 Sessler D. Complications and treatment of mild hypothermia. *Anesthesiology* 2001; 95: 531–43.

53 Bock M, Muller J, Bach A et al. Effects of preinduction and intraoperative warming during major laparotomy. *Br J Anaesth* 1998; 80: 159–63.

54 Schmied H, Kurz A, Sessler DI et al. Mild intraoperative hypothermia increases blood loss and allogeneic transfusion requirements during total hip arthroplasty. *Lancet* 1996; 347: 289–92.

55 Schmied H, Schiferer A, Sessler D, Meznik C. The effects of red-cell scavenging, hemodilution and active warming on allogenic blood requirements in patients undergoing hip or knee arthorplasty. *Anesth Analg* 1998; 86: 387–91.

56 Frank S, Higgins M, Breslow M et al. The catecholamine, cortisol and hemodynamic responses to mild perioperative hypothermia – a randomised controlled trial. *Anesthesiology* 1995; 82: 83–93.

57 Frank SM, Fleisher LA, Breslow MJ et al. Perioperative maintenance of normothermia reduces the incidence of morbid cardiac events. *JAMA* 1997; 277: 1127–34.

58 Lenhardt R, Marker E, Goll V et al. Mild intraoperative hypothermia prolongs post-anesthetic recovery. *Anesthesiology* 1997; 87: 1318–23.

59 De Witte J, Sessler D. Perioperative shivering. *Anesthesiology* 2002; 96: 467–84.

60 Sharkey A, Lipton J, Murphy M, Geisecke A. Inhibition of post-anesthetic shivering with radiant heat. *Anesthesiology* 1987; 66: 249–52.

61 Kranke P, Eberhart L, Roewer M, Tramer M. Pharmacological treatment of postoperative shivering: a quantitative systematic review of randomized controlled trials. *Anesth Analg* 2002; 94: 453–60.

62 Eagle K, Berger P, Calkins H et al. ACC/AHA guideline update for perioperative cardiovascular evaluation for noncardiac surgery – executive summary a report of the American College of Cardiology/American Heart Association Task Force on Practice Guidelines. *Circulation* 2002; 105: 1257–67.

63 Juul A. Randomized blinded trial on perioperative metoprolol versus placebo for diabetic patients undergoing noncardiac surgery. Presented at *Late-Breaking Clinical Trials I, American Heart Association Scientific Sessions* (abstract), New Orleans, USA, November 7–10, 2004.

64 Jakobsen CJ, Bille S, Ahlburg P, Rybro L, Pedersen KD, Rasmussen B. Preoperative metoprolol improves cardiovascular stability and reduces oxygen consumption after thoracotomy. *Acta Anaesthesiol Scand* 1997; 41: 1324–30.

65 Wallace A, Layug B, Tateo I, Li J, Hollenberg M, Browner W et al. Prophylactic atenolol reduces postoperative myocardial ischemia. *Anesthesiology* 1998; 88: 7–17.

66 Bayliff CD, Massel DR, Inculet RI, Malthaner RA, Quinton SD, Powell FS et al. Propranolol for the prevention of postoperative arrhythmias in general thoracic surgery. *Ann Thorac Surg* 1999; 67: 182–6.

67 Poldermans D, Boersma E, Bax JJ, Thompson IR, van de Ven LL, Blankensteijn JD et al. The effect of bisoprolol on perioperative mortality and myocardial infarction in high-risk patients undergoing vascular surgery. *N Engl J Med* 1999; 341: 1789–94.

68 Raby KE, Brull SJ, Timimi F, Akhtar S, Rosenbaum S, Naimi C et al. The effect of heart rate control on myocardial ischemia among high-risk patients after vascular surgery. *Anesth Analg* 1999; 88: 477–82.

69 Zaugg M, Tagliente T, Lucchinetti E, Jacobs E, Krol M, Bodian C et al. Beneficial effects from beta-adrenergic blockade in elderly patients undergoing noncardiac surgery. *Anesthesiology* 1999; 91: 1674–86.

70 Urban MK, Markowitz SM, Gordon MA, Urquhart BL, Kligfield P. Postoperative prophylactic administration of beta-adrenergic blockers in patients at risk for myocardial ischemia. *Anesth Analg* 2000; 90: 1257–61.

71 Yang H, Raymer K, Butler R, Parlow J, Roberts R. Metoprolol after vascular surgery (MaVS). *Can J Anesth* 2004; 51: A7.

72 Nishana K, Mikawa K, Uesugi T et al. Efficacy of clonidine for prevention of perioperative myocardial ischemia. *Anesthesiology* 2002; 96: 323–9.

73 Mangram A, Horan T, Pearson M et al. Guideline for prevention of surgical site infection, 1999. *Infect Cont Hosp Epidemiol* 1999; 20: 247–77.

74 Catarci M, Mancini S, Gentileschi P et al. Antibiotic prophylaxis in elective laparoscopic cholecystectomy. *Surg Endosc* 2004; 18: 638–41.

75 Andersen B, Kallehave F, Andersen H. Antibiotics versus placebo for prevention of postoperative infection after appendicectomy. *Cochrane Database Syst Rev* 2005; 3: 1–74.

76 Qiang W, Jianchen W, MacDonald R, Monga M, Wilt TJ. Antibiotic prophylaxis for transurethral prostatic resection in men with preoperative urine containing less than 100 000 bacteria per ml: a systematic review. *J Urol* 2005; 173: 1175–81.

77 Gutt C, Oniu T, Wolkener F et al. Prophylaxis and treatment of deep venous thrombosis in general surgery. *Am J Surg* 2005; 189: 14–22.

78 Mismetti P, Laporte S, Darmon J et al. Meta-analysis of low molecular weight heparin in the prevention of venous thromboembolism in general surgery. *Br J Surg* 2001; 88: 913–30.

79 Wille-Jørgensen P, Rasmussen MS, Andersen BR, Borly L. Heparins and mechanical methods for thromboprophylaxis in colorectal surgery. *The Cochrane Database Syst Rev* 2004, Issue 1, Art. No.: CD001217. DOI: 10.1002/14651858.

80 Oates-Whitehead R, D'Angelo A, Mol B. Anticoagulant and aspiring prophylaxis for preventing thromboembolism after major gynaecological surgery. *The Cochrane Database Sys Rev* 2003, Issue 4. Art. No.: CD0033679. DOI: 10.1002/14651858.

81 Cheatham ML, Chapman WC, Key SP, Sawyers JL. A meta-analysis of selective versus routine nasogastric decompression after elective laparotomy. *Ann Surg* 1995; 221: 469–76.

82 Nelson R, Edwards S, Tse B. Prophylactic nasogastric decompression after abdominal surgery. *The Cochrane Database Syst Rev* 2005, Issue 1. Art. No.: CD004929. DOI: 10.1002/14651858.

83 Lewis SJ, Egger M, Sylvester PA, Thomas S. Early enteral feeding versus "nil by mouth" after gastrointestinal surgery: systematic review and meta-analysis of controlled trials. *BMJ* 2001; 323: 773–6.

84 Bozzetti F, Braga M, Gianotti L, Gavazzi C, Mariani L. Postoperative enteral versus parenteral nutrition in malnourished patients with gastrointestinal cancer: a randomised multicentre trial. *Lancet* 2001; 358: 1487–92.

85 Braga M, Gianotti L, Gentilini O et al. Early postoperative enteral nutrition improves gut oxygenation and reduces costs compared with total parenteral nutrition. *Crit Care Med* 2001; 29: 242–8.

86 Malhotra V. Transurethral resection of the prostate. *Anesthesiol Clin N Am* 2000; 18: 883–97.

87 Reeves MD, Myles PS. Does anaesthetic technique affect the outcome after transurethral resection of the prostate? *Br J Urol Int* 1999; 84: 982–6.

20

Anaesthesia for paediatric surgery

Neil S Morton

Department of Paediatric Anaesthesia and Pain Management, Royal Hospital for Sick Children, Glasgow, Scotland

This chapter covers selected topics which illustrate the basis for modern general paediatric anaesthesia practices. Sub-specialty topics have not been covered. It is generally agreed that detailed preparation of children and families is vital for success. This includes providing better information upon which consent and assent is gained. Behavioural management decreases psychological upset and reduces the need for sedative premedication. Parental involvement in the pre- and post-operative periods is usually helpful. Many paediatric procedures can be undertaken on a day case basis which has tremendous benefits for children and families. Fasting rules for elective surgery are generally accepted. Topical local anaesthesia prior to venous cannulation for intravenous induction is well-established practice. Sedative premedication has a place and oral midazolam is the most commonly used. Inhalational induction of anaesthesia has undergone a renaissance with the introduction of sevoflurane, although maintenance with sevoflurane can result in emergence delirium. Desflurane maintenance may be particularly useful for neonates. Intravenous induction with propofol is also very common practice and total intravenous anaesthesia (TIVA) and TCI techniques are still being developed for children. Tracheal intubation can be performed safely and effectively in children without muscle relaxants and cuffed tracheal tubes are now more widely used. The laryngeal mask airway (LMA) is very commonly used in paediatric anaesthesia for elective cases and can also be useful in children with difficult airways. New muscle relaxants have been evaluated in children and rocuronium is particularly useful for modified rapid sequence induction. Local and regional analgesia techniques are now routinely used in paediatric practice and ultrasound guidance may be useful. New local anaesthetics such as levo-bupivacaine and ropivacaine have improved the safety of both single injection blocks and continuous infusion techniques. The adjuncts clonidine and ketamine have been evaluated for caudal epidural blockade and are now in common use. Safe dosing regimens for opioids, non-steroidal anti-inflammatory drugs (NSAIDs) and paracetamol have evolved for use in children and are the basis for

Key words: Anaesthesia, analgesia, paediatric, children, neonate, infant.

analgesia plans organised by acute paediatric pain teams. Postoperative nausea and vomiting (PONV) prevention by 5HT3 antagonists and steroids has proven to be very effective for children at high risk.

Preparation and premedication of children

Information and consent

Preparation begins at the initial outpatient clinic visit. Clear written, verbal and pictorial information concerning fasting, surgery, anaesthesia, analgesia and post-operative care are an essential part of obtaining informed consent from parents and children. Children are much more involved in consent and assent processes nowadays and so information must be provided in a form appropriate to their developmental stage and cognitive abilities [1].

Behavioural preparation

A pre-admission programme is very useful in allaying fears and anxieties. Toys, games, computer games, colouring books, videos and play therapy can all be employed depending on the child's age and maturity. Visits to the anaesthetic induction room and recovery area are very helpful and the types of anaesthesia, pain relief and postoperative care can be discussed with the parents and child. Pre-admission clinics where physical examination, preoperative screening checks and blood tests are carried out can be useful in reducing cancellation of cases but the vast majority of paediatric day cases do not need preoperative investigations or tests. Telephone contact on the day before surgery is useful and gives an opportunity to re-emphasise preoperative instructions, to confirm attendance and to rule out last minute reasons for postponement such as infections, travel difficulties or family problems.

Parental involvement

Parental involvement in the induction of anaesthesia can be very helpful, particularly for the pre-school age group. Parents should not be forced to be present if they do not wish as there is evidence that many parents find this experience very stressful and excessively anxious parents may transmit this anxiety to their child [2–7].

Day care

The multidisciplinary report "Just for the Day" [8] set out 12 quality standards for care of paediatric day cases. These apply whether children are managed in a specialist paediatric unit or in an adult unit which has been adapted for children.

Quality standards for care of paediatric cases

1 Integrate the admission plan to include pre-admission, day of admission and post-admission care with planned transfer of care to primary care and/or community services.
2 Prepare the child and parents before and during the day of admission.
3 Give specific written information to parents.
4 Admit the child to an area designated for day cases and do not mix with acutely ill inpatients.
5 Do not admit or treat children alongside adults.
6 Specifically designated day case staff should care for the child.
7 Trained paediatric staff should be used.
8 Organise care so that every child is likely to be discharged within the day.
9 Ensure that the building, equipment and furnishings comply with paediatric safety standards.
10 Ensure that the environment is child friendly.
11 Complete essential documents before each child goes home to ensure after care and follow-up are seamless.
12 Establish paediatric nursing support for the child at home.

The important principles which can be drawn from these standards are that children should be managed by staff trained in their care, in appropriate child friendly and child safe facilities with free parental access to the conscious child. Pre-school paediatric patients gain particular benefit from well planned and conducted day care because separation from parents is reduced [9]. For older children and parents the disruption to schooling and work is minimised.

Fasting

The following paediatric fasting rules for elective surgery are widely accepted [10]:
• 6 h for solids, milk or milky drinks,
• 4 h for breast fed infants,
• 2 h for clear fluids, including non-particulate fruit juices, carbonated drinks, water, tea and coffee without milk.

The risk of aspiration pneumonitis is low in healthy children [11,12]. Although many have residual gastric volumes $>0.4 \, mL \, kg^{-1}$ with pHs <2.5, this is unaffected by prolonged fasting [10]. Breast milk leaves the stomach twice as rapidly as formula (25 versus 51 min) [13,14]. Fasting reduces gastric volumes in children presenting for emergency surgery but does not affect pH. The lowest risk of aspiration is in those over 10 years of age with superficial injuries [15].

Pharmacological premedication

Use of topical local anaesthesia

The use of topical local anaesthesia of the skin with EMLA cream or amethocaine gel allows painless venous access after 60 and 45 min, respectively [16–18].

Anxiolytics and sedatives

Sedative premedication can be very helpful for selected cases where the child is very anxious, has previously had a traumatic experience with the induction of anaesthesia, has a needle phobia or is inconsolable. Oral midazolam, 0.5 mg kg^{-1} is very effective when given 20–30 min prior to induction. The standard formulation of midazolam is very acidic and tastes very bitter so must be disguised by a sweet liquid either by preparation of a syrup in the pharmacy or by adding the midazolam to a small volume (1–2 mL kg^{-1}) of cola, lemonade, or other sweet drink or by mixing with paracetamol syrup [19,20]. This presupposes that the child will cooperate in drinking this solution. The same limitation applies to oral ketamine (up to 10 mg kg^{-1}). Other options such as intranasal midazolam, rectal induction or intramuscular ketamine are not very satisfactory as they involve a degree of restraint of the child to administer them, which many find unacceptable. Most children find these routes of administration unpleasant and upsetting. Oral midazolam does not delay discharge and may ameliorate postoperative behavioural changes [21]. Recently, melatonin has been shown to be an effective premedicant [22,23] as has clonidine [24]. Oral transmucosal fentanyl is associated with a high risk of emesis [25,26].

Induction and maintenance of anaesthesia

Inhalational induction and maintenance

Sevoflurane [27] is now the most often used agent for induction in children because it is more pleasant and less irritant than the other volatile agents [28–30]. The incidence of PONV is lower than with halothane [31]. Onset is rapid due to low blood: gas partition (0.66) [32–35]. The minimum alveolar concentration (MAC) varies with age (<6 months old, MAC is 3.3; >6 months, 2.5; adults, 2.0) [36,37]. Emergence is rapid [38–40] but may be complicated by delirium [41]. A recent double-blinded randomised controlled trial showed the same incidence and severity of behavioural changes after halothane as after sevoflurane anaesthesia [42]. Cardiovascular stability is good with sevoflurane [31,37,43–47]. Sevoflurane can be used in children with airway difficulties [48,49] although is less potent than halothane and attaining and maintaining a sufficient depth of anaesthesia may be a practical problem in children with severe airway obstruction. Sevoflurane may be used for insertion of a laryngeal mask [50] or for tracheal intubation [51,52]. Sevoflurane can precipitate malignant hyperthermia [53] and may induce seizures in epileptic patients [54] and epileptiform EEG changes in healthy children [55].

Desflurane [56] has an extremely low blood:gas solubility coefficient (0.42) but is not suitable for induction as it is very pungent and irritant, commonly causing severe coughing, laryngospasm or breath-holding [57–59]. It may increase heart rate and systolic and pulmonary blood pressures if the inspired concentration is rapidly increased [59]. Desflurane is useful for maintenance of anaesthesia in neonates, babies and children and maintains haemodynamic stability during surgery [58]. Recovery is rapid [60], but emergence delirium has been reported [61]. In ex-premature babies, desflurane may be associated with lower incidence of postoperative apnoea compared with halothane or sevoflurane [62].

Intravenous induction and maintenance

Intravenous induction is thought to be less psychologically disturbing to children than inhalational induction [63,64]. Intravenous induction with propofol, 4 mg kg^{-1} with added lignocaine, 0.2 mg kg^{-1} [65–68] is very effective and results in a slightly earlier recovery than thiopentone induction [69]. TIVA may be used in children [70–73] but the dose of propofol is twice that of adults (ED95 of 10.5 mg kg^{-1}h^{-1} compared with 5 mg kg^{-1}h^{-1}) when combined with an alfentanil infusion at 50 μg kg^{-1}h^{-1} [74]. TCI systems have been used successfully in children [75–79].

Airway control

Tracheal intubation

Recent evidence supports various techniques of tracheal intubation without muscle relaxants in children [33,51,52,80–83] and the use of cuffed tracheal tubes in infants and children [84–86].

The laryngeal mask airway

The airway anatomy of babies and children makes LMA insertion and positioning more problematic than in adults [87–91]. The LMA is particularly useful in children with abnormalities of the airway in whom intubation is difficult. It can be used in place of a tracheal tube or to facilitate intubation by acting as a conduit for fibre-optic bronchoscopy and delivery of oxygen and volatile agents during intubation of the trachea [48,92]. The reinforced LMA is very useful in paediatric surgery of the head and neck and for dental, ophthalmology and ENT procedures.

Newer non-depolarising muscle relaxants in children

Cisatracurium has an onset time of 2 min and a duration of action of 30 min after a dose of 80–100 μg kg^{-1} [93]. Rocuronium 0.6 mg kg^{-1}, produces good intubating conditions at 90 s and has a duration of action of 24 min. Increasing the dose to 0.8 mg kg^{-1} allows earlier intubation (at about 28 s) but prolongs the duration of block to 32 min [94]. The onset of action is more rapid in children compared with babies or adults. Rocuronium can be used for rapid sequence induction, providing intubating conditions comparable to suxamethonium at 1 min [95].

Analgesia

Local and regional analgesia

Regional anaesthesia produces excellent postoperative analgesia and attenuation of the stress response in infants and children [96–101]. Epidural anaesthesia can decrease the need for postoperative ventilation after tracheo-esophageal fistula repair [102] and reduce the complications and costs following open fundoplication [103,104].

An overall incidence of complications of 0.9 in 1000 blocks, with no complications of peripheral techniques has been reported [105,106]. Descriptions of the technical aspects of regional anaesthesia and management of the child with a block are readily available [107–112]. Pharmacokinetics of local anaesthetics in infants and children have been comprehensively reviewed recently [113]. The technique of threading catheters from the sacral hiatus to position the tip at thoracic or lumbar level [114] reported success rates of 85–96%, particularly in small children but a review of radiographs in babies younger than six months of age [115] found that only 58 catheter tips were considered optimal (67%); 10 were too high (12%) and 17 were coiled at the lumbo-sacral level (20%). Alternatives are use of electrocardiography [116] or stimulating epidural catheters and evaluating muscle contractions.

Ultrasound guidance can be helpful for infraclavicular brachial plexus blockade [117], lumbar plexus block [118], caudal and epidural blocks [118,119].

Continuous catheter techniques are becoming popular in children for femoral, brachial plexus, fascia iliaca, lumbar plexus and sciatic blockade [120–123].

Safe dosing guidelines for racemic bupivacaine in children have been defined [124,125] although racemic bupivacaine is gradually being replaced by ropivacaine or levo-bupivacaine. There is now sufficient paediatric data to recommend either of the new agents [120,126–137]. For continuous epidural levo-bupivacaine the use of a 0.0625% solution appears optimal [130]. For single injection caudal blockade ropivacaine and levo-bupivacaine provide similar postoperative analgesia compared to racemic bupivacaine with slightly less early postoperative motor blockade [126,138,139] with no discernable differences between ropivacaine and levo-bupivacaine [126,132,139]. The esterase systems in tissues, plasma and red blood cells are mature in early life and ester local anaesthetics such as amethocaine (tetracaine) and 2-chloroprocaine are particularly applicable in neonates [18,140–142].

A recent systematic review of paediatric caudal adjuncts has been published [143]. Caution is required in neonates as sedation and apnoea have been noted. Caudally administered preservative-free S(+)-ketamine is more potent than racemate and may reduce neuro-psychiatric effects [144–147]. The same dose given systemically produces a much shorter duration of analgesia [148]. When used for single injection S(+)-ketamine has been found to be more effective in prolonging postoperative pain relief than clonidine [149]. The combination of S(+)-ketamine $1\,mg\,kg^{-1}$ and clonidine $1\,\mu g\,kg^{-1}$ without the concomitant use of local anaesthetics for caudal blockade produced approximately 24 h of adequate postoperative analgesia compared to only 12 h for plain S(+)-ketamine [150]. Adjunct clonidine in the dose range of $1–2\,\mu g\,kg^{-1}$ for single injection caudal blockade will typically double the duration of analgesia compared with plain local anaesthetics [151,152] and addition of approximately $0.1\,\mu g\,kg^{-1}h^{-1}$ will enhance the effect of continuous epidural blockade [153]. The systemic effect of clonidine might be more important than the local action [154]. The routine use of opioids as additives for postoperative analgesia has recently been critically challenged [155]. Although there is a risk of respiratory depression, less dramatic side effects such as itching, nausea and vomiting, urinary retention, and decrease gastrointestinal motility are more troublesome [156,157]. A recent comparison of plain levo-bupivacaine with levo-bupivacaine combined with fentanyl for postoperative epidural analgesia in children, failed to show any major benefit of adjunct fentanyl [130]. Neuraxial administration of opioids still has a place where extensive analgesia is needed, for example after spinal surgery or liver transplantation [158,159] or when adequate spread of local anaesthetic blockade cannot be achieved within dosage limits [140].

The potential benefits and risks of regional anaesthesia for paediatric cardiac surgery have recently been investigated and reviewed [160–163]. Single doses of intrathecal opioids with or without local anaesthetic or continuous spinal anaesthesia using a micro-catheter technique appear particularly promising for open heart surgery, while epidural or paravertebral techniques seem to offer benefit for closed procedures. The main concern is that of local bleeding at the site of subarachnoid or epidural puncture in the heparinised child [160].

Systemic analgesia

Recent evidence has produced more logical dosing guidelines for opioids, NSAIDs and acetaminophen (paracetamol) in children [164–175].

Morphine infusions of between $10–30\,\mu g\,kg^{-1}h^{-1}$ provide adequate analgesia with an acceptable level of side effects when administered with the appropriate level of monitoring [110]. Morphine clearance in-term infants >1 month of age is comparable to children from 1–17 years old. In neonates aged 1–7 days, the clearance of morphine is one-third that of older infants and elimination half-life approximately 1.7 times longer [176,177]. In appropriately selected cases, the subcutaneous route of administration is a useful alternative to the intravenous route [178,179]. The subcutaneous route is contraindicated when the child is hypovolemic or has significant ongoing fluid compartment shifts [180]. Patient-controlled analgesia (PCA) is now widely used in children as young as age 5 years and compares favourably with continuous morphine infusion in the older child [181]. A low dose background infusion is useful in the first 24 h of PCA in children, and has been shown to improve sleep pattern without increasing the adverse effects seen with higher background infusions in children and in adults [182]. Most regimens for nurse or parent-controlled analgesia use a higher level of background infusion with a longer lockout time of around 30 min [110,150,183–186].

Tramadol, oxycodone, hydromorphone may have applicability as alternatives to morphine in the postoperative period [164,187,188]. Pethidine (meperidine) is not recommended in children due to the adverse effects of its main metabolite, norpethidine. Fentanyl, sufentanil, alfentanil and remifentanil may have a role for major surgery and in intensive care practice. Remifentanil is very titrateable, has a context-insensitive half-time with extremely rapid recovery due to esterase clearance but transition to the postoperative phase is difficult to manage and may be complicated by acute tolerance. It may have a particular role in intraoperative stress control and in neonatal anaesthesia [189–193]. Sufentanil and fentanyl have long context-sensitive half-times but give a smoother transition to maintenance analgesia. Alfentanil has a rapid onset, is titrateable, and is relatively context-insensitive after 90 min with a relatively smooth transition in the postoperative phase. The potent opioids may be best delivered by target-controlled infusion devices and paediatric pharmacokinetic programs have now been developed.

NSAIDs are important in the treatment and prevention of mild or moderate pain in children [194]. NSAIDs are highly effective in combination with a local or regional nerve block, particularly in day case surgery [194,195]. NSAIDs are often used in combination with opioids and the "opioid sparing" effect of NSAIDs is 30–40%, as reported for adults [196,197]. This produces a reduction in opioid-related adverse effects, especially ileus, bladder spasms and skeletal muscle spasms, and facilitates more rapid weaning from opioid infusions or PCA [110,183,198–200]. NSAIDs in combination with acetaminophen (paracetamol) produce better analgesia than either alone [194,197,201]. Novel formulations of NSAIDs as eyedrops have found application after strabismus correction or laser surgery to the eye [174]. Pharmacokinetic studies of NSAIDs have revealed a higher than expected dose requirement if scaled by body weight from adult doses [165,202]. NSAIDs should be avoided in infants <6 months of age [194,203], children with aspirin or NSAID allergy, those with dehydration or hypovolemia, children with renal or hepatic failure, coagulation disorders or peptic ulcer disease and where there is a significant risk of haemorrhage. Concurrent administration of NSAIDs with anticoagulants, steroids and nephrotoxic agents is not recommended. The most commonly reported adverse effects of NSAIDs are bleeding, followed by gastrointestinal, skin, central nervous system, pulmonary, hepatic and renal toxic effects. Other serious side effects have been reported, including oedema, bone marrow suppression, and Stevens-Johnson syndrome [175,194,204].

NSAIDs and tonsillectomy

Two recent meta-analyses have considered the role of NSAIDs in post-tonsillectomy haemorrhage [205,206]. One included studies of aspirin which is not recommended in children [206]. The other showed a small increased risk of re-operation for bleeding in patients receiving NSAIDs [205]. However, the authors discuss why clear recommendations cannot be drawn from the evidence as the patients receiving NSAIDs benefited from good pain control and reduced PONV [205]. Thus, for every 100 patients, 2 more will require re-operation if they receive a NSAID than if they do not but 11 will not have PONV who otherwise would [205]. These meta-analyses also did not include studies of COX-2 inhibitors.

NSAIDs and asthma

Provocation of bronchospasm by NSAIDs is thought to be due to a relative excess of leukotriene production. Aspirin sensitivity is present in about 2% of children with asthma and around 5% of these patients are cross-sensitive to other NSAIDs [194]. Caution is required in those with severe eczema or multiple allergies and in those with nasal polyps. It is important to check for past exposure to NSAIDs as many asthmatic children take these agents with no adverse effects [204]. A recent study found no change in lung function in a group of known asthmatic children given a single dose of diclofenac under controlled conditions [207].

NSAIDs and bone healing

Concerns have been raised by animal studies showing impaired bone healing in the presence of NSAIDs [194]. For most orthopaedic surgery in children, the benefits of short-term perioperative use of NSAIDs outweigh the risks but limitation of use is recommended in fusion operations, limb-lengthening procedures and where bone healing has previously been difficult [194].

COX-2 inhibitors in paediatrics

Several COX-2 inhibitors have recently been evaluated in paediatrics although the situation has been complicated by the withdrawal of rofecoxib from worldwide markets [208]. Some early studies used too low a dose [209] and pharmacokinetic studies are now informing dosing schedules and intervals in children [210–212]. The studies show equal efficacy to other analgesic interventions with non-selective NSAIDs or acetaminophen (paracetamol) and a morphine-sparing effect, but trials have not been large enough to confirm reduced adverse effects such as bleeding [213–215].

Acetaminophen (paracetamol)

On its own, acetaminophen can be used to treat or prevent most mild and some moderate pain. In combination with either NSAIDs or weak opioids, such as codeine, it can be used to treat or prevent most moderate pain [197,216]. A morphine-sparing effect has been demonstrated with higher doses in day cases [197,217].

Although the site of action of acetaminophen is central, dosing is often based on a putative "therapeutic plasma concentration" of $10-20 \, mg \, mL^{-1}$. It is important to realise that the time to peak analgesia even after intravenous administration is between 1 and 2 h. The time-concentration profile of acetaminophen in cerebrospinal fluid lags behind that in plasma, with an equilibration half-time of around 45 min. There is evidence that a plasma concentration of $11 \, \mu g \, mL^{-1}$ or more is associated with lower pain scores. In a computer simulation, a plasma concentration of $25 \, \mu g \, mL^{-1}$ was predicted to result in good pain control in up to 60% of children undergoing tonsillectomy [166–169,197,218]. Dosing regimens for acetaminophen have been revised in the last few years on the basis of age, route of administration, loading dose, maintenance dose and duration of therapy to ensure a reasonable balance between efficacy and safety. In younger infants, sick children, and the pre-term neonate, considerable downward dose adjustments are needed.

Analgesic doses for children

Table 20.1 shows suggested maximum dosages of bupivacaine, levo-bupivacaine, and ropivacaine in infants and children, Table 20.2 shows opioids: relative potency and

Table 20.1. Dosages of bupivacaine, levo-bupivacaine, and ropivacaine

Single bolus injection	*Maximum dosage*
Neonates	$2 \, mg \, kg^{-1}$
Children	$2.5 \, mg \, kg^{-1}$
Continuous postoperative infusion	*Maximum infusion rate*
Neonates	$0.2 \, mg \, kg^{-1} h^{-1}$
Children	$0.4 \, mg \, kg^{-1} h^{-1}$

dosing, Table 20.3 shows context-sensitive half-times of opioids in children, and Table 20.4 shows acetaminophen (paracetamol) dosing guide.

Table 20.2. Opioids: relative potency and dosing

Drug	Potency relative to morphine	Single dose	Continuous infusion
Tramadol	0.1	$1\text{--}2\,\text{mg}\,\text{kg}^{-1}$	
Morphine	1	$0.05\text{--}0.2\,\text{mg}\,\text{kg}^{-1}$	$10\text{--}40\,\mu\text{g}\,\text{kg}^{-1}\text{h}^{-1}$
Hydromorphone	5	$0.01\text{--}0.03\,\text{mg}\,\text{kg}^{-1}$	
Alfentanil	10	$5\text{--}10\,\mu\text{g}\,\text{kg}^{-1}$	$\cdot\text{--}4\,\mu\text{g}\,\text{kg}^{-1}\text{min}^{-1}$ or use TCI system
Fentanyl	50–100	$0.5\text{--}1\,\mu\text{g}\,\text{kg}^{-1}$	$0.1\text{--}0.2\,\mu\text{g}\,\text{kg}^{-1}\text{min}^{-1}$
Remifentanil	50–100	$0.1\text{--}1\,\mu\text{g}\,\text{kg}^{-1}$	$0.05\text{--}4\,\mu\text{g}\,\text{kg}^{-1}\text{min}^{-1}$ or use TCI system
Sufentanil	500–1000	$0.25\text{--}0.5\,\mu\text{g}\,\text{kg}^{-1}$	Use TCI system

Table 20.3. Context-sensitive half-times of opioids in children (minutes)

Infusion Duration (min)	10	100	200	300	600
Remifentanil	3–6	3–6	3–6	3–6	3–6
Alfentanil	10	45	55	58	60
Sufentanil		20	25	35	60
Fentanyl	12	30	100	200	

Table 20.4. Acetaminophen (paracetamol) dosing guide

Age	Oral		Rectal		Maximum daily dose oral or rectal	Duration at maximum dose
	Loading dose	Maintenance dose	Loading dose	Maintenance dose		
Pre-term 28–32 w	$20\,\text{mg}\,\text{kg}^{-1}$	$15\,\text{mg}\,\text{kg}^{-1}$ up to 12 hourly	$20\,\text{mg}\,\text{kg}^{-1}$	$15\,\text{mg}\,\text{kg}^{-1}$ up to 12 hourly	$35\,\text{mg}\,\text{kg}^{-1}\text{day}^{-1}$	48 h
Pre-term 32–38 w	$20\,\text{mg}\,\text{kg}^{-1}$	$20\,\text{mg}\,\text{kg}^{-1}$ up to 8 hourly	$30\,\text{mg}\,\text{kg}^{-1}$	$20\,\text{mg}\,\text{kg}^{-1}$ up to 12 hourly	$60\,\text{mg}\,\text{kg}^{-1}\text{day}^{-1}$	48 h
0–3 m	$20\,\text{mg}\,\text{kg}^{-1}$	$20\,\text{mg}\,\text{kg}^{-1}$ up to 8 hourly	$30\,\text{mg}\,\text{kg}^{-1}$	$20\,\text{mg}\,\text{kg}^{-1}$ up to 12 hourly	$60\,\text{mg}\,\text{kg}^{-1}\text{day}^{-1}$	48 h
>3 m	$20\,\text{mg}\,\text{kg}^{-1}$	$15\,\text{mg}\,\text{kg}^{-1}$ up to 4 hourly	$40\,\text{mg}\,\text{kg}^{-1}$	$20\,\text{mg}\,\text{kg}^{-1}$ up to 6 hourly	$90\,\text{mg}\,\text{kg}^{-1}\text{day}^{-1}$	72 h

Postoperative nausea and vomiting

Ondansetron $100\,\mu g\,kg^{-1}$ prevents nausea and vomiting more effectively than placebo or droperidol [219–222]. Granisetron is more effective in children than droperidol or metoclopramide especially when given with dexamethasone [223–225].

Practice points

- Oral midazolam is the most commonly used as premedication.
- Inhalational induction of anaesthesia has undergone a renaissance with the introduction of sevoflurane.
- Desflurane maintenance may be particularly useful for neonates.
- Tracheal intubation can be performed safely and effectively in children without muscle relaxants and cuffed tracheal tubes are now more widely used.
- The LMA is very commonly used in paediatric anaesthesia for elective cases and can also be useful in children with difficult airways.
- New muscle relaxants have been evaluated in children and rocuronium is particularly useful for modified rapid sequence induction.
- Local and regional analgesia techniques are now routinely used in paediatric practice and ultrasound guidance may be useful.
- New local anaesthetics such as levo-bupivacaine and ropivacaine have improved the safety of both single injection blocks and continuous infusion techniques.
- The adjuncts clonidine and ketamine have been evaluated for caudal epidural blockade and are now in common use.
- Safe dosing regimens for opioids, NSAIDs and paracetamol have evolved for use in children.
- PONV prevention by 5HT3 antagonists and steroids has proven to be very effective for children at high risk.

Conclusion

The topics selected in this review have been chosen to illustrate changes in clinical practice in the last 15 years. Although formal evidence-based systematic reviews or meta-analyses are relatively few, there is now a fairly robust basis for modern paediatric anaesthesia techniques and practices.

REFERENCES

1 RCA (2003) Raising the standard: information for patients. London, Royal College of Anaesthetists.

2 Bevan J, Johnston C, Haig M et al. Preoperative parental anxiety predicts behavioural and emotional responses to induction of anaesthesia in children. *Can J Anaesth* 1990; 37: 177–82.

3 Hannallah RS. Who benefits when parents are present during anaesthesia induction in their children? *Can J Anaesth* 1994; 41: 271–5.

4 Hannallah RS, Rosales JK. Experience with parents' presence during anaesthesia induction in children. *Can Anaesth Soc J* 1983; 30: 286–9.

5 Thompson N, Irwin MG, Gunawardene WMS et al. Pre-operative parental anxiety. *Anaesthesia* 1996; 51: 1008–12.

6 Kain ZN, Ferris CA, Mayes LC et al. Parental presence during induction of anaesthesia: practice differences between the United States and Great Britain. *Paediatr Anaesth* 1996; 6: 187–93.

7 McCormick ASM, Spargo PM. Parents in the anaesthetic room: a questionnaire survey of departments of anaesthesia. *Paediatr Anaesth* 1996; 6: 183–6.

8 Thornes R (1991). Caring for Children in the Helath Services Just for the Day. NAWCH, London: Action for Sick Children.

9 Campbell IR, Scaife JM, Johnstone JMS. Psychological effects of day case surgery compared with inpatient surgery. *Arch Dis Child* 1988; 63: 415–17.

10 Phillips S, Daborn AK, Hatch DJ. Preoperative fasting for paediatric anaesthesia. *Br J Anaesth* 1994; 73: 529–31.

11 Cote CJ, Goudsouian NG, Liu LMP et al. Assessment of risk factors related to the acid aspiration syndrome in paediatric patients – gastric pH and residual volume. *Anesthesiology* 1982; 56: 70–2.

12 Manchikanti L, Colliver JA, Marrero TC et al. Assessment of age-related acid aspiration risk factors in pediatric, adult and geriatric patients. *Anesth Analg* 1985; 64: 11–17.

13 Cavell B. Gastric emptying in preterm infants. *Acta Paediatr Scand* 1979; 68: 527–31.

14 Cavell B. Gastric emptying in infants fed human milk or infant formula. *Acta Paediatr Scand* 1981; 70: 639–41.

15 Schurizek BA, Rybro L, Boggild-Madsen NB et al. Gastric volume and pH in children for emergency surgery. *Acta Anaesthesiol Scand* 1986; 30: 404–8.

16 Freeman JA, Doyle E, Ng TI et al. Topical anaesthesia of the skin: a review. *Paediatr Anaesth* 1993; 3: 129–38.

17 Lawson RA, Morton NS. Amethocaine gel for percutaneous local anaesthesia. In: Bernard Dalens and Isabelle Murat(eds). *Hosp Med* July 1998; 59: 564–6.

18 Lawson RA, Smart NG, Gudgeon AC, Morton NS. Evaluation of an amethocaine gel preparation for percutaneous analgesia before venous cannulation in children. *Br J Anaesth* 1995; 75: 282–5.

19 McCluskey A, Meakin GH. Oral administration of midazolam as a premedicant for paediatric day-case anaesthesia. *Anaesthesia* 1994; 49: 782–5.

20 Cray SH, Dixon JL, Heard CMB et al. Oral midazolam premedication for paediatric day case patients. *Paediatr Anaesth* 1996; 6: 265–70.

21 McGraw T. Oral midazolam and postoperative behaviour in children. *Can J Anaesth* 1993; 40: 682–3.

22 Acil M, Basgul E, Celiker V, Karagoz AH, Demir B, Aypar U. Perioperative effects of melatonin and midazolam premedication on sedation, orientation, anxiety scores and psychomotor performance. *Eur J Anaesthesiol* 2004; 21: 553–7.

23 Samarkandi A, Naguib M, Riad W, Thalaj A, Alotibi W, Aldammas F, Albassam A. Melatonin vs. midazolam premedication in children: a double-blind, placebo-controlled study. *Eur J Anaesthesiol* 2005; 22: 189–96.

24 Bergendahl HT, Lonnqvist PA, Eksborg S, Ruthstrom E, Nordenberg L, Zetterqvist H, Oddby E. Clonidine vs. midazolam as premedication in children undergoing adeno-tonsillectomy: a prospective, randomized, controlled clinical trial. *Acta Anaesthesiol Scand* 2004; 48: 1292–300.

25 Friesen RH, Carpenter E, Madigan CK et al. Oral transmucosal fentanyl citrate for preanaesthetic medication of paediatric cardiac surgery patients. *Paediatr Anaesth* 1995; 5: 29–31.

26 Binstock W, Rubin R, Bachman C, Kahana M, Mcdade W, Lynch JP. The effect of premedication with OTFC, with or without ondansetron, on postoperative agitation, and nausea and vomiting in pediatric ambulatory patients. *Paediatr Anaesth* 2004; 14: 759–67.

27 Patel SS, Goa KL. Sevoflurane. A review of its pharmacodynamic and pharmacokinetic properties and its clinical use in general anaesthesia. *Drugs* 1996; 51: 658–700.

28 Dubois MC, Piat V, Constant I, Lamblin O, Murat I. Comparison of three techniques for induction of anaesthesia with sevoflurane in children. *Paediatr Anaesth* 1999; 9: 19–23.

29 Epstein RH, Stein AL, Marr AT, Lessin JB. High concentration versus incremental induction of anesthesia with sevoflurane in children: a comparison of induction times, vital signs, and complications. *J Clin Anesth* 1998; 10: 41–5.

30 Morimoto Y, Mayhew JF, Knox SL, Zornow MH. Rapid induction of anesthesia with high concentrations of halothane or sevoflurane in children. *J Clin Anesth* 2000; 12: 184–8.

31 Kataria B, Epstein RH, Bailey A et al. A comparison of sevoflurane to halothane in paediatric surgical patients: results of a multicentre international study. *Paediatr Anaesth* 1996; 6: 283–92.

32 Ho KY, Chua WL, Lim SS, Ng AS. A comparison between single- and double-breath vital capacity inhalation induction with 8% sevoflurane in children. *Paediatr Anaesth* 2004; 14: 457–61.

33 Wappler F, Frings DP, Scholz J, Mann V, Koch C, Schulte Am Esch J. Inhalational induction of anaesthesia with 8% sevoflurane in children: conditions for endotracheal intubation and side-effects. *Eur J Anaesthesiol* 2003; 20: 548–54.

34 Fernandez M, Lejus C, Rivault O, Bazin V, Le Roux C, Bizouarn P, Pinaud M. Single-breath vital capacity rapid inhalation induction with sevoflurane: feasibility in children. *Paediatr Anaesth* 2005; 15: 307–13.

35 Yurino M, Kimura H. Vital capacity rapid inhalational induction technique: comparison of sevoflurane and halothane. *Can J Anaesth* 1993; 40: 440–3.

36 Katoh T, Ikeda K. Minimum alveolar concentration of sevoflurane in children. *Br J Anaesth* 1992; 68: 139–41.

37 Lerman J, Sikich N, Kleinman S et al. The pharmacology of sevoflurane in infants and children. *Anesthesiology* 1994; 80: 814–24.

38 Kihara S, Inomata S, Yaguchi Y, Toyooka H, Baba Y, Kohda Y. The awakening concentration of sevoflurane in children. *Anesth Analg* 2000; 91: 305–8.

39 Sury MR, Black A, Hemington L et al. A comparison of the recovery characteristics of sevoflurane and halothane in children. *Anaesthesia* 1996; 51: 543–6.

40 Landais A, Saint-Maurice CP, Hamza J, Al E. Sevoflurane elimination kinetics in children. *Paediatr Anaesth* 1995; 5: 297–301.

41 Beskow A, Westrin P. Sevoflurane causes more postoperative agitation in children than does halothane. *Acta Anaesthesiol Scand* 1999; 43: 536–41.

42 Kain ZN, Caldwell-Andrews AA, Weinberg ME, Mayes LC, Wang SM, Gaal D, Saadat H, Maranets I. Sevoflurane versus halothane: postoperative maladaptive behavioral changes: a randomized, controlled trial. *Anesthesiology* 2005; 102: 720–6.

43 Kawana S, Wachi J, Nakayama M, Namiki A. Comparison of haemodynamic changes induced by sevoflurane and halothane in paediatric patients. *Can J Anaesth* 1995; 42: 603–7.

44 Lerman J, Davis PJ, Welborn LG, Orr RJ, Rabb M, Carpenter R, Motoyama E, Hannallah R, Haberkern CM. Induction, recovery, and safety characteristics of sevoflurane in children undergoing ambulatory surgery. A comparison with halothane. *Anesthesiology* 1996; 84: 1332–40.

45 Sarner JB, Levine M, Davis PJ, Lerman J, Cook DR, Motoyama EK. Clinical characteristics of sevoflurane in children. A comparison with halothane. *Anesthesiology* 1995; 82: 38–46.

46 Mori N, Suzuki M. Sevoflurane in paediatric anaesthesia: effects on respiration and circulation during induction and recovery. *Paediatr Anaesth* 1996; 6: 95–102.

47 Kern C, Erb T, Frei FJ. Haemodynamic responses to sevoflurane compared with halothane during inhalational induction in children. *Paediatr Anaesth* 1997; 7: 439–40.

48 Walker RWM, Allen DL, Rothera MR. A fibreoptic intubation technique for children with mucopolysaccharidoses using the laryngeal mask airway. *Paediatr Anaesth* 1997; 7: 421–6.

49 Meretoja OA, Taivainen T, Raiha L, Al E. Sevoflurane-nitrous oxide or halothane-nitrous oxide for paediatric bronchoscopy or gastroscopy. *Br J Anaesth* 1996a; 76: 767–71.

50 Kwek TK, Ng A. Laryngeal mask insertion following inhalational induction in children: a comparison between halothane and sevoflurane. *Anaesth Intens Care* 1997; 25: 413–16.

51 O'Brien K, Kumar R, Morton NS. Sevoflurane compared with halothane for tracheal intubation in children. *Br J Anaesth* 1998a; 80: 452–5.

52 Inomata S, Yamashita S, Toyooka H, Al E. Anaesthetic induction time for tracheal intubation using sevoflurane or halothane in children. *Anaesthesia* 1998; 53: 440–5.

53 Otsuka H, Komura Y, Mayumi T, Al E. Malignant hyperthermia during sevoflurane anaesthesia in a child with central core disease. *Anesthesiology* 1994; 75: 699–701.

54 Komatsu H, Taie DS, Endo S, Al E. Electrical seizures during sevoflurane anesthesia in two pediatric patients with epilepsy. *Anesthesiology* 1994; 81: 1535–7.

55 Constant I, Seeman R, Murat I. Sevoflurane and epileptiform EEG changes. *Paediatr Anaesth* 2005; 15: 266–74.

56 Johr M, Berger TM. Paediatric anaesthesia and inhalation agents. *Best Prac Res Clin Anaesthesiol* 2005; 19: 501–22.

57 Fisher DM, Zwass MS. MAC of desflurane in 60% nitrous oxide in infants and children. *Anesthesiology* 1992; 76: 354–6.

58 Taylor RH, Lerman J. Induction, maintenance and recovery characteristics of desflurane in infants and children. *Can J Anaesth* 1992; 39: 6–13.

59 Zwass MS, Fisher DM, Welborn LG, Cote CJ, Davis PJ, Dinner M, Hannallah RS, Liu LM, Sarner J, Mcgill WA et al. Induction and maintenance characteristics of anesthesia with desflurane and nitrous oxide in infants and children. *Anesthesiology* 1992; 76: 373–8.

60 Davis PJ, Cohen IT, Mcgowan FXJ, Latta K. Recovery characteristics of desflurane versus halothane for maintenance of anesthesia in pediatric ambulatory patients. *Anesthesiology* 1994; 80: 298–302.

61 Lerman J. Inhalational anesthetics. *Paediatr Anaesth* 2004; 14: 380–3.

62 O'Brien K, Robinson DN, Morton NS. Induction and emergence in infants less than 60 weeks post-conceptual age: comparison of thiopental, halothane, sevoflurane and desflurane. *Br J Anaesth* 1998b; 80: 456–9.

63 Kotiniemi LH, Ryhanen PT, Moilanen IK. Behavioural changes following routine ENT operations in two to ten year old children. *Paediatr Anaesth* 1996; 6: 45–9.

64 Kotiniemi LH, Ryhanen PT. Behavioural changes and children's memories after intravenous, inhalational and rectal induction of anaesthesia. *Paediatr Anaesth* 1996; 6: 201–7.

65 Cameron E, Johnston G, Crofts S, Morton NS. The minimum effective dose of lignocaine to prevent injection pain due to propofol in children. *Anaesthesia* 1992; 47: 604–6.

66 Morton NS. Abolition of injection pain due to propofol in children. *Anaesthesia* 1990; 45: 70.

67 Morton NS, Wee M, Christie G, Gray IG, Grant IS. Propofol for induction of anaesthesia in children. A comparison with thiopentone and halothane inhalational induction. *Anaesthesia* 1988; 43: 350–5.

68 Purcell-Jones G, Yates A, Baker JR, James IG. Comparison of the induction characteristics of thiopentone and propofol in children. *Br J Anaesth* 1987; 59: 1431–6.

69 Runcie CJ, Mackenzie SJ, Arthur DS, Morton NS. Comparison of recovery from anaesthesia induced in children with either propofol or thiopentone. *Br J Anaesth* 1993; 70: 192–5.

70 Morton NS. Total intravenous anaesthesia (TIVA) in paediatrics: advantages and disadvantages. [see comment]. *Paediatr Anaesth* 1998b; 8: 189–94.

71 Grundmann U, Uth M, Eichner A, Wilhelm W, Larsen R. Total intravenous anaesthesia with propofol and remifentanil in paediatric patients: a comparison with a desflurane-nitrous oxide inhalation anaesthesia. *Acta Anaesthesiol Scand* 1998; 42: 845–50.

72 Laycock GJ, Mitchell IM, Paton RD, Donaghey SF, Logan RW, Morton NS. EEG burst suppression with propofol during cardiopulmonary bypass in children: a study of the haemodynamic, metabolic and endocrine effects. *Br J Anaesth* 1992; 69: 356–62.

73 Usher AG, Kearney RA, Tsui BC. Propofol total intravenous anesthesia for MRI in children. [see comment]. *Paediatr Anaesth* 2005; 15: 23–8.

74 Browne BL, Prys-Roberts C, Wolf AR. Propofol and alfentanil in children: infusion technique and dose requirements for total intravenous anaesthesia. *Br J Anaesth* 1992; 69: 570–6.

75 Kataria BK, Ved SA, Nicodemus HF, Hoy GR, Lea D, Dubois MY, Mandema JW, Shafer SL. The pharmacokinetics of propofol in children using three different data analysis approaches. [see comment]. *Anesthesiology* 1994; 80: 104–22.

76 Doyle E, Mcfadzean W, Morton NS. IV anaesthesia with propofol using a target-controlled infusion system: comparison with inhalation anaesthesia for general surgical procedures in children. *Br J Anaesth* 1993b; 70: 542–5.

77 Varveris DA, Morton NS. Target controlled infusion of propofol for induction and maintenance of anaesthesia using the paedfusor: an open pilot study. *Paediatr Anaesth* 2002; 12: 589–93.

78 Marsh B, White M, Morton N, Kenny GN. Pharmacokinetic model driven infusion of propofol in children. [see comment]. *Br J Anaesth* 1991; 67: 41–8.

79 Munoz HR, Cortinez LI, Ibacache ME, Altermatt FR. Estimation of the plasma effect site equilibration rate constant (ke0) of propofol in children using the time to peak effect: comparison with adults. *Anesthesiology* 2004; 101: 1269–74.

80 Robinson DN, O'Brien K, Kumar R, Morton NS. Tracheal intubation without neuromuscular blockade in children: a comparison of propofol combined either with alfentanil or remifentanil. *Paediatr Anaesth* 1998; 8: 467–71.

81 Senel AC, Akturk G, Yurtseven M. Comparison of intubation conditions under propofol in children–alfentanil vs atracurium. *Middle East J Anesthesiol* 1996; 13: 605–11.

82 Crawford MW, Hayes J, Tan JM. Dose-response of remifentanil for tracheal intubation in infants. *Anesth Analg* 2005; 100: 1599–604.

83 Steyn MP, Quinn AM, Gillespie JA, Miller DC, Best CJ, Morton NS. Tracheal intubation without neuromuscular block in children. [see comment]. *Br J Anaesth* 1994; 72: 403–6.

84 Newth CJ, Rachman B, Patel N, Hammer J. The use of cuffed versus uncuffed endotracheal tubes in pediatric intensive care. *J Pediatr* 2004; 144: 333–7.

85 Dullenkopf A, Gerber A, Weiss M. The Microcuff tube allows a longer time interval until unsafe cuff pressures are reached in children. *Can J Anaesth* 2004; 51: 997–1001.

86 Weiss M, Gerber AC, Dullenkopf A. Appropriate placement of intubation depth marks in a new cuffed paediatric tracheal tube. *Br J Anaesth* 2005; 94: 80–7.

87 O'Neill B, Josephine B, Caramico L et al. The laryngeal mask airway in pediatric patients: factors affecting ease of use during insertion and emergence. *Anesth Analg* 1994; 78: 659–62.

88 Rowbottom SJ, Simpson DL, Grubb D. The laryngeal mask airway in children. A fibreoptic assessment of positioning. *Anaesthesia* 1991; 46: 659–62.

89 Goudzouzian NG, Denman W, Cleveland R et al. Radiologic localization of the laryngeal mask airway in children. *Anesthesiology* 1992; 77: 1085–9.

90 Lopez-Gil M, Brimacombe J. Safety and efficacy of the laryngeal mask airway. A prospective study of 1400 children. *Anaesthesia* 1996; 51: 969–72.

91 Vergese C, Smith TGC, Young E. Prospective survey of the use of the laryngeal mask airway in 2359 patients. *Anaesthesia* 1993; 48: 58–60.

92 Hasan MA, Black AE. A new technique for fibreoptic intubation in children. *Anaesthesia* 1994; 49: 1031–4.

93 Meretoja OA, Taivainen T, Wirtavuori K. Cisatracurium during halothane and balanced anaesthesia in children. *Paediatr Anaesth* 1996b; 6: 373–8.

94 Kelly O, Frossard J, Meistelman C, Al E. Neuromuscular blockade following Org 9426 in children during nitrous oxide-halothane anaesthesia. *Anesthesiology* 1991; 75: A787.

95 Stoddart PA, Mather SJ. Onset of neuromuscular blockade and intubating conditions one minute after the administration of rocuronium in children. *Paediatr Anaesth* 1998; 8: 37–40.

96 Ross AK, Eck JB, Tobias JD. Pediatric regional anesthesia: beyond the caudal. *Anesth Analg* 2000; 91: 16–26.

97 De Negri P, Ivani G, Tirri T, Favullo L, Nardelli A. New drugs, new techniques, new indications in pediatric regional anesthesia. *Minerva Anestesiol* 2002; 68: 420–7.

98 Dalens B. Some open questions in pediatric regional anesthesia. *Minerva Anestesiol* 2003; 69: 451–6.

99 Bosenberg A. Pediatric regional anesthesia update. *Paediatr Anaesth* 2004; 14: 398–402.

100 Wolf AR, Eyres RL, Laussen PC, Edwards J, Stanley IJ, Rowe P, Simon L. Effect of extradural analgesia on stress responses to abdominal surgery in infants. *Br J Anaesth* 1993; 70: 654–60.

101 Wolf AR, Doyle E, Thomas E. Modifying infant stress responses to major surgery: spinal vs extradural vs opioid analgesia. *Paediatr Anaesth* 1998; 8: 305–11.

102 Bosenberg AT, Hadley GP, Wiersma R. Oesophageal atresia: caudo-thoracic epidural anaesthesia reduces the need for post-operative ventilatory support. *Pediatr Surg* 1992; 7: 289–91.

103 McNeely JK, Farber NE, Rusy LM, Hoffman GM. Epidural analgesia improves outcome following pediatric fundoplication. A retrospective analysis. *Reg Anesth Pain Med* 1997; 22: 16–23.

104 Wilson GA, Brown JL, Crabbe DG, Al E. Is epidural analgesia associated with an improved outcome following open Nissen fundoplication? *Paediatr Anaesth* 2001; 11: 65–70.

105 Giaufre E, Dalens B, Gombert A. Epidemiology and morbidity of regional anesthesia in children: a one-year prospective survey of the French-Language Society of Pediatric Anesthesiologists. *Anesth Analg* 1996; 83: 904–12.

106 Dalens B. Complications in paediatric regional anaesthesia. In: Dalens B, Murat I, G, B. (eds). *Proceedings of 4th European Congress of Paediatric Anaesthesia*. Paris: ADARPEF, FEAPA, 1997.

107 Cupples P, McNicol R. Common local anaesthetic techniques in children. *Anaesth Intensive Care Med* 2001; 1: 132–7.

108 Dalens B. Regional Anesthesia in Infants, Children and Adolescents. London: Williams & Wilkins Waverly Europe, 1995.

109 Peutrell JM, Mather SJ. *Regional Anaesthesia in Babies and Children*. Oxford, UK: Oxford University Press, 1997.

110 Morton NS. Acute Paediatric Pain Management – a practical guide. London: WB Saunders, 1998a.

111 Morton NS, Peutrell JM. Paediatric anaesthesia and critical care in the district hospital: a practical guide. Oxford: Butterworth-Heinemann Medical, 2003.

112 Morton NS. Local and regional anaesthesia in infants. Continuing Education in Anaesthesia. *Crit Care Pain* 2004; 4: 148–51.

113 Mazoit JX, Dalens BJ. Pharmacokinetics of local anaesthetics in infants and children. *Clin Pharmacokinetic* 2004; 43: 17–32.

114 Bosenberg AT, Bland BA, Schulte-Steinberg O, Al E. Thoracic epidural anesthesia via caudal route in infants. *Anesthesiology* 1988; 69: 265–9.

115 Valairucha S, Seefelder C, Houck C. Thoracic epidural catheters placed by the caudal route in infants: the importance of radiographic confirmation. *Paediatr Anaesth* 2002; 12: 424–8.

116 Tsui BCH, Seal R, Koller J. Thoracic epidural catheter placement via the caudal approach in infants by using electrocardiographic guidance. *Anesth Analg* 2002; 95: 326–30.

117 Kirchmair L, Enna B, Mitterschiffthaler G, Moriggl B, Greher M, Marhofer P, Kapral S, Gassner I. Lumbar plexus in children. A sonographic study and its relevance to pediatric regional anesthesia. *Anesthesiology* 2004; 101: 445–50.

118 Marhofer P, Greher M, Kapral S. Ultrasound guidance in regional anaesthesia. *Br J Anaesth* 2005; 94(1): 1–3.

119 Chawathe MS, Jones RM, Koller J. Detection of epidural catheters with ultrasound in children. *Paediatr Anaesth* 2003; 13: 681–4.

120 Ivani G, Tonetti F. Postoperative analgesia in infants and children: new developments. *Minerva Anestesiol* 2004; 70: 399–403.

121 Dadure C, Raux O, Troncin R, Rochette A, Capdevila X. Continuous infraclavicular brachial plexus block for acute pain management in children. *Anesth Analg* 2003; 97: 691–3.

122 Dadure C, Acosta C, Capdevila X. Perioperative pain management of a complex orthopedic surgical procedure with double continuous nerve blocks in a burned child. *Anesth Analg* 2004a; 98: 1653–5.

123 Dadure C, Raux O, Gaudard P, Sagintaah M, Troncin R, Rochette A, Capdevila X. Continuous psoas compartment blocks after major orthopedic surgery in children: a prospective computed tomographic scan and clinical studies. *Anesth Analg* 2004b; 98: 623–8.

124 Berde CB. Toxicity of local anesthetics in infants and children. *J Pediatrics* 1993; 122: S14–20.

125 Wolf AR, Valley RD, Fear DW, Roy WL, Lerman J. Bupivacaine for caudal analgesia in infants and children: the optimal effective concentration. *Anesthesiology* 1988; 69: 102–6.

126 Ivani G, Denegri P, Conio A, Grossetti R, Vitale P, Vercellino C, Gagliardi F, Eksborg S, Lonnqvist PA. Comparison of racemic bupivacaine, ropivacaine, and levo-bupivacaine for pediatric caudal anesthesia: effects on postoperative analgesia and motor block. *Reg Anesth Pain Med* 2002; 27: 157–61.

127 Ivani G. Ropivacaine: is it time for children? *Paediatr Anaesth* 2002; 12: 383–7.

128 Morton NS. Ropivacaine in children. *Br J Anaesth* 2000; 85: 344–6.

129 Taylor R, Eyres R, Chalkiadis GA, Austin S. Efficacy and safety of caudal injection of levobupivacaine 0.25% in children under 2 years of age undergoing inguinal hernia repair, circumcision or orchidopexy. *Paediatr Anaesth* 2003; 13: 114–21.

130 Lerman J, Nolan J, Eyres R, Schily M, Stoddart P, Bolton CM, Mazzeo F, Wolf AR. Efficacy, safety, and pharmacokinetics of levobupivacaine with and without fentanyl after continuous epidural infusion in children: a multicenter trial. *Anesthesiology* 2003; 99: 1166–74.

131 Chalkiadis GA, Eyres RL, Cranswick N, Taylor RH, Austin S. Pharmacokinetics of levobupivacaine 0.25% following caudal administration in children under 2 years of age. *Br J Anaesth* 2004; 92: 218–22.

132 Ivani G, Mereto N, Lamgpugnani E, De Negri P, Torre M, Mattioloi G, Jasonni V, Lonnqvist PA. Ropivacaine in paediatric surgery: preliminary results. *Paediatr Anaesth* 1998; 8: 127–130.

133 Ivani G, De Negri P, Lonnqvist PA, L'Erario M, Mossetti V, Difilippo A, Rosso F. Caudal anesthesia for minor pediatric surgery: ropivacaine 0.2% vs. levobupivacaine 0.2%. *Paediatr Anaesth* 2005; 15(6): 491–4.

134 Rapp HJ, Molnar V, Austin S, Krohn S, Gadeke V, Motsch J, Boos K, Williams DG, Gustafsson J, Huledal G, Larsson LE. Ropivacaine in neonates and infants: a population pharmacokinetic evaluation following single caudal block. *Paediatr Anaesth* 2004; 14: 724–32.

135 Bosenberg AT, Cronje L, Thomas J, Lopez T, Crean PM, Gustafsson U, Huledal G, Larsson LE. Ropivacaine plasma levels and postoperative analgesia in neonates and infants during 48–72 h continuous epidural infusion following major surgery. *Paediatr Anaesth* 2003; 13: 851–2.

136 Yaster M, Berde CB, Meretoja O, Huledal G, Lybeck A, Larsson LE. Pharmacokinetics, safety and efficacy of 24–72 h epidural infusion of ropivacaine in 1–9 year old children. *Paediatr Anaesth* 2002; 12: 98–9.

137 Dalens B, Ecoffey C, Joly A, Giaufre E, Gustafsson U, Huledal G, Larsson LE. Pharmacokinetics and analgesic effect of ropivacaine following ilioinguinal/iliohypogastric nerve block in children. *Paediatr Anaesth* 2001; 11: 415–20.

138 Da Conceicao MJ, Coelho L, Khalil M. Ropivacaine 0.25% compared with bupivacaine 0.25% by the caudal route. *Paediatr Anaesth* 1999; 9: 229–33.

139 De Negri P, Ivani G, Tirri T, Modano P, Reato C, Eksborg S, Lonnqvist PA. A comparison of epidural bupivacaine, levobupivacaine, and ropivacaine on postoperative analgesia and motor blockade. *Anesth Analg* 2004; 99: 45–8.

140 Berde C. Local anaesthetics in infants and children: an update. *Paediatr Anaesth* 2004; 14: 387–93.

141 Watson DM. Topical amethocaine in strabismus surgery. *Anaesthesia* 1991; 46: 368–70.

142 Long CP, McCafferty DF, Sittlington NM, Halliday HL, Woolfson AD, Jones DS. Randomized trial of novel tetracaine patch to provide local anaesthesia in neonates undergoing venepuncture. *Br J Anaesth* 2003; 91: 514–18.

143 Ansermino M, Basu R, Vandebeek C, Montgomery C. Nonopioid additives to local anaesthetics for caudal blockade in children: a systematic review. *Paediatr Anaesth* 2003; 13: 561–73.

144 Naguib M, Sharif AMY, Seraj M, El-Gammal M, Dawlatly AA. Ketamine for caudal analgesia in children: comparison with caudal bupivacaine. *Br J Anaesth* 1991; 67: 559–64.

145 Cook B, Grubb DJ, Aldridge LA, Doyle E. Comparison of the effects of adrenaline, clonidine and ketamine on the duration of caudal analgesia produced by bupivacaine in children. *Br J Anaesth* 1995; 75: 698–701.

146 Koinig H, Marhofer P. S(+)-ketamine in paediatric anaesthesia. *Paediatr Anaesth* 2003; 13: 185–7.

147 Marhofer P, Krenn CG, Plochl W, Wallner T, Glaser C, Koinig H, Fleischmann E, Hochtl A, Semsroth M. S(+)-ketamine for caudal block in paediatric anaesthesia. *Br J Anaesth* 2000; 84: 341–5.

148 Martindale SJ, Dix P, Stoddart PA. Double-blind randomized controlled trial of caudal versus intravenous S(+)- ketamine for supplementation of caudal analgesia in children. *Br J Anaesth* 2004; 92: 344–7.

149 De Negri P, Ivani G, Visconti C, De Vivo P. How to prolong postoperative analgesia after caudal anaesthesia with ropivacaine in children: S-ketamine versus clonidine. *Paediatr Anaesth* 2001a; 11: 679–83.

150 Hager H, Marhofer P, Sitzwohl C, Adler L, Kettner S, Semsroth M. Caudal clonidine prolongs analgesia from caudal S(+)-ketamine in children. *Anesth Analg* 2002; 94: 1169–72.

151 Lee JJ, Rubin AP. Comparison of a bupivacaine-clonidine mixture with plain bupivacaine for caudal analgesia in children. *Br J Anaesth* 1994; 72: 258–62.

152 Jamali S, Monin S, Begon C, Dubousset AM, Ecoffey C. Clonidine in pediatric caudal anesthesia. *Anesth Analg* 1994; 78: 663–6.

153 De Negri P, Ivani G, Visconti C, De Vivo P, Lönnqvist PA. The dose-response relationship for clonidine added to a postoperative continuous epidural infusion of ropivacaine in children. *Anesth Analg* 2001b; 93: 71–6.

154 Hansen TG, Henneberg SW, Walther-Larsen S, Lund J, Hansen M. Caudal bupivacaine supplemented with caudal or intravenous clonidine in children undergoing hypospadias repair: a double-blind study. *Br J Anaesth* 2004; 92: 223–7.

155 Lonnqvist PA, Ivani G, Moriarty T. Use of caudal-epidural opioids in children: still state of the art or the beginning of the end? *Paediatr Anaesth* 2002; 12: 747–9.

156 Lloyd-Thomas AR, Howard RF. A pain service for children. *Paediatr Anaesth* 1994; 4: 3–15.

157 Kim TW, Harbott M. The use of caudal morphine for pediatric liver transplantation. *Anesth Analg* 2004; 99: 373–4.

158 De Beer DA, Thomas ML. Caudal additives in children-solutions or problems? *Br J Anaesth* 2003; 90: 487–98.

159 Tobias JD. A review of intrathecal and epidural analgesia after spinal surgery in children. *Anesth Analg* 2004; 98: 956–65.

160 Bosenberg A. Neuraxial blockade and cardiac surgery in children. *Paediatr Anaesth*, 2003; 13: 559–60.

161 Humphreys N, Bays SMA, Pawade A, Parry A, Wolf AR. Prospective randomized controlled trial of high dose opioid vs high spinal anaesthesia in infant heart surgery with cardiopulmonary bypass: effects on stress and inflammation. *Paediatr Anaesth* 2004a; 14: 705.

162 Humphreys N, Bays SMA, Sim D, Wolf AR. Spinal anaesthesia with an indwelling catheter for cardiac surgery in children: description and early experience of the technique. *Paediatr Anaesth* 2004b; 14: 704.

163 Drover DR, Hammer GB, Williams GD, Boltz MG, Ramamoorthy C. A comparison of patient state index (PSI) changes and remifentanil requirements during cardiopulmonary bypass in infants undergoing general anesthesia with or without spinal anaesthesia. *Anesthesiology* 2004; 101: A1453.

164 Lundeberg S, Lonnqvist PA. Update on sytemic postoperative analgesia in children. *Paediatr Anaesth* 2004; 14: 394–7.

165 Dix P, Prosser DP, Streete P. A pharmacokinetic study of piroxicam in children. *Anaesthesia* 2004; 59: 984–7.

166 Anderson BJ, Holford NHG. Rectal paracetamol dosing regimens: determination by computer simulation. *Paediatr Anaesth* 1997; 7: 451–5.

167 Anderson B, Lin YC, Sussman H, Benitz WE. Paracetamol pharmacokinetics in the premature neonate; the problem with limited data. *Paediatr Anaesth* 1998; 8: 442–3.

168 Anderson B. What we don't know about paracetamol in children. *Paediatr Anaesth* 1998; 8: 451–60.

169 Autret EDJ, Jonville AP, Furet Y, Laugier J. Pharmacokinetics of paracetamol in the neonate and infant after administration of propacetamol chlorhydrate. *Dev Pharmacol Therap* 1993; 20: 129–34.

170 Granry JC, Rod B, Monrigal JP, Merckx J, Berniere J, Jean N, Boccard E. The analgesic efficacy of an injectable prodrug of acetaminophen in children after orthopaedic surgery. *Paediatr Anaesth* 1997; 7: 445–9.

171 Hartley R, Levene MI. Opioid pharmacology in the newborn. *Bailliere's Clin Paediatr* 1995; 3: 467–93.

172 Lin YC, Sussman HH, Benitz WE. Plasma concentrations after rectal administration of acetaminophen in preterm neonates. *Paediatr Anaesth* 1997; 7: 457–9.

173 Montgomery C, McCormack JP, Reichert CC, Marshland CP. Plasma concentrations after high dose (45 mg/kg) rectal acetaminophen in children. *Can J Anaesth* 1995; 42: 982–6.

174 Morton NS, Benham SW, Lawson RA, McNicol LR. Diclofenac vs oxybuprocaine eyedrops for analgesia in paediatric strabismus surgery. *Paediatr Anaesth* 1997a; 7: 221–6.

175 RCPCH *Medicines for Children 2003*. London: RCPCH, 2003.

176 Anderson BJ, Meakin GH. Scaling for size: some implications for paediatric anaesthesia dosing. *Paediatr Anaesth* 2002; 12: 205–19.

177 Berde CB, Sethna NF. Drug therapy: analgesics for the treatment of pain in children. *New Engl J Med* 2002; 347: 1094–1103.

178 Semple D, Aldridge L, Doyle E. Comparison of i.v and s.c. diamorphine infusions for the treatment of acute pain in children. *Br J Anaesth* 1996; 76: 310–2.

179 McNicol LR. Post-operative analgesia in children using continuous subcutaneous morphine. *Br J Anaesth* 1993; 71: 752–6.

180 Wolf AR, Lawson RA, Fisher S. Ventilatory arrest after a fluid challenge in a neonate receiving sc morphine. *Br J Anaesth* 1995; 75: 787–9.

181 Bray R, Woodhams AM. A double-blind comparison of morphine infusion and patient controlled analgesia in children. *Paediatr Anaesth* 1996; 6: 121–7.

182 Doyle E, Harper I, Morton NS. Patient controlled analgesia with low dose background infusions after lower abdominal surgery in children. *Br J Anaesth* 1993a; 71: 818–22.

183 Howard RF. Planning for pain relief. *Bailliere's Clin Anaesthesiol* 1996; 10: 657–75.

184 Lloyd-Thomas A. Assessment and control of pain in children. *Anaesthesia* 1995; 50: 753–5.

185 McKenzie I, Gaukroger PB, Ragg P, Brown TCK. *Manual of Acute Pain Management in Children*. London: Churchill Livingstone, 1997.

186 Morton NS. Paediatric postoperative analgesia. *Curr Opin Anaesthesiol* 1996; 9: 309–12.

187 Zwaveling J, Bubbers S, Van Meurs AHJ, Schoemaker RC, Ruijs-Dudok Van Heel I, Vermeij P, Burggraaf J. Pharmacokinetics of rectal tramadol in postoperative paediatric patients. *Br J Anaesth* 2004; 93: 224 7.

188 Engelhardt T, Steel E, Johnston G, Veitch DY. Tramadol for pain relief in children undergoing tonsillectomy: a comparison with morphine. *Paediatr Anaesth* 2003; 13: 249–52.

189 Ross AK, Davis PJ, Dear GL, Ginsberg B, McGowan FX, Stiller RD, Henson LG, Huffman C, Miuir KT. Pharmacokinetics of remifentanil in anesthetized pediatric patients undergoing elective surgery or diagnostic procedures. *Anesth Analg* 2001; 93: 1393–401.

190 Prys-Roberts C, Lerman J, Murat I, Taivainen T, Lopez T, Lejus C, Spahr-Scopfer I, Splinter W, Kirkham AJ. Comparison of remifentanil versus regional anaesthesia in children anaesthetised with isoflurane/nitrous oxide. *Anaesthesia* 2000; 55: 870–6.

191 Davis PJ, Wilson A S, Siewers RD, Pigula F A, Landsman IS. The effects of cardiopulmonary bypass on remifentanil kinetics in children undergoing atrial septal defect repair. *Anesth Analg* 1999; 89: 904–8.

192 Davis PJ, Lerman J, Suresh S, Mcgowan FX, Cote CJ, Landsman I, Henson LG. A randomized multicenter study of remifentanil compared with alfentanil, isoflurane, or propofol in anesthetized pediatric patients undergoing elective strabismus surgery. *Anesth Analg* 1997; 84: 982–9.

193 Lynn AM. Remifentanil: the paediatric anaesthetist's opiate? *Paediatr Anaesth* 1996; 6: 433–5.

194 Kokki H. Nonsteroidal anti-inflammatory drugs for postoperative pain: a focus on children. *Paediatr Drugs* 2003; 5: 103–23.

195 Morton NS. Practical paediatric day case anaesthesia and analgesia. In: Millar J (ed.). *Practical Day Case Anaesthesia*. Oxford: Bios Scientific Publications Ltd, 1997.

196 Morton NS, O'Brien K. Analgesic efficacy of paracetamol and diclofenac in children receiving PCA morphine. *Br J Anaesth* 1999; 83: 715–17.

197 Anderson BJ. Comparing the efficacy of NSAIDs and paracetamol in children. *Paediatr Anaesth* 2004; 14: 201–17.

198 Howard RF, Lloyd-Thomas A. Pain management in children. In: Sumner E, Hatch D (eds). *Paediatric Anaesthesia*. London: Arnold, 1999.

199 Vetter TR, Heiner EJ. Intravenous ketorolac as an adjuvant to pediatric patient-controlled analgesia with morphine. *J Clin Anesth* 1994; 6: 110–13.

200 Park JM, Houck CS, Sethna NF, Al E. Ketorolac suppresses postoperative bladder spasms after pediatric ureteral reimplantation. *Anesth Analg* 2000; 91: 11–15.

201 Hiller A, Taivainen T, Korpela R, Satu P, Meretoja O. Combination of acetaminophen and ketoprofen for postoperative analgesia in children. *Anesthesiology* 2004; 101: A-1477.

202 Romsing J, Ostergaard D, Senderovitz T, Drozdziewicz D, Sonne J, Ravn G. Pharmacokinetics of oral diclofenac and acetaminophen in children after surgery. *Paediatr Anaesth* 2001; 11: 205–13.

203 Morris JL, Rosen DA, Rosen KR. Nonsteroidal anti-inflammatory agents in neonates. *Paediatr Drugs* 2003; 5: 385–405.

204 RCA *Guidelines for the use of non-steroidal anti-inflammatory drugs in the perioperative period*. London: Royal College of Anaesthetists, 1998.

205 Moiniche S, Romsing J, Dahl J, Tramer MR. Nonsteroidal anti-inflammatory drugs and the risk of operative site bleeding after tonsillectomy: a quantitative systematic review. *Anesth Analg* 2003; 96: 68–77.

206 Krishna S, Hughes LF, Lin SY. Postoperative hemorrhage with nonsteroidal anti-inflammatory drug use after tonsillectomy. *Arch Otolaryngol Head Neck Surg* 2003; 129: 1086–9.

207 Short JA, Barr CA, Palmer CD, Al E. Use of diclofenac in children with asthma. *Anaesthesia* 2000; 55: 334–7.

208 Turner S, Ford V. Role of the selective cyclooxygenase 2 (COX-2) inhibitors in children. *Arch Dis Child Educ Pract Ed* 2004; 89: ep46–49.

209 Pickering AE, Bridge HS, Nolan J, Al E. Double-blind, placebo-controlled analgesic study of ibuprofen or rofecoxib in combination with paracetamol for tonsillectomy in children. *Br J Anaesth* 2002; 88: 72–7.

210 Stempak D, Gammon J, Klein J, Al E. Single-dose and steady-state pharmacokinetics of celecoxib in children. *Clin Pharmacol Ther* 2002; 72: 490–7.

211 St Rose E, Fernandiz M, Kiss M, Al E. Steady-state plasma concentrations of rofecoxib in children (ages 2–5 years) with juvenile rheumatoid arthritis. *Arthritis Rheum* 2001; 44: S291.

212 Edwards DJ, Prescella RP, Fratarelli DA, Al E. Pharmacokinetics of rofecoxib in children. *Clin Pharmacol Ther* 2004; 75: 73.

213 Joshi W, Connelly NR, Reuben SS, Al E. An evaluation of the safety and efficacy of administering rofecoxib for postoperative pain management. *Anesth Analg* 2003; 97: 35–8.

214 Vallee E, Lafrenaye S, Dorion D. Rofecoxib in pain control after tonsillectomy in children. *Pain* 2004; 5: S84.

215 Sheeran PW, Rose JB, Fazi LM, Chiavacci R, Mccormick L. Rofecoxib administration to paediatric patients undergoing adenotonsillectomy. *Paediatr Anaesth* 2004; 14: 579–83.

216 McQuay H, Moore A. An evidence-based resource for pain relief. Oxford: Oxford Medical Publications, 1998.

217 Korpela R, Korvenoja P, Meretoja O. Morphine-sparing effect of acetaminophen in pediatric day-case surgery. *Anesthesiology* 1999; 91: 442–7.

218 Arana A, Morton NS, Hansen TG. Treatment with paracetamol in infants. *Acta Anaesthesiol Scand* 2001; 45: 20–9.

219 Goodarzi M. A double blind comparison of droperidol and ondansetron for prevention of emesis in children undergoing orthopaedic surgery. *Paediatr Anaesth* 1998; 8: 325–9.

220 Morton NS, Camu F, Dorman T, Knudsen KE, Kvalsvik O, Nellgard P, Saint-Maurice CP, Wilhelm W, Cohen LA. Ondansetron reduces nausea and vomiting after paediatric adenotonsillectomy. *Paediatr Anaesth* 1997b; 7: 37–45.

221 Splinter WM, Rhine EJ. Prophylactic antiemetics in children undergoing tonsillectomy: high-dose vs low-dose ondansetron. *Paediatr Anaesth* 1997; 7: 125–9.

222 Rose JB, Martin TM. Posttonsillectomy vomiting. Ondansetron or metoclopramide during paediatric tonsillectomy: are two doses better than one? *Paediatr Anaesth* 1996; 6: 39–44.

223 Fujii Y, Tanaka H. Prophylactic therapy with granisetron in the prevention of vomiting after paediatric surgery. A randomized, double-blind comparison with droperidol and metoclopramide. *Paediatr Anaesth* 1998; 8: 149–53.

224 Fujii Y, Tanaka H, Toyooka H. Granisetron and dexamethasone provide more improved prevention of postoperative emesis than granisetron alone in children. *Can J Anaesth* 1996; 43: 1229–32.

225 Fujii Y, Tanaka H. Granisetron decreases postoperative vomiting in children. *Eur J Anaesthesiol* 1999; 16: 62–5.

21

Anaesthesia for eye, ENT and dental surgery

Mathew Zacharias and Robyn Chirnside

Department of Anaesthesia and Intensive Care, Dunedin Hospital, Dunedin, Otago, New Zealand

We endeavoured to look at the best available evidence to support some of our current practices in areas of ENT (ear, nose and throat), eye and dental anaesthesia.

- Endotracheal anaesthesia has been the standard for anaesthesia for tonsillectomy. Laryngeal mask airway (LMA) is used more often for the procedure than in the past. We look at the safety of this transition.
- Many surgeons use local anaesthesia for better postoperative analgesia after tonsillectomy. In spite of lack of supportive evidence this practice is still common.
- There is a belief that non-steroidal anti-inflammatory drugs (NSAIDs) might increase posttonsillectomy bleeding and newer COX2 inhibitors are devoid of this problem. We look at the evidence for such contention.
- We explore for any generally accepted way of providing safe anaesthesia for surgery for the human papilloma virus (HPV) of the larynx.
- There is considerable difference of opinion on fasting before cataract surgery under local anaesthetic blocks and on the indications for sedation during eye blocks.
- Opinion varies on the use of LMA for outpatient dental surgery. Evidence is sought for all the above from available literature.

Anaesthesia for ENT surgery

Anaesthesia for ENT surgery has to specifically address the problems of a shared airway, perioperative bleeding and postoperative pain and discomfort.

Endotracheal tube or LMA for tonsillectomy?

Tonsillectomy is one of the common operations. Endotracheal anaesthesia has been the standard for many years, but this trend has changed since the introduction of

Key words: Laryngeal mask airway, tonsillectomy, posttonsillectomy bleeding, HPV of the larynx, fasting and cataract surgery, sedation for eye blocks, dental anaesthesia.

reinforced LMAs. Avoiding endotracheal intubation in favour of a LMA can minimise some of the problems of tracheal intubation in the mainly paediatric population, but often the question is raised, "*Is this a safe practice*"?

Two surveys looked at the frequency of use of LMA for tonsillectomy. In 1996 in a French survey [1], only 2% respondents used LMA for tonsillectomy whereas later in 1999 a British survey [2] found that 16% of anaesthetists routinely used LMA for tonsillectomies in children and 33% had used LMA for tonsillectomies at some time. There are also some useful reviews on this topic [3]. One study in 1993 commented on the ease of insertion of a prototype armoured LMA in a paediatric population undergoing tonsillectomy [4] and reported difficulty in 18% of cases. However it is unlikely that such high incidence is seen now since LMA is used much more frequently for anaesthesia.

Incidence of conversion from LMA to an endotracheal tube (ETT) is reported in three studies [4–6] as around 9.5%. These studies were mostly in the paediatric population though one of the studies included adults [6]. Conversion was usually at the time of insertion, or because of ongoing obstruction by the Boyle Davis gag. Some studies commented on the ease of surgical access, but failed to state how this was assessed [4,5]. One study [6] used a visual analogue scale to assess this, and found that there was better surgical access with the ETT than with the LMA.

A fibreoptic scope has been used to look for evidence of tracheal soiling during tonsillectomy using LMA. Two studies in children [5,7] looked for blood in the larynx (LMA group) or in the trachea (ETT group). Prior to emergence from anaesthesia there was evidence of blood in the larynx in two patients in the LMA group and in the trachea in 20 patients in the ETT groups (odds ratio, OR: 0.16, 95% confidence intervals, CIs: 0.06, 0.38, $P = 0.0001$). This was supported by another study [4], which found no evidence of laryngeal contamination in 18/19 patients in the LMA group that were subjected to endoscopy prior to emergence from anaesthesia.

The use of LMAs avoids the dilemma of extubation either under deep anaesthesia with an unprotected airway, or with the patient awake, with increased potential risk of coughing, laryngospasm or postoperative bleeding. Recovery room problems appear to be lower in patients who have LMA for tonsillectomy rather than an ETT [4,5,7]. The incidence of laryngospasm during the immediate recovery period was significantly lower in the LMA group (OR: 0.31, 95% CIs: 0.15, 0.63, $P = 0.001$). The presence of blood in the lower airway of children with ETTs may be associated with the increase in coughing during recovery period (OR: 0.01, 95% CIs: 0.04, 0.25, $P < 0.0001$). In children, maintenance of an unobstructed airway may be easier with the LMA [5] and recovery room nurses were happier with the airway control ($P < 0.05$) with the LMA. Currently there are a number of anaesthetists who routinely and successfully use the reinforced LMA for tonsillectomy both in adults and children; they resort to the use of ETT when they cannot get in LMA to fit or where the Boyle Davis gag obstructs the airway. This practice has supporting evidence in the literature.

Local anaesthesia for pain control following tonsillectomy

Posttonsillectomy pain is regarded as the primary cause of failure to discharge paediatric day case tonsillectomy patients, as it results in reluctance to swallow and may result in inadequate oral fluid intake. Some surgeons advocate the administration of local anaesthetic agents into the operative field either just before or after the removal of the tonsils.

The Cochrane Ear Nose and Throat Disorders group published a systematic review on this topic in 1999. This review [8] analysed six randomised controlled trials of mostly adult patients, undergoing tonsillectomy and concluded that there was no evidence for the use of perioperative local anaesthetics in patients undergoing tonsillectomy to improve postoperative pain control. A number of other studies have been reported in the literature since 1999 with differing methodology. Injection of local anaesthetic agents was studied in the adult population [9–12] and in children [13,14]. Topical application of local anaesthetic was also used in some studies [15–17]. Injection of local anaesthetic either before or at the end of tonsillectomy did not give any significant advantage except in the immediate period following the operation. Similar findings were noted in children. Topical application of local anaesthetic also offered some benefit, but only in the immediate postoperative period.

There is no evidence supporting the use of perioperative local anaesthetic to improve pain control after tonsillectomy.

Use of NSAIDs for tonsillectomy

The common drugs used for pain control following tonsillectomy are opioids (parenteral or oral), paracetamol (oral or rectal) and NSAIDs (parenteral or oral). The Royal College of Anaesthetists' *Guidelines for the Use of Non-steroidal Anti-inflammatory Drugs in the Peri-operative Period* concludes that NSAIDs are effective alternative to opioids with less nausea and vomiting. This guideline has recommended that NSAIDs should be avoided for patients undergoing tonsillectomy where increased blood loss or reduced platelet function pose particular risk [18]. This raises the question, *"Is it safe to give NSAIDs to patients undergoing tonsillectomy"*?

There are a number of reports in the literature addressing this issue. Of note are one meta-analysis [19] and two systematic reviews [20,21]. The meta-analysis [19] identified seven trials but the authors used a somewhat limited search of MEDLINE publications. This report included data on 1368 patients, mostly children. The results suggested that overall risk for posttonsillectomy bleeding was not different for NSAIDs (diclofenac, ibuprofen or aspirin) compared to control treatments. But aspirin (which the majority of the subjects received as an analgesic) gave a statistically significant increase in bleeding compared to the control treatments, which included tramadol, paracetamol, codeine or placebo (OR: 1.94, 95% CIs: 1.09–3.42).

A Cochrane Review [20] (updated 2005) identified 13 trials having met the inclusion criteria (955 children comparing NSAIDs with another analgesic or placebo). The results suggested no significant alteration in the perioperative bleeding requiring surgical intervention (OR: 1.46, 95% CIs: 0.49–4.40). Another systematic review [21] did a similar database search and used 25 randomised controlled trials (1853 patients, 970 receiving NSAIDs and others receiving other analgesics such as codeine, paracetamol or placebo). This review did not identify any differences between the two treatments in terms of intraoperative or postoperative bleeding after tonsillectomy.

There are only a few randomised controlled trials in the literature attempting to compare non-specific NSAIDs (COX1 inhibitors) and COX2-specific NSAIDs. Refocoxib was compared to placebo in 45 children undergoing tonsillectomy in one study [22]; there were no differences in the intraoperative blood loss. Another study of 118 adult patients undergoing tonsillectomy [23] compared celecoxib with either ketoprofen or placebo. Even though there were no significant differences between the groups in intraoperative blood loss, larger number of patients who received ketoprofen as a postoperative analgesic required surgery for secondary haemorrhage ($P = 0.026$) compared to patients who received celecoxib. However the methodological quality of these trials may be questioned. Both these studies looked at pain control as the main outcome of interest and hence further studies are required to establish any benefit for COX2 inhibitors in reducing posttonsillectomy bleeding.

It may be concluded that there is insufficient evidence that NSAIDs may increase posttonsillectomy bleeding.

Anaesthesia for surgery for recurrent respiratory papillomatosis

Infection of larynx and the respiratory tract with HPV is a rare condition, but anaesthetists are called to provide anaesthesia for surgical removal of the warts. This condition is the most common benign neoplasm of the larynx in children. The disease is often diagnosed at 2–3 years of age [24,25]. Surgery is the mainstay of treatment for this condition and repeated surgical interventions are necessary because of the high incidence of recurrence of this condition.

There are no randomised controlled trials on the best form of anaesthesia for this condition. A survey of Pediatric Otolaryngology Members' experience of this condition [26] describes the practice amongst the members in USA, France, Canada and Australia who were dealing with 700 active patients. Microdebrider and carbon dioxide laser were the two main surgical methods used, microdebrider being a slightly more preferred option than carbon dioxide laser by the participants of this survey (53%). The majority (64%) chose a spontaneous breathing or apnoeic ventilation technique. Twenty-four per cent chose jet ventilation and a small number (10%) chose laser safe ETTs. Tracheostomy is indicated in patients with extensive spread in the respiratory tract.

The choice of anaesthetic technique varies with the experience of the team. There are only case reports on anaesthesia for surgery for recurrent respiratory papillomatosis. The aim of surgery is to provide removal of as much lesion as possible, whilst at the same time minimising the damage to the surrounding normal tissues.

Tubeless spontaneous respiration anaesthesia [27] involves a spontaneously breathing patient, but with the vocal cords sprayed with local anaesthetic agent. The anaesthetic agents are delivered at the end of the laryngoscope, but fire risk and lack of scavenging of both anaesthetic gases and surgical plume are problems. This may be minimised by total intravenous anaesthesia [28]. The apnoeic anaesthesia method [29] uses anaesthesia with the smallest possible ETT, and intermittent removal of the tube during the use of the laser. The patient is paralysed and hyperventilated before the periods of apnoea. Anaesthesia may also be delivered via the intravenous route. This allows 2–3 min of operation time before further ventilation. Jet ventilation with intravenous anaesthesia is popular for microsurgery of the larynx [30], supraglottic jet ventilation being a popular technique, with minimal fire hazard. However there is a theoretical risk that it may deliver the laser plume deeper into the lung and cause pulmonary spread of the papilloma, though clinical evidence for this is lacking.

There is insufficient evidence in the literature to recommend any one way of anaesthetising for this procedure. It appears that jet ventilation is gaining popularity, anaesthesia being maintained with intravenous propofol, with or without a short acting opoids and non-depolarising muscle relaxant. What is generally appreciated is the fact that an experienced team gets better results, with minimal complications.

> The reinforced LMA is safe in tonsillectomy. There is no evidence for use of local anaesthesia for tonsillectomy and NSAIDs do not affect posttonsillectomy blood loss. There is little information regarding anaesthetic technique for laser surgery for HPV of the larynx.

Anaesthesia for eye surgery

Cataract surgery is one of the main areas where anaesthetists are involved in ophthalmic surgery. The majority of patients presenting for cataract surgery are elderly, with multiple co-morbidities requiring multiple medications. Cataract surgery is usually done under a regional block.

Is there a need to starve before cataract surgery under local anaesthesia?

Unfortunately there are no controlled trials addressing this topic, even though this subject has been discussed in the literature. It is important to recognise that many patients undergoing cataract surgery have multiple medical conditions, including diabetes mellitus. In 1993 a correspondence in the *British Journal of Anaesthesia* [31] reported that the authors and their colleagues followed a regimen of no change in dietary or medication routine prior to cataract surgery in 30 000 patients with no incidence of any adverse outcomes, even though 14 of their patients lost consciousness during the procedure due to a number of reasons. None of their patients received heavy sedation or required conversion to general anaesthesia.

A survey of the anaesthetic practice for cataract surgery in the UK [32] suggested that the majority of hospitals surveyed (84%) had a fasting policy before cataract surgery under local anaesthesia and nearly half of these (44%) involved no restrictions of food or drink. However, the majority (74%) was not prepared to supplement the local anaesthetic block with sedation in patients who were not fasted. The general consensus was that critical incidents were rare in non-fasting patients undergoing cataract surgery under local anaesthesia. A document by the Royal College of Anaesthetists and the Royal College of Ophthalmologists [33] in 2001 agrees with the practice of continuing usual preoperative medications and diet in patients undergoing cataract surgery under local anaesthesia, especially those with diabetes.

It appears that there is really no need for fasting before cataract surgery done under local anaesthesia. The evidence for this is based on case reports and experience of anaesthetists and ophthalmologists involved with this procedure.

Is intravenous sedation useful for cataract surgery under local anaesthetic block?

Pain and consequent movement during the block, particularly during retrobulbar or peribulbar blocks is not desirable. A number of randomised controlled trials are identified in the recent literature in an attempt to address this issue, but the methodological quality of the trials is not high. Four trials compared sedative drugs (midazolam, propofol, alfentanil or remifentanil or a combination) with controls during the placement of the block [34–37]. Deep sedation or respiratory depression was recorded in 20/138 treated cases and none in 72 controls (OR: 5.33, 95% CIs: 1.79, 15.87, $P = 0.003$). A drop in oxygen saturation (below 90%) was noted in 11/200 sedated cases and in none of the 77 controls (OR: 4.19, 95% CIs: 1.04,

$16.82, P = 0.04$). Many other studies looked at combinations of drugs, had various premedications, differing depths of sedation or lacked control groups, thus making it difficult to compare them. None of the sedation techniques described appear to cause major risks to the patients, though the reasons for such sedation techniques is found wanting. The increasing use of the sub-Tenon's block, which is relatively pain free and is devoid of some of the risks of retrobulbar or peribulbar blocks such as haemorrhage and accidental subdural injection, have made sedation during cataract surgery under local anaesthesia somewhat unnecessary.

The increasing use of topical anaesthesia for cataract extraction has caused renewed interest in analgesia and sedation during cataract surgery. A recent study has showed that small doses of fentanyl compared to placebo improved patient comfort during cataract surgery performed under local anaesthesia and reduced the need for supplemental intraoperative fentanyl [38]. Yet another study [39] suggested that intravenous midazolam did not significantly alter patient satisfaction for those having cataract surgery under topical anaesthesia.

There is some evidence that low-dose benzodiazepine premedication prior to cataract surgery may be useful to reduce anxiety without compromising the safety [40,41]. It is important to recall the recommendations of the Royal College of Anaesthetists and the Royal College of Ophthalmologists [33] that conscious sedation during cataract surgery should not be a tool to deal with an inadequate block.

Intravenous sedation during local anaesthetic blocks cataract surgery is not routinely practised, but it may have a role in a selected group of patients when used appropriately.

> There is probably no need to fast patients prior to cataract surgery done under local anaesthesia. There may be a limited role for sedation in some patients undergoing cataract surgery.

Dental anaesthesia

The majority of dental anaesthesia is done as a day case procedure and have similar problems to anaesthesia for ENT surgery. Dental anaesthesia aims to provide an unrestricted operating field, a safe stable airway and protection from aspiration of blood and fluid from the mouth.

Has LMA replaced ETT in day case dental anaesthesia?

Oral surgery with a LMA can challenge anaesthetic requirements for a secure airway and adequate surgical access and requires co-operation between the anaesthetist and the surgeon. The reinforced LMA was specifically designed for use in oral surgery, and has extra flexibility and increased length than the classic LMA.

There are only few randomised controlled trials comparing the reinforced LMA with nasal or oral ETTs for dental surgical procedures, though there are a number of reports on the topic in the literature. A randomised, prospective trial [42] of 100 patients found no difference in the ease of positioning of the LMA and ETT (OR: 1.71, 95% CIs: 0.41, 7.21, $P = 0.46$). There was however an increase in partial obstruction to breathing due to the LMA (OR: 8.04, 95% CIs: 1.34, 48.12, $P = 0.02$).

In a large case report [43] of 1201 intellectually handicapped patients (predominantly young adults) undergoing dental comprehensive treatment, 249 had an ETT, 826 had a LMA and 122 had a nasal mask. It is unclear whether the ETT was placed nasally or orally. The mean duration of procedure was approximately 60 min. Of those with a LMA 1.7% had low oxygen saturation during the procedure, whereas none with ETT had low oxygen saturations. It is of note that 38.5% of those who had a nasal mask technique had low oxygen saturations during the procedure. Two patients who had ETTs and none who had a LMA, experienced laryngeal spasm following the surgery. Even though this report is a review of cases, it points out to the fact that LMA is reasonably safe in dental anaesthesia.

Some studies have looked for evidence of tracheal soiling following oral surgery by observing for any evidence of aspiration using a bronchoscope. One trial [42] showed no evidence of laryngeal soiling in the LMA group, whereas blood was found in three cases after endotraceal intubation, but without any negative outcome (OR: 0.13, 95% CIs: 0.01, 1.28, $P = 0.08$). Another study [44] in 51 patients looked only at evidence of laryngeal soiling following LMA using a coloured dye. Twenty per cent cases showed some evidence of soiling at the end of operation, but the methodological quality of this study was poor, with no control group. There were no adverse postoperative sequelae in any patient.

> Many anaesthetists currently use reinforced LMA successfully for common dental procedures.

Summary

We endeavoured to look at the best available evidence to support some of the common practices in the areas of ENT, ophthalmological and dental anaesthesia. The use of the reinforced LMA for tonsillectomy has supporting evidence in the literature. There is no evidence to support the use of perioperative local anaesthetic to improve pain control after tonsillectomy or for the avoidance of NSAIDs for the fear of increasing posttonsillectomy bleeding. There is no clearly superior way of anaesthetising patients with HPV of the larynx, though it appears that jet ventilation is gaining popularity. There is no need for fasting before cataract surgery done under local anaesthesia. Intravenous sedation during local anaesthetic blocks for cataract surgery is not routinely recommended, but it may have a role in a selected group of patients. There is only limited evidence regarding the use of reinforced LMAs for dental procedures.

Most anaesthetists are called upon to provide anaesthesia for ENT, eye and dental cases. We plan to look at a few common issues in these areas and look for the available evidence for specific management strategies. A broad search strategy of MEDLINE, EMBASE and EBM databases was used for this purpose.

Future research options
- Safe anaesthetic techniques for treatment of HPV of the larynx.
- Fasting prior to cataract surgery under local anaesthesia.
- Role of sedation for cataract surgery done under topical anaesthesia.

REFERENCES

1 Ecoffey C, Auroy Y, Pequignot F, Jougla E, Clergue F, Lazenaire M-C et al. A French survey of paediatric airway management use in tonsillectomy and appendicectomy. *Paediatr Anaesth* 2003; 13: 584–8.

2 Hatcher IS, Stack CG. Postal survey of the anaesthetic techniques used for paediatric tonsillectomy surgery. *Paediatr Anaesth* 1999; 9: 311–15.

3 Kretz F-J, Reimann B, Stelzner J, Heumann H, Lange-Stumpf U. Die Larynxmaske bei adenostonsillektomie bei kindern. *Der Anaesthesist* 2000; 49: 706–11.

4 Webster AC, Morley-Forster PK. Anaesthesia for adenotonsillectomy: a comparison between tracheal intubation and the armoured laryngeal mask airway. *Can J Anaesth* 1993; 40: 1171–7.

5 William PJ, Bailey PM. Comparison of the reinforced laryngeal mask airway and tracheal intubation for adenotonsillectomy. *Br J Anaesth* 1993; 70: 30–3.

6 Hern JD, Jayaraj SM, Sidhu VS, Almeyda JS, O'Neill G, Tolley NS. The laryngeal mask airway in tonsillectomy: the surgeons's perspective. *Clin Otolaryngol* 1999; 24: 122–5.

7 Boisson-Bertrand D. Amygdalectomies et masque larynge reinforce. *Can J Anaesth* 1995; 42: 857–61.

8 Hollis LJ, Burton MJ, Miller JM. Perioperative local anaesthesia for reducing pain following tonsillectomy. *The Cochrane Database of Syst Rev* 1999, Issue 4. Art. No.: CD0018174. DOI: 10.1002/14651858.

9 Nordahl SHG, Aalbrektsen G, Guttormsen AB, Pedersen IL, Breidablikk H-J. Effect of bupivacaine on pain after tonsillectomy: a randomized clinical trial. *Acta Otolaryngol* 1999; 119: 369–76.

10 Kountakis SE. Effectiveness of perioperative bupivacaine infiltration in tonsillectomy patients. *Am J Otolaryngol* 2002; 23: 76–80.

11 Vasan NR, Stevenson S, Ward M. Preincisional bupivacaine in posttonsillectomy pain relief: a randomized prospective study. *Arch Otolaryngol – Head Neck Surg* 2002; 128: 145–9.

12 Sorensen WT, Wagner N, Aarup AT, Bonding P. Beneficial effect of low-dose peritonsillar injection of lidocaine-adrenaline before tonsillectomy. A placebo-controlled clinical trial. *Auris Nasus Larynx* 2003; 30: 159–62.

13 Ozmen S, Tuk M, Eroglu F, Uygur K, Dogru H. The effect of peritonsillar lidocaine infiltration for postoperative pain relief in the immediate postoperative period after pediatric adenotonsillectomy. *Pain Clinic* 2002; 13: 339–42.

14 Somdas MA, Senturk M, Ketenci I, Erkorkmaz U, Unlu T. Efficacy of bupivacaine for posttonsillectomy pain: a study with the intra-individual design. *Int J Pediatr Otorhinolaryngol* 2004; 68: 1391–5.

15 Hung T, Moore-Gillon V, Hern J, Hinton A, Patel N. Topical bupivacaine in paediatric daycare tonsillectomy: a prospective randomized controlled trial. *J Laryngol Otol* 2002; 116: 33–6.

16 Kaygusuz I, Susaman N. The effect of dexamethasone, bupivacaine and topical lidocainne spray on pain after tonsillectomy. *Int J Pediatr Otorhinolaryngol* 2003; 67: 737–42.

17 Egeli E, Harputluoglu U, Oghan F, Demiraran Y, Guclu E, Oztruk O. Does topical lidocaine with adrenaline have an effect on morbidity in pediatric tonsillectomy? *Int J Pediatr Otorhinolaryngol* 2005; 69: 811–15.

18 The Royal College of Anaesthetists. Guidelines for the use of non-steroidal anti-inflammatory drugs in the peri-operative period, March 1998.

19 Krishna S, Hughes LF, Lin SY. Postoperative haemorrhage with non-steroidal anti-inflammatory drug use after tonsillectomy. A meta-analysis. *Arch Otolaryngol – Head Neck Surg* 2003; 129: 1086–9.

20 Cardwell M, Siviter G, Smith A. Non-steroidal anti-inflammatory drugs and perioperative bleeding in paediatric tonsillectomy. *The Cochrane Database of Syst Rev* 2005, Issue 2. Art. No.: CD003591. DOI: 10.1002/14651858.

21 Moiniche S, Romsing J, Dahl JB, Tramer MR. Non-steroidal anti-inflammatory drugs and the risk of operative site bleeding after tonsillectomy: a quantitative systematic review. *Anesth Analg* 2003; 96: 68–77.

22 Sheehan PW, Rose JB, Fazi LM, Chiavacci R, McCormick L. Rofocoxib administration to paediatric patients undergoing adenotonsillectomy. *Pediatr Anesth* 2004; 14: 579–83.

23 Nikanne E, Kokki H, Salo J, Linna T-J. Celecoxib and ketoprofen for pain management during tonsillectomy: a placebo-controlled clinical trial. *Otolaryngol – Head Neck Surg* 2005; 132: 287–94.

24 Derkay CS. Recurrent respiratory papillomatosis. *Laryngoscope* 2001; 111: 57–69.

25 Reeves WC, Puparelia SS, Swanson KI, Derkay CS, Marcus A, Unger ER for RRP Task Force. National registry for juvenile-onset recurrent respiratory papillomatosis. *Arch Otolaryngol – Head Neck Surg* 2003; 129: 976–82.

26 Schraff S, Derkay CS, Burke B, Lawson L. American Society of Pediatric Otolaryngology members' experience with recurrent respiratory papillomatosis and the use of adjuvant therapy. *Arch Otolaryngol – Head Neck Surg* 2004; 130: 1039–42.

27 McCall JE, Willging JP, Mueller KL, Cotton RT. Spontaneous respiration anesthesia for respiratory papillomatosis. *Ann Otol Rhinol Laryngol* 2000; 109: 72–6.

28 Quintal M-C, Cunningham MJ, Ferrari LR. Tubeless spontaneous respiration technique for pediatric microlaryngeal surgery. *Arch Otolaryngol – Head Neck Surg* 1997; 123: 209–14.

29 Weisberger EC, Miner JD. Apneic anesthesia for improved endoscopic removal of laryngeal papillomata. *Laryngoscope* 1988; 98: 693–7.

30 Werkhaven JA. Microlaryngoscopy-airway management with anesthetic techniques for CO_2 laser. *Pediatr Anesth* 2004; 14: 90–4.

31 Maltby JR, Hamilton RC. Preoperative fasting guidelines for cataract surgery under regional anaesthesia. *Br J Anaesth* 1993; 71: 167.

32 Morris EAJ, Mather SJ. A survey of pre-operative fasting regimens before regional ophthalmic anaesthesia in three regions of United Kingdom. *Anaesthesia* 1999; 54: 1204–19.

33 Royal College of Anaesthetists and the Royal College of Ophthalmologists. Local Anaesthesia for Intraocular Surgery, 2001.

34 Herrick IA, Gelb AW, Nichols B, Kirby J. Patient-controlled propofol sedation for elderly patients: safety and patient attitude towards control. *Can J Anaesth* 1996; 43: 1114–18.

35 Pac-Soo CK, Deacock S, Lockwood G, Carr C, Whitwam JG. Patient-controlled sedation for cataract surgery using peribulbar block. *Br J Anaesth* 1996; 77: 370–4.

36 Wong DHW, Merrick PM. Intravenous sedation prior to peribulbar anaesthesia for cataract surgery in the elderly patients. *Can J Anaesth* 1996; 43: 1115–20.

37 Rewari V, Madan R, Kaul HL, Kumar L. Remifentanil and propofol sedation for retrobulbar nerve block. *Anaesth Intens Care* 2002; 30: 433–7.

38 Aydin ON, Ugur B, Kir E, Ozkan SB. Effect of single-dose fentanyl on the cardiorespiratory system in elderly patients undergoing cataract surgery. *J Clin Anesth* 2004; 16: 98–103.

39 Habib NE, Mandour NM, Balmer HGR. Effect of midazolam on anxiety level and pain perception in cataract surgery with topical anesthesia. *J Cataract Refr Surg* 2004; 30: 437–43.

40 Kiefer RT, Weindler J, Ruprecht KW. Oral low-dose midazolam as premedication for intraocular surgery in retrobulbar anesthesia: cardiovascular effects and relief of perioperative anxiety. *Eur J Ophthalmol* 1997; 7: 185–92.

41 Bellan L, Gooi A, Rehsia S. The Misericordia Health Centre cataract comfort study. *Can J Ophthalmol* 2002; 37: 155–60.

42 Quinn AC, Samaan A, McAteer EM, Moss E, Vucevic M. The reinforced laryngeal mask airway for dento-alveolar surgery. *Br J Anaesth* 1996; 77: 185–8.

43 Hung W-T, Liao S-M, Ko W-R, Chau M-Y. Anesthetic management of dental procedures in mentally handicapped patients. *Acta Anaesthesiol Sin* 2003; 41: 65–70.

44 Chen C-C, Hung W-T, Liou C-M. Evaluation of airway leakage using reinforced laryngeal mask during dental anesthesia with spontaneous breathing. *Acta Anaesthesiol Sin* 2002; 40: 21–4.

22

Anaesthesia for neurosurgery

Divya Chander and Adrian W Gelb

Department of Anesthesia and Perioperative Care, University of California, San Francisco, USA

The practice of neuroanaesthesia is unique in that the target organ of both the surgeon and the anaesthetist is one and the same. Thus, the surgical goals have a profound impact on the constraints that the anaesthesiologist must work within. In order to appropriately anaesthetise the patient for neurosurgery, an understanding of the interrelationships of neurophysiology, pathophysiology and pharmacology is important. This chapter will review: (1) basic neurophysiological principles, (2) specific approaches to the management of intracranial pressure (ICP) as they relate to clinical neuroanaesthesia, and (3) intraoperative management of the patient with a supratentorial mass lesion.

Basic principles of neurophysiology

There are six interrelated components that are important to the practice of neuroanaesthesia. They are maintenance of cerebral perfusion pressure (CPP), cerebral blood flow (CBF), cerebral blood volume (CBV), intracranial pressure (ICP), CO_2 responsiveness (CO_2R) and cerebral oxygen metabolism ($CMRO_2$).

Cerebral perfusion pressure

CPP is the difference between mean arterial pressure (MAP) and intracranial pressure (ICP) (CPP = MAP − ICP), although in the occasional patient where central venous pressure (CVP) is higher than ICP, CPP = MAP − CVP. Both intracranial pathology and drugs may compromise CPP through effects on MAP and/or ICP. CPP is usually >70 mmHg. An optimal CPP has not been defined but in the context of head trauma, a CPP <60 is associated with a poorer outcome; a benefit of higher CPP has not been shown [1].

Key words: Cerebral blood flow, autoregulation, mannitol, hyperventilation, traumatic brain injury, brain tumour, barbiturate coma, anaesthetic effects.

Cerebral blood flow

The average CBF is ~40–50 mL/100 g min^{-1} with grey matter having a higher flow than white matter (60 mL/100 g min^{-1} and 20 mL/100 g min^{-1} respectively). CBF is autoregulated – that is, blood flow is maintained over a wide range (~50–150 mmHg) of perfusion pressures in order to avoid ischaemia when blood pressure is reduced and oedema or haemorrhage at higher blood pressures. Static autoregulation refers to changes in flow that occur slowly (minutes) in response to changes in blood pressure and dynamic autoregulation is used to describe changes that occur within seconds. The autoregulatory range and the relationship between CBF and perfusion pressure can change rapidly as one would want from a homeostatic response. When sympathetic tone is reduced the entire response can shift to lower pressures and when tone is increased such as during stress it moves to a higher-pressure range. With hyperventilation the response shifts to lower CBF and covers a wider perfusion pressure range while an increased CO_2 results in a narrower range at a higher CBF.

Volatile anaesthetics affect CBF both indirectly and directly. When cerebral metabolism ($CMRO_2$) is decreased, vasoconstriction occurs to appropriately reduce CBF. However, direct vasodilation also occurs in a dose-dependent fashion [2–5] but may not manifest as increased CBF except at higher concentrations. Evidence from both animal and humans suggest that the increase in CBF is more pronounced with desflurane and least with sevoflurane [2, 6–8].

Both static and dynamic autoregulation remain essentially intact with both sevoflurane and isoflurane up to 1 MAC [9,10] but preservation is better and persists to a higher concentration with sevoflurane [11]. Desflurane >1 MAC abolishes autoregulation [10]. Static autoregulation also appears to be intact in children undergoing non-neurosurgical procedures with doses of sevoflurane up to 1.5 MAC [12]. The effect of volatile anaesthetics on cerebral haemodynamics including CBF and autoregulation has been well reviewed [6,8].

Propofol, barbiturates and etomidate are potent cerebral vasoconstrictors reducing CBF secondary to decreasing $CMRO_2$ [13–15]. The effect on CBF is greater with propofol and thiopental than etomidate. Propofol and thiopental do not alter autoregulation [10].

Opioids have minimal effect on CBF [16].

Cerebral blood volume

Approximately 15% of CBV is in the arterial tree and ~15% in the major venous sinuses. The remainder is in the capillary and venous systems. CBF is often incorrectly used as a surrogate for blood volume, probably because it has been easier to measure. Changes in CBF and CBV are generally proportional to one another but, for instance, changes in head position from standing to supine to head down can increase CBV without changing CBF.

Propofol decreases CBV in humans and sevoflurane increases it but less than isoflurane [17,18].

Intracranial pressure

Maintenance or reduction of ICP (normal value $\sim$10 mmHg) of ICP is one of the important aims of neuroanaesthesia. ICP is a critical determinant of CPP and by extension CBF and brain function. As ICP increases above $\sim$20 mmHg, focal reductions in CBF occur and further increases eventually result in global cerebral ischaemia. The three major components of the intracranial cavity are brain ($\sim$80%), cerebrospinal fluid (CSF) ($\sim$10%) and CBV ($\sim$10%). If one component increases its volume, it must be compensated for by a decrease in another to prevent ICP from increasing.

CO$_2$ responsiveness

CO$_2$R of the cerebral arterial tree is important in that hypercarbia results in vasodilation and increased CBV. Conversely, hyperventilation causes cerebral arterial vasoconstriction, decreased CBF & CBV and a decreased ICP. While the reduction in ICP is beneficial, the reduced CBF can result in ischaemia so that caution must be exercised with the extent and duration of hyperventilation (see below).

CO$_2$ reactivity is maintained with both sevoflurane and isoflurane up to 1.5 MAC in adults [3,19,20] and with sevoflurane, isoflurane and halothane up to 1.0 MAC in children [21,22]. Intravenous (IV) anaesthetics do not influence CO$_2$R significantly.

Cerebral oxygen metabolism

CMRO$_2$ is a key determinant of the risk of ischaemic insult. If metabolic rate is high, then a reduced CBF is more likely to disrupt neuronal function and integrity. This is the rationale behind decreasing CMRO$_2$ in order to prevent ischaemia. While this notion is appealing in its simplicity, there are no clinical trials in neuroanaesthesia to support such a practice and animal studies indicate that any benefit from anaesthetics probably reflects both intra- and extra-cellular effects [23].

IV anaesthetics potently reduce CMRO$_2$. As CBF is closely coupled to CMRO$_2$, CBF is reduced in parallel with an associated reduction in CBV and ICP which makes them very useful agents in patients with intracranial hypertension. Volatile anaesthetics in contrast reduce CMRO$_2$ but increase CBF through direct effects on the vasculature. Although often referred to as "uncoupled," experimental studies in rats suggest that flow and metabolism continue to track in the same direction but with CBF at a higher "set point" [24].

Clinical neuroanaesthesia

The common types of neurosurgery can be divided into excision of intracranial mass lesions, especially supratentorial tumours, decompressive procedures in major head trauma and aneurysm clipping. This review will focus on managing elevated ICP as this is a problem common to all types of intracranial surgery and then specifically the management of supratentorial masses.

Management of intracranial pressure

ICP may be affected by four major variables in the operating room – hyperventilation, anaesthetic drugs, diuretics such as mannitol, and head position.

Hyperventilation

Hyperventilation constricts the cerebral arterioles with concomitant decreases in CBF and CBV. The effect takes place rapidly and may be especially useful for decreasing ICP in situations in which ICP is critically elevated or the surgeon is having difficulty with brain bulk. However, cerebral vasoconstriction may lead to critical hypoperfusion and brain ischaemia with no improvement or worsened outcomes especially with prolonged use [25–28].

Therefore, current recommendations are that hyperventilation: (1) Should not be used prophylactically in the traumatically brain injured patient and should only be used for brief periods to manage significant increases in ICP not responsive to alternate treatments [25,26]. (2) Similar concerns prevail in the operating room although no trials have addressed outcomes in this context. In either case, unless neurosurgical conditions demand it, ventilation to moderate levels of hypocapnia ($PaCO_2$ 32–35 mmHg) rather than severe ($PaCO_2 < 32$ mmHg) should be used.

Anaesthetic drugs

Volatile anaesthetics produce direct vasodilation and thus have the potential to increase ICP. However the effect on ICP, in both paediatric and adult patients with space-occupying lesions is clinically insignificant when anaesthetic concentrations are maintained below 1.2 MAC and if the ICP is not critically elevated [4,29–32].

Propofol, barbiturates (thiopental) and etomidate have minimal effect or decrease ICP [32]. Few randomised controlled trials have compared IV and inhalation agents and their effect on ICP. In a trial of 117 patients with supratentorial tumours undergoing elective resection, subjects received propofol or isoflurane or sevoflurane as well as a fentanyl infusion (2–3 $\mu g\,kg^{-1}h^{-1}$). ICP was lower, brain swelling less, and CPP better preserved in the propofol group [33]. An earlier trial on 121 patients undergoing elective removal of supratentorial tumours found no difference in mean ICP amongst propofol/fentanyl, fentanyl/nitrous oxide, or isoflurane/nitrous oxide [34]. However, there were significantly more patients in the isoflurane/nitrous oxide group that had an intraoperative ICP ≥ 24 mmHg.

The benefits of high dose barbiturate coma in the management of elevated ICP have not been demonstrated while deleterious outcomes including increased mortality have been shown [35].

Opioids do not increase or decrease ICP [36]. However, when blood pressure decreases, the cerebral vasculature dilates to maintain CBF; this dilation may increase ICP if it is critically increased [16].

Mannitol

Mannitol has become the mainstay of ICP management protocols. An osmotic diuretic, mannitol draws water from the brain and other tissues into the intravascular compartment. Mannitol may also lower ICP by decreasing blood viscosity and expanding plasma volume which increase CBF. When autoregulation is intact this prompts vasoconstriction to restore CBF towards normal [37].

A small, randomised trial concluded that there may be a mortality benefit to using mannitol instead of barbiturate infusion in cases of elevated ICP [35]. Other prospective, randomised studies evaluated long-term outcomes in TBI patients. In each study, one group received early, preoperative treatment of high-dose mannitol whereas the other group did not. The early, high-dose mannitol groups had clinical reversal of impending signs of brain death, better postoperative control of ICP, and better cerebral perfusion [38–41]. Thus current guidelines advocate use of high-dose mannitol boluses for elevated ICP as long as hypovolaemia and excessive serum osmolalities (>320 mOsm) are avoided. The use of mannitol to reduce brain bulk in the OR has not been as well investigated; current practice guidelines are drawn from the head trauma literature.

Hypertonic saline is being investigated as an alternative to mannitol [42]. It has been suggested that by using a hypertonic saline solution, a similar ICP lowering effect to mannitol may be achieved with better outcomes, better preservation of MAP and a potentially longer duration of effect [42,43].

Head-up position

Head-up position is an effective intervention to reduce ICP although there is concern that MAP and consequently CPP would drop. There have been two cohort craniotomy trials examining 10 degree head-up position. One involved 40 patients, the other 15. Head-up position of 10 degrees significantly decreased ICP and MAP but left CPP unaffected [44]. Similar results have been found in head trauma patients subjected to 30 degree head up [45].

Anaesthesia for a patient with a supratentorial mass

The most common mass is a supratentorial tumour. Resection of the tumour requires maintenance of adequate cerebral perfusion to prevent ischaemia while ensuring that ICP is not dangerously elevated. Timely wake-up is desirable in order to facilitate neurological evaluation soon after surgery.

Preoperative evaluation

Besides the routine assessments the patient should be assessed for signs of elevated ICP (nausea/vomiting, papilloedema, headache, visual changes, altered mental status, altered breathing patterns, hypertension, bradycardia) and the neurological deficits documented. It is better if the anaesthesiologist does his/her own examination but the neurologist or neurosurgeon's examination may be more complete. The diagnostic imaging should be seen so as to identify the type of tumour, its location, vascularity, evidence of midline shift and presence of hydrocephalus. Often, patients are taking steroids and anti-epileptic medications which can have an impact on glucose homeostasis and pharmacodynamics of neuromuscular blockers respectively. Pre-medication for anxiolysis may be offset by sedation which may hamper neurological assessment and hypercarbia which may increase ICP. In most patients, a carefully titrated dose of IV benzodiazepine can safely be given if needed.

Monitors

Monitors consist of standard monitors. Continuous blood pressure measurement, preferably via peripheral artery catheter is useful in detecting and treating abrupt haemodynamic changes that might compromise CPP or ICP. Core temperature should be monitored and kept in the normal range. A Foley catheter is important if diuretics are to be used or the surgery will be long.

Induction of anaesthesia

Induction of anaesthesia is a critical time because of the highly stimulating effects of direct laryngoscopy and intubation which is followed a short time later with pinning the head for optimal positioning which is painful. Excessive increases in blood pressure and coughing should be avoided. The most common induction agents are propofol or thiopental with etomidate or ketamine occasionally used in the haemodynamically unstable patient. These are supplemented with an opioid such as fentanyl $2-3\,\mu g\,kg^{-1}$ or a remifentanil infusion [46]. In addition $1-1.5\,mg\,kg^{-1}$ lidocaine IV or esmolol $5-10\,mg$ IV may help blunt the haemodynamic effect on ICP but the effect may be incomplete [47]. Either succinylcholine or a non-depolarising muscle relaxant may be used. There has been controversy about succinylcholine in patients with elevated ICP but the effects are usually of short duration and can be buffered by some additional propofol. The efficacy of lidocaine has not been demonstrated [48]. Level 2 evidence exists to support use of a defasciculating dose of a non-depolarising relaxant to blunt the increase in ICP with succinylcholine [49]. Expeditious intubation followed by oxygenation and hyperventilation is much preferred to the avoidance of succinylcholine but with a delayed and problematic intubation. Neuromuscular blockade may not be needed during the procedure but should be used during positioning and head pinning.

Maintenance of anaesthesia

There needs to be constant attention to the balance between ICP and CPP together with adequacy of anaesthetic depth. Attention to ICP is especially important before the dura is opened; once the dura is open, ICP is effectively zero. Another important consideration is the need for neuromonitoring, for example, somatosensory or motor evoked potentials which are used with increasing frequency during neurosurgical procedures. Good communication between anaesthesiologist, neurosurgeon and monitoring technician is essential as local preferences tend to dictate drug choices. This is especially true for direct stimulation of the motor cortex as there is a paucity of clinical studies to support the use of one drug over another. Somatosensory evoked potentials (SSEPs) are only minimally influenced by total intravenous anaesthesia (TIVA) and are suppressed by inhalational agents in a dose dependent manner although good signals can be obtained with <0.75 MAC vapour.

A typical maintenance anaesthetic might consist of a vapour anaesthetic at <1 MAC and an opioid (fentanyl, sufentanil or remifentanil) infusion or alternatively a TIVA. The latter is especially appropriate where ICP is markedly elevated or there is acute decompensation.

Recovery

If the patient is to be extubated at the end of surgery, the anaesthetic drugs should be appropriately tapered as the scalp is sutured. If fentanyl or sufentanil have been used by infusion, these are usually terminated at dural closure. Remifentanil should be continued until scalp closure and transitional analgesia such as fentanyl 50–100 μg is given [46]. The goal is a comfortable patient in whom a neurological examination can be conducted early after the surgery.

Summary and recommendations

Management of the patient for neurosurgery requires a good understanding of the interrelationships of neurophysiology, pathophysiology and pharmacology. Good data (mostly level 1) exist to describe the effects of volatile and IV anaesthetics on cerebral haemodynamics (CBF, autoregulation, CBV, CO_2 reactivity). Based on this data, one would recommend using <1 MAC sevoflurane or isoflurane over desflurane in adults with elevated ICP with a slight preference for sevoflurane. In children, a similar recommendation can be made. For patients with critically elevated ICP, a TIVA anaesthetic may be preferred. Most studies, however, have used physiological measurements such as CBF or ICP intraoperatively. No level 1 study exists which measured clinical outcomes.

Induction of anaesthesia may be achieved with IV agents normally used (e.g. propofol, thiopental or etomidate). There is level 2 data to support pre-treatment with lidocaine to minimise elevation in ICP (Grade B recommendation). There is also level 2 data to support the use of a defasciculating dose of non-depolarising muscle relaxant if succinylcholine is to be used.

The clinical data for management of ICP come mostly from studies of patients with head trauma. Level 2 data (Grade B recommendation) support the use of the head-up position for significantly reducing ICP without compromising CPP. With respect to hyperventilation and mannitol, this data has been subjected to formal Cochrane reviews and review by the Brain Trauma Foundation. There are Grade A recommendations for the use of: (1) brief, moderate hyperventilation ($PaCO_2$ 32–35 mmHg) in cases of acutely elevated ICP, and (2) high-dose mannitol (1.2–$1.4\,g\,kg^{-1}$) in place of conventional dose mannitol ($\leqslant 1\,g\,kg^{-1}$) for the treatment of acutely elevated ICP (in comatose patients). These guidelines can be applied to the OR for non-head trauma patients. More randomised control trials that explore these interventions for elevated ICP specifically in this setting are needed.

REFERENCES

1 Juul, N et al. Intracranial hypertension and cerebral perfusion pressure: influence on neurological deterioration and outcome in severe head injury. The Executive Committee of the International Selfotel Trial. *J Neurosurg* 2000; 92(1): 1–6.

2 Matta, B.F. et al. Direct cerebral vasodilatory effects of sevoflurane and isoflurane. *Anesthesiology* 1999; 91(3): 677–80.

3 Bundgaard H et al. Effects of sevoflurane on intracranial pressure, cerebral blood flow and cerebral metabolism. A dose-response study in patients subjected to craniotomy for cerebral tumours. *Acta Anaesthesiol Scand* 1998; 42(6): 621–7.

4 Cold GE et al. ICP during anaesthesia with sevoflurane: a dose-response study. Effect of hypocapnia. *Acta Neurochir Suppl* 1998; 71: 279–81.

5 Matta BF, Mayberg TS, Lam AM. Direct cerebrovasodilatory effects of halothane, isoflurane, and desflurane during propofol-induced isoelectric electroencephalogram in humans. *Anesthesiology* 1995; 83(5): 980–5; discussion 27A.

6 De Deyne C, Joly LM, Ravussin P. Newer inhalation anaesthetics and neuro-anaesthesia: what is the place for sevoflurane or desflurane? *Ann Fr Anesth Reanim* 2004; 23(4): 367–74.

7 Monkhoff M et al. The effects of sevoflurane and halothane anaesthesia on cerebral blood flow velocity in children. *Anesth Analg* 2001; 92(4): 891–6.

8 Duffy CM, Matta BF. Sevoflurane and anaesthesia for neurosurgery: a review. *J Neurosurg Anesthesiol* 2000; 12(2): 128–40.

9 Gupta S, Heath K, Matta BF. Effect of incremental doses of sevoflurane on cerebral pressure autoregulation in humans. *Br J Anaesth* 1997; 79(4): 469–72.

10 Strebel S et al. Dynamic and static cerebral autoregulation during isoflurane, desflurane, and propofol anaesthesia. *Anesthesiology* 1995; 83(1): 66–76.

11 Summors AC, Gupta AK, Matta BF. Dynamic cerebral autoregulation during sevoflurane anaesthesia: a comparison with isoflurane. *Anesth Analg* 1999; 88(2): 341–5.

12 Fairgrieve R et al. The effect of sevoflurane on cerebral blood flow velocity in children. *Acta Anaesthesiol Scand* 2003; 47(10): 1226–30.

13 Petersen KD et al. ICP is lower during propofol anaesthesia compared to isoflurane and sevoflurane. *Acta Neurochir Suppl* 2002; 81: 89–91.

14 Roberts I. Barbiturates for acute traumatic brain injury. *The Cochrane Database Syst Rev*, 2000, Issue 2, CD000033.

15 Bazin JE. Effects of anesthetic agents on intracranial pressure. *Ann Fr Anesth Reanim* 1997; 16(4): 445–52.

16 Werner C et al. Effects of sufentanil on cerebral hemodynamics and intracranial pressure in patients with brain injury. *Anesthesiology* 1995; 83(4): 721–6.

17 Kaisti KK et al. Effects of sevoflurane, propofol, and adjunct nitrous oxide on regional cerebral blood flow, oxygen consumption, and blood volume in humans. *Anesthesiology* 2003; 99(3): 603–13.

18 Lorenz IH et al. Subanesthetic concentration of sevoflurane increases regional cerebral blood flow more, but regional cerebral blood volume less, than subanesthetic concentration of isoflurane in human volunteers. *J Neurosurg Anesthesiol* 2001; 13(4): 288–95.

19 Nishiyama T et al. Cerebrovascular carbon dioxide reactivity during general anaesthesia: a comparison between sevoflurane and isoflurane. *Anesth Analg* 1999; 89(6): 1437–41.

20 Mielck F et al. Effects of one minimum alveolar anesthetic concentration sevoflurane on cerebral metabolism, blood flow, and CO_2 reactivity in cardiac patients. *Anesth Analg* 1999; 89(2): 364–9.

21 Leon JE, Bissonnette B. Cerebrovascular responses to carbon dioxide in children anaesthetized with halothane and isoflurane. *Can J Anaesth* 1991; 38(7): 817–25.

22 Rowney DA, Fairgrieve R, Bissonnette B. Cerebrovascular carbon dioxide reactivity in children anaesthetized with sevoflurane. *Br J Anaesth* 2002; 88(3): 357–61.

23 Gelb AW, Wilson JX, Cechetto DF. Anesthetics and cerebral ischemia – should we continue to dream the impossible dream? *Can J Anaesth* 2001; 48(8): 727–31.

24 Hansen TD et al. The role of cerebral metabolism in determining the local cerebral blood flow effects of volatile anesthetics: evidence for persistent flow-metabolism coupling. *J Cereb Blood Flow Metab* 1989; 9(3): 323–8.

25 The Brain Trauma Foundation. The American Association of Neurological Surgeons. The Joint Section on Neurotrauma and Critical Care. Hyperventilation. *J Neurotrauma* 2000; 17(6–7): 513–20.

26 The Brain Trauma Foundation. The American Association of Neurological Surgeons. The Joint Section on Neurotrauma and Critical Care. Initial management. *J Neurotrauma* 2000; 17(6–7): 463–9.

27 Muizelaar JP et al. Adverse effects of prolonged hyperventilation in patients with severe head injury: a randomized clinical trial. *J Neurosurg* 1991; 75(5): 731–9.

28 Roberts I, Schierhout G. Hyperventilation therapy for acute traumatic brain injury. *The Cochrane Database Syst Rev* 1997, Issue 4, Art. No.: CD000566. DOI: 10.1002/14651858.

29 Sponheim S et al. Effects of 0.5 and 1.0 MAC isoflurane, sevoflurane and desflurane on intracranial and cerebral perfusion pressures in children. *Acta Anaesthesiol Scand* 2003; 47(8): 932–8.

30 Kaye A et al. The comparative effects of desflurane and isoflurane on lumbar cerebrospinal fluid pressure in patients undergoing craniotomy for supratentorial tumors. *Anesth Analg* 2004; 98(4): 1127–32.

31 Fraga M et al. The effects of isoflurane and desflurane on intracranial pressure, cerebral perfusion pressure, and cerebral arteriovenous oxygen content difference in normocapnic patients with supratentorial brain tumors. *Anesthesiology* 2003; 98(5): 1085–90.

32 Ravussin P et al. Effect of propofol on cerebrospinal fluid pressure and cerebral perfusion pressure in patients undergoing craniotomy. *Anaesthesia* 1988; 43(Suppl): 37–41.

33 Petersen KD et al. Intracranial pressure and cerebral hemodynamic in patients with cerebral tumors: a randomized prospective study of patients subjected to craniotomy in propofol-fentanyl, isoflurane-fentanyl, or sevoflurane-fentanyl anaesthesia. *Anesthesiology* 2003; 98(2): 329–36.

34 Todd MM et al. A prospective, comparative trial of three anesthetics for elective supratentorial craniotomy. Propofol/fentanyl, isoflurane/nitrous oxide, and fentanyl/nitrous oxide. *Anesthesiology* 1993; 78(6): 1005–20.

35 Schwartz ML et al. The University of Toronto head injury treatment study: a prospective, randomized comparison of pentobarbital and mannitol. *Can J Neurol Sci* 1984; 11(4): 434–40.

36 Guy J et al. Comparison of remifentanil and fentanyl in patients undergoing craniotomy for supratentorial space-occupying lesions. *Anesthesiology* 1997; 86(3): 514–24.

37 Bouma GJ Muizelaar JP. Cerebral blood flow in severe clinical head injury. *New Horiz* 1995; 3(3): 384–94.

38 Cruz J, Minoja G, Okuchi K, Improving clinical outcomes from acute subdural hematomas with the emergency preoperative administration of high doses of mannitol: a randomized trial. *Neurosurgery* 2001; 49(4): 864–71.

39 Cruz J, Minoja G, Okuchi K. Major clinical and physiological benefits of early high doses of mannitol for intraparenchymal temporal lobe hemorrhages with abnormal pupillary widening: a randomized trial. *Neurosurgery* 2002; 51(3): 628–37; discussion 637–8.

40 Cruz J et al. Successful use of the new high-dose mannitol treatment in patients with Glasgow Coma Scale scores of 3 and bilateral abnormal pupillary widening: a randomized trial. *J Neurosurg* 2004; 100(3): 376–83.

41 Wakai A, Roberts I, Schierhout G. Mannitol for acute traumatic brain injury. *The Cochrane Database Syst Rev* 2005, Issue 4, Art. No.: CD001049. DOI: 10.1002/14651858.pub2.

42 Vialet R et al. Isovolume hypertonic solutes (sodium chloride or mannitol) in the treatment of refractory posttraumatic intracranial hypertension: 2 mL/kg 7.5% saline is more effective than 2 mL/kg 20% mannitol. *Crit Care Med* 2003; 31(6): 1683–7.

43 Mirski AM et al. Comparison between hypertonic saline and mannitol in the reduction of elevated intracranial pressure in a rodent model of acute cerebral injury. *J Neurosurg Anesthesiol* 2000; 12(4): 334–44.

44 Haure P et al. The ICP-lowering effect of 10 degrees reverse Trendelenburg position during craniotomy is stable during a 10-minute period. *J Neurosurg Anesthesiol*, 2003; 15(4): 297–301.

45 Ng I, Lim J, Wong HB. Effects of head posture on cerebral hemodynamics: its influences on intracranial pressure, cerebral perfusion pressure, and cerebral oxygenation. *Neurosurgery* 2004; 54(3): 593–7; discussion 598.

46 Gelb AW et al. Remifentanil with morphine transitional analgesia shortens neurological recovery compared to fentanyl for supratentorial craniotomy. *Can J Anaesth* 2003; 50(9): 946–52.

47 Samaha T et al. Prevention of increase of blood pressure and intracranial pressure during endotracheal intubation in neurosurgery: esmolol versus lidocaine. *Ann Fr Anesth Reanim*, 1996; 15(1): 36–40.

48 Robinson N, Clancy M. In patients with head injury undergoing rapid sequence intubation, does pretreatment with intravenous lignocaine/lidocaine lead to an improved neurological outcome? A review of the literature. *Emerg Med J* 2001; 18(6): 453–7.

49 Clancy M et al. In patients with head injuries who undergo rapid sequence intubation using succinylcholine, does pretreatment with a competitive neuromuscular blocking agent improve outcome? A literature review. *Emerg Med J* 2001; 18(5): 373–5.

23

Cardiothoracic anaesthesia and critical care

R Peter Alston

Department of Anaesthesia, Critical Care and Pain Medicine, Royal Infirmary of Edinburgh, Edinburgh, UK

Much of the practice of cardiothoracic anaesthesia and critical care developed without an evidence base. However, in recent years there have been an increasing number of randomised controlled trials (RCTs). In some areas their findings have been inconclusive often because their sample size has been too small. Where there are a sufficient number of such studies, some areas of research have been subjected to meta-analysis. Some of these have been inconclusive because of a lack of good quality studies upon which to base them. Others, such as atrial fibrillation (AF) prophylaxis, have clearly identified efficacious therapy yet they have been found to have no influence on important clinical outcomes. Remarkably, there are yet others that have been ignored whilst researchers continue to undertake trials to establish the veracity of that which is already known, as is the case with aprotinin to reduce blood loss and transfusion. Finally, there are those, such as the use of epidural analgesia, where meta-analysis has informed us of its efficacy in reducing complications but do not and can never answer the key question "What is the incidence of epidural haematoma"? However, whilst the literature on evidence practice is steadily increasing, the great majority of cardiothoracic anaesthesia and critical care remains without any.

Introduction

Not unlike the surgery that it serves, for most of the last 50 years cardiothoracic anaesthesia, and the associated postoperative critical care, developed largely without any evidence base [1]. Although there was much research in the area, it was often focused on surrogate rather than important clinical outcomes. However, the publication in 1989 of what was to become a seminal RCT, which revealed that the choice

Key words: Surgery, heart valve, coronary artery, thoracic, aortic aneurysm; angioplasty; cardiopulmonary bypass, hypothermia; colloids; bleeding; blood transfusion; plasma transfusion; erythropoietin; fluid, colloid, crystalloid; antibiotic; analgesia, postoperative, epidural drug administration, spinal anaesthesia; glucose; potassium; insulin; cerebral spinal fluid, drainage; arrhythmias, atrial, ventricular; aprotinin, traneximic acid; aminocaproic acid; desmopressin; endotracheal intubation; physiotherapy.

of anaesthetic agent had no influence on cardiac outcome, led to a sea change in research direction [2]. Since then, studies of cardiothoracic anaesthesia and critical care have been far more clearly focused on clinical outcomes.

Robustly designed and adequately powered RCTs are required to definitively answer key questions. Notable recent examples concern the use of the COX2 inhibitor, valdecoxib and its pro-drug parecoxib for analgesia in patients undergoing coronary artery bypass grafting (CABG) surgery. The first study confirmed their analgesic efficacy but identified an increased incidence of serious adverse effects [3]. As there were a number of limitations to the design including its population size, a second adequately powered study was undertaken that confirmed the association with serious adverse events, in particular thrombotic events [4]. Clearly, valdecoxib and parecoxib should not be used after CABG surgery.

Unfortunately, many of the RCTs undertaken have been underpowered to definitively answer the question posed. Meta-analysis and systematic reviews are a tool that may provide insight where a number of such studies exist. As there have now been a considerable number of such reviews, this chapter will focus on those that address adult cardiothoracic anaesthesia and critical care and assess their impact on practice. As a result, many important aspects, for example trans-oesophageal echocardiography, which have fundamentally changed the character of cardiothoracic anaesthesia will not be covered. In addition, where relevant, reference will be made to the quality of the meta-analyses in regard to the soundness of their methodology as this is fundamental to their interpretation.

Finally, without a clear understanding of the research that drives surgical innovation and technique, it is not possible to provide a high quality of cardiothoracic anaesthesia. Therefore, no apology is offered for the inclusion in this chapter of many areas that might be considered surgical rather than anaesthetic.

Thoracic surgery

Video-assisted thoracic surgery

Remarkably, for a speciality as complex as thoracic anaesthesia, only one relevant meta-analysis could be identified. Any surgery requiring thoracotomy is a major form of physiological trespass and video-assisted thorascopic surgery (VATS) greatly reduces the degree of trespass. A recent meta-analysis found that, in the treatment of pneumothorax or for minor resections, VATS was associated with a shorter hospital stay, less pain and less analgesic administration than conventional thoracotomy [5]. The findings were more equivocal for lobectomy and further research is required. Nevertheless, anaesthetists can expect that, at least for the treatment of pneumothorax or minor resections, VATS will become the standard surgical approach.

Cardiac surgery

Coronary artery angioplasty and stenting

Stenting has dramatically increased angioplasty's effectiveness in the treatment of coronary artery disease and this, combined with the interventionalist's increasing ability to tackle more complex patterns of disease, means that the role of CABG surgery is increasingly being questioned. However, meta-analysis would suggest that, whilst there is no difference in survival between treatments, CABG surgery is associated with fewer repeat myocardial re-vascularisations [6,7]. At least for the near future, CABG surgery will continue to be undertaken, albeit less frequently and probably for the more complex patterns of coronary artery disease.

Off-pump CABG surgery

Although cardiopulmonary bypass (CPB) was the keystone that enabled CABG surgery to be undertaken on millions of patients, it has also been blamed for many of the complications of CABG surgery, including stroke, systemic inflammatory response syndrome and renal dysfunctions. So as to avoid CPB, surgeons are increasingly undertaking off-pump or beating heart CABG surgery. Many extravagant claims have been made as to the benefits of off-pump over conventional CABG surgery. Often, these have been made on the basis of non-randomised, cohort studies using historical controls and with limited attempts to address the many biases that may result (see Chapter 8). On the other side of the debate, concerns have been raised that it is not possible, off-pump, to obtain the same quality of coronary anastomosis and that, consequently, the incidence of graft thrombosis is higher.

Several meta-analyses and systematic reviews of off- versus on-pump CABG surgery have been undertaken in recent years. However, the reliability of their conclusions depends on the robustness of their methodology (see Chapter 7). For example, off-pump CABG surgery has been associated with a significantly lower incidence of AF. Yet, if only high-quality studies are analysed, the difference in incidence becomes non-significant [8]. Meta-analysis has found off-pump to be associated with a number of benefits over conventional CABG surgery including reduced hospital stay and lower incidences of myocardial infarction (MI), stroke, re-operation for bleeding, renal failure, wound infection and AF [9]. However, all of these findings should be interpreted with caution as non-RCTs were included.

Another important limitation of these meta-analyses is that, when only RCTs are included, they have small populations and so have to use composite outcomes. Even then, most have – at best – only identified beneficial "trends" that do not reach statistical significance [10,11]. Reassuringly, off-pump CABG surgery appears to be no worse than conventional surgery with CPB and, as such, it can be assumed that the technique is here to stay. However, complete reassurance requires further research and, in particular, consideration of equivalent long-term outcomes.

Cardiac anaesthesia

Antibiotic prophylaxis

Surgical site infections (SSI) are a common complication of heart surgery and, importantly, deep mediastinal infection is associated with a high mortality. Prophylactic antibiotics have been found to confer up to a five-fold reduction in the incidence of SSI [12]. Traditionally, beta-lactams have been used for prophylaxis, but growing concern about drug resistance has led to the increased use of glycopeptide antibiotics. However, meta-analysis found no overall difference between the antibiotic groups in incidence of SSI and therefore, in most circumstances, the standard antibiotic prophylaxis should continue to be beta-lactams [12].

Spinal and epidural analgesia

Currently, by far the most controversial aspect of cardiac anaesthesia is the use of spinal or epidural analgesia. Many positive benefits, often extrapolated from their use in other settings, have been claimed for such regional techniques. On the negative side, there is the unquantified risk of epidural haematoma, and consequent paraplegia, following high-dose heparin administration and coagulopathy induced by CPB.

A meta-analysis found that, whilst it modestly decreased systemic morphine use and pain scores, spinal analgesia had no effect on the incidence of mortality, MI, supra-ventricular arrhythmias, nausea and vomiting or duration of tracheal intubation [13]. Therefore, although it is an effective analgesic technique, spinal analgesia confers no other outcome benefits and, given the unknown risk of epidural haematoma, cannot be routinely recommended.

In contrast, thoracic epidural analgesia influences, at least, the short-term outcomes by reducing the incidences of supra-ventricular arrhythmias and pulmonary complications as well as allowing earlier tracheal extubation and improved pain relief [13]. Importantly, epidural analgesia did not lower mortality or reduce the incidence of MI. The lack of effect on mortality and MI may be because the sample size was too small to detect differences in such low-incidence adverse events. Even if it has no true effect on mortality and MI, epidural analgesia is clearly an effective analgesic technique that facilitates faster tracheal extubation whilst limiting the incidences of chest infection and supra-ventricular arrhythmias.

What meta-analysis has not established is whether or not epidural analgesia is associated with an increased incidence of epidural haematoma as even a very low incidence of this devastating complication would outweigh any of the short-term benefits. To establish whether or not it is associated with an increased incidence of haematoma does not require meta-analysis but, given the very low incidence, the establishment of a database of epidurals undertaken for heart surgery and epidural haematomas that occur in order to quantify the numerator and denominator of this complication.

Glucose, potassium and insulin

Combinations of glucose, potassium and insulin (GKI) have long been advocated to improve outcome from heart surgery. In recent years there has been a resurgence of interest in the influence of tightly controlled blood glucose levels in critical care patients. A recent meta-analysis indicates that GKI improves cardiac index and reduces the incidence of AF following heart surgery [14]. However, weak methodology greatly impairs the quality of this meta-analysis and thus any interpretation of the findings. Consequently, GKI cannot be currently recommended for routine use.

Cerebral spinal fluid drainage

Paraplegia has a devastating effect on quality of life and is a dreaded complication of thoraco-abdominal aortic aneurysm surgery. The drainage of cerebrospinal fluid (CSF) so as to improve blood flow in the spinal cord during aortic cross-clamping is an approach to reducing paraplegia. There are two published meta-analyses on this technique and, whilst they agree to its effectiveness for Type I and II aneurysms, one extends this to Type III and IV as well [15,16]. There are important differences in the approaches that were used to identify trials and in how the meta-analyses were undertaken and these are likely to account for the minor discrepancies in their conclusions (C. Cina, Personal Communication, 2005). So whilst there may be factors about the technique and how it is combined with other treatments that need further investigation, CSF drainage is effective and should be used in Type I and II and most probably, Type III and IV as well.

CPB

Hypothermia

Hypothermia has traditionally been combined with CPB for organ protection. The move towards "fast-tracking" patients in recent years has led to an increasing use of normothermia so as to avoid the postoperative complications associated with hypothermia including shivering, haemodynamic instability and coagulopathy. However, there has been concern that this approach might lead to more neurological damage. Meta-analysis of pooled adverse events found no evidence to suggest that either technique was superior in this respect [17]. Therefore, there is currently insufficient evidence to advocate one form of thermal management over another.

Prime

To initiate CPB, the circuit has to be primed with fluid. Over the years, there has been ongoing debate as to the relative merits of different priming solutions and most hotly debated, has been the difference between colloid and crystalloid solutions. Whilst meta-analysis indicates that using crystalloid solution results in a more positive fluid balance, it was not able to determine if this translated into meaningful outcomes such as mortality, adverse events or prolonged stay in critical care units [18].

The choice of colloid solutions has also been debated. Albumin has traditionally been the preferred colloid but it is expensive and may be a vector for prion transmission. For this reason, the synthetic colloid hydroxyethyl starch has been used in some centres as an inexpensive alternative colloid. However, there are reasonable concerns that these solutions may impair coagulation and lead to increased blood loss and, consequently, more blood transfusion. Indeed, meta-analysis indicates that hydroxyethyl starch increases blood loss by an average of 14% [19]. Again, this difference had no effect on important clinical outcomes including re-exploration, duration of mechanical ventilation, intensive care unit (ICU) stay or blood products usage. Thus, although there are measurable differences between crystalloids and colloids and between colloids, the current information is insufficient to inform a change in practice.

Blood loss and transfusion

Considerable blood loss can occur during and after heart surgery and transfusion with red blood cells and blood products is frequently required, with the attendant risks of infection, reactions and transfusion related lung injury. For this reason, pharmacological and mechanical approaches to reducing blood loss and transfusion have been extensively investigated.

Erythropoietin

Preoperative use of erythropoietin to stimulate marrow production of red blood cells is one approach to reducing the need for blood transfusion. Meta-analysis indicates that, for heart surgery, it is effective in reducing blood transfusion when it is combined with autologous predonation of blood, but not when used alone [20]. There are also practical limitations to preoperative administration of erythropoietin and autologous blood donation and the clinical effectiveness, cost effectiveness and safety, compared to other therapies, needs to be evaluated before it could be recommended for routine clinical use.

Fresh frozen plasma

Fresh frozen plasma (FFP) is frequently administered to patients undergoing heart surgery to reduce bleeding. A meta-analysis found that there had been no therapeutic trials of FFP and that the prophylactic intraoperative administration of FFP was not associated with reduced blood loss [21]. Thus, the administration of FFP, which is an everyday occurrence, lacks an evidence base.

Aprotinin

One of the most fascinating meta-analysis in this area is on the use of aprotinin [22]. Cumulative meta-analysis indicates that after the twelfth study of aprotinin, published in June of 1992, aprotinin was found to effectively reduce blood transfusion (Figure 23.1). Results were similar irrespective of whether patients were, or were not taking aspirin or whether the sternotomy was first-time or re-do surgery. If only good quality studies were included then the effectiveness of aprotinin was established by 1990. Despite this, a remarkable 31 good quality but redundant trials were published between 1990 and 2001.

The motivation for undertaking these additional trials is unclear. Although there were concerns that aprotinin might cause graft thrombosis, much larger sample sizes would have been required to investigate this outcome. Perhaps a more likely reason that so many redundant trials were undertaken is a consistent and unethical failure to undertake an adequate literature search [22].

Another recent meta-analysis allays concerns regarding graft occlusion, as aprotinin has been associated with a lower mortality and incidence of MI [23]. So, whilst there may remain arguments for using other means, there can be no dubiety that aprotinin can safely be used to reduce blood loss and transfusion.

Other pharmacological agents

Tranexemic acid is of similar efficacy as aprotinin, but is far cheaper [24]. Epsilon aminocaproic acid (EACA) may also be effective but meta-analysis was inconclusive because of scarcity of RCTs. By contrast, meta-analysis of desmopressin found no associated reduction in blood loss or red blood cell transfusion [25]. Therefore, the current evidence base means that desmopressin should not be routinely used to reduce blood transfusion and that there is insufficient evidence to use EACA. Tranexemic acid should be used to reduce blood transfusion especially where cost is a factor.

Cell salvage

Cell salvage is a mechanical approach to minimising transfusion and involves re-infusion of the patient's own blood following salvage of red blood cells. Washed cell salvage, that is when the non-cellular matter is removed by centrifuging, but not unwashed cell salvage effectively reduces blood transfusion [26]. However, the relative

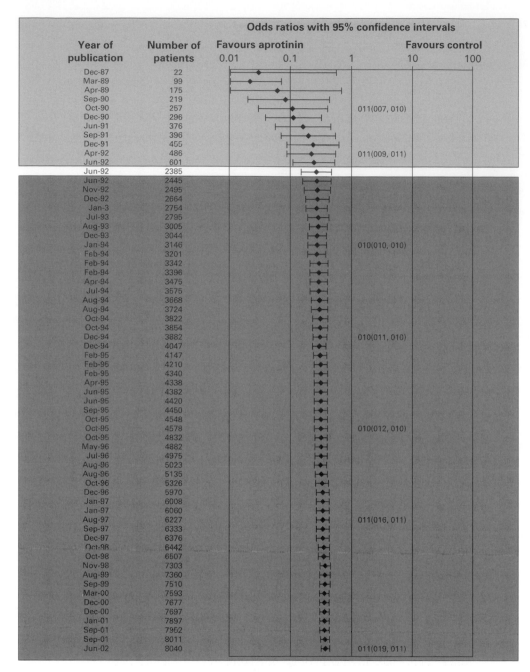

Figure 23.1 A cumulative meta-analysis of 64 randomised controlled trials investigating the effect of aprotonin on the proportion of patients transfused of one or more units of allogeneic red blood cells. By twelfth study published in June 1992, it is clear that aprotinin greatly decreased the need for perioperative blood transfusion with an odds ratio stabilising at 0.25 ($P < 10^{-6}$) [22]. In the next decade, a further 52 trials were undertaken which were *redundant* as the efficacy of aprotinin had clearly been previously established. Figure modified from the original generously supplied by Dean Fergusson and reproduced with permission of the publisher, Holder and Co

merits of cell salvage compared to pharmacological methods to reduce blood loss, or the potential of a combined approach, requires further investigation.

Postoperative care

Fast tracking

Traditionally, elective mechanical ventilation until, at least, the first postoperative day was the norm. In part, this was a necessity given the widespread use of high-dose opioid anaesthesia [1]. Burgeoning costs of critical care, most especially in the USA, combined with the recognition that such high-dose opioid anaesthesia did not influence outcome [2], led to the concept of "fast-tracking" patients through the critical care area. Early tracheal extubation, that is within a few hours of surgery, is a fundamental component of "fast tracking". A major concern was that fast tracking would increase adverse events, but meta-analysis has found no evidence of an increased mortality or morbidity with early tracheal extubation [27]. However, early tracheal extubation did significantly reduce the average time spent in critical care and the total hospital stay. Therefore, techniques of anaesthesia and systems of critical care that facilitate early extubation should be used. The definition of early extubation as 4–8 h was used in the meta-analysis, which some might now consider conservative, and research is required to establish safety of tracheal extubation immediately after or within an hour or two of surgery.

Chest drains

Cardiac tamponade is a life-threatening complication of heart surgery. Tamponade is a consequence of blood collecting in the pericardial space compressing the heart and so reducing cardiac output. For this reason, mediastinal chest drains are routinely inserted to assist the clearance of blood from the pericardial space. To prevent chest tubes from blocking with clots, and so precipitating tamponade, a variety of manipulations are used including milking, stripping, fan folding and tapping. Unfortunately, meta-analysis could give no insight as to the best approach because there were an insufficient number of studies comparing the different methods [28]. Thus, we have no evidence base to inform or guide a common clinical practice.

Physiotherapy

Respiratory physiotherapy is widely used to prevent pulmonary complications, yet meta-analysis indicates that the usefulness of physical therapy, incentive spirometry, continuous positive pressure and intermittent positive pressure breathing all remain unproven [29]. Large RCTs are needed to establish whether any of these costly therapies have a place following heart surgery.

Arrhythmias

AF is a frequent complication of heart surgery, occurring in about 35% of patients. Observational studies have associated AF with stroke, prolonged hospital stay and increased costs. There are a remarkably large number of meta-analyses, many of high quality, regarding pharmacological prophylaxis that have established that beta-blockers, sotalol, amiodarone, magnesium and the rate-limiting calcium channel blockers all reduce the incidence of AF by a similar magnitude [30,31,8,32,33,34,35]. In addition, electrical pacing of the heart has also been found to be effective [36,37].

Given its reputed effectiveness, one might expect prophylaxis to be universally used, but this is not the case. Indeed, the most recent meta-analyses have failed to establish an association between prophylaxis and shorter hospital stays, economic benefits or the reduced incidence of stroke [37,33,35]. Many of the pro-prophylaxis meta-analyses are based on RCTs from the last 30 years. During this time there have been major changes in surgery and postoperative care. In particular, pharmacological treatments, such as amiodarone and sotalol, have been introduced and they rapidly control the heart rate if not always convert AF to sinus rhythm. Thus any benefits in preventing AF and the associated adverse outcomes are matched by fast-acting treatments. Therefore, despite the large volume of high-quality evidence of efficacy, routine prophylaxis against AF cannot be recommended.

Ventricular arrhythmias are far less frequent than supra-ventricular arrhythmias, but ventricular tachycardia (VT) and fibrillation (VF) are associated with a very high in-hospital mortality [33]. However, patients who are successfully resuscitated have a good long-term prognosis. Only magnesium has been found by meta-analysis to significantly reduce the incidence of ventricular arrhythmias, but this does not translate into reduced mortality, incidence of MI or hospital stay [33]. Therefore, magnesium is not routinely recommended for prophylaxis of ventricular arrhythmias and early detection and defibrillation must remain paramount to salvage those patients who will experience VF/VT.

Summary

Meta-analyses have informed change in the practice of some important areas of cardiothoracic anaesthesia and critical care, such as pharmacological and mechanical reduction of blood loss and transfusion. They have also clearly established that some treatments are highly effective, such as the prophylaxis of AF, yet are of questionable value. In addition, meta-analyses have failed in other areas because the studies upon which they are based are too few, poor quality or not focused on important clinical outcomes, as for example is the case with the choice of prime for CPB. Finally, there are many important aspects of cardiothoracic anaesthesia and critical care that have not been subjected to RCTs far less meta-analysis. These aspects remain without an evidence base and practice is based on individual and institutional clinical experience, which is always prone to idiosyncrasy.

Practice points

- VATS is the technique of choice for minor resection.
- Off-pump has equivalent outcomes to conventional on-pump CABG surgery.
- Beta-lactams and not glycopeptides, should be the routine antibiotics used for prophylaxis of SSI.
- Spinal analgesia improves the quality of pain relief but has not been shown to confer outcome benefits.
- Epidural analgesia reduces adverse effects following CABG surgery but the incidence of epidural haematoma remains unknown.
- CSF drainage reduces the incidence of paraplegia associated with thoraco-abdominal aortic aneurysm surgery.
- Aprotinin, tranexemic acid or washed cell salvage, but not desmopressin, should be used to reduce blood loss and transfusion.
- Tracheal extubation with 4–8 h of surgery is safe.
- Routine prophylaxis of atrial fibrillation is unwarranted.

Research agenda

- Comparison of long-term outcomes after on- and off-pump CABG surgery.
- Comparison of outcomes for lobectomy using VATS and open thoracotomy.
- Combination of pharmacological and cell salvage techniques to reduce blood loss and transfusion.
- Establishment of a database to define the incidence of haematoma after epidural analgesia.
- High-quality studies of GKI regimes.
- Safety of tracheal extubation immediately after, or within 2 h of heart surgery.
- Effectiveness of manipulations to facilitate chest drainage.
- Efficacy and cost effectiveness of physiotherapy techniques to prevent pulmonary complications.
- Future studies into the prophylaxis of AF should be powered on outcomes such as stroke, and not its incidence.
- Further research of the safety and efficacy of aprotinin is *not* required.

REFERENCES

1 Alston RP. Anaesthesia and cardiopulmonary bypass: an historical review. *Perfusion* 1992; 7: 77–88.

2 Slogoff S, Keats AS. Randomized trial of primary anesthetic agents on outcome of coronary artery bypass operations. *Anesthesiology* 1989; 70: 179–88.

3 Ott E, Nussmeier NA, Duke PC et al. Efficacy and safety of the cyclooxygenase 2 inhibitors parecoxib and valdecoxib in patients undergoing coronary artery bypass surgery. *J Thorac Cardiovasc Surg* 2003; 125: 1481–92.

4 Nussmeier NA, Whelton AA, Brown MT et al. Complications of the COX-2 inhibitors parecoxib and valdecoxib after cardiac surgery. *New Engl J Med*; 352: 1081–91.

5 Sedrakyan A, van der Meulen J, Lewsey J et al. Video assisted thoracic surgery for treatment of pneumothorax and lung resections: systematic review of randomised clinical trials. *BMJ* 2004; 329: 1008–10.

6 Biondi-Zoccai GG, Abbate A, Agostoni P et al. Stenting versus surgical bypass grafting for coronary artery disease: systematic overview and meta-analysis of randomized trials. *Ital Heart J* 2003; 4: 271–80.

7 Bakhai A, Hill RA, Dundar Y et al. Percutaneous transluminal coronary angioplasty with stents versus coronary artery bypass grafting for people with stable angina or acute coronary syndromes. *The Cochrane Database of Syst Rev*, Issue 1, 2005. Art. No. CD004588. DOI: 10.1002/14651858.CD004588.pub3.

8 Athanasiou T, Aziz O, Mangoush O et al. Does off-pump coronary artery bypass reduce the incidence of post-operative atrial fibrillation? A question revisited. *Eur J Cardiothorac Surg* 2004a; 26: 701–10.

9 Reston JT, Tregear SJ, Turkelson CM. Meta-analysis of short-term and mid-term outcomes following off-pump coronary artery bypass grafting. *Ann Thorac Surg* 2003; 76: 1510–5.

10 Parolari A, Alamanni F, Cannata A et al. Off-pump versus on-pump coronary artery bypass: meta-analysis of currently available randomized trials. *Ann Thorac Surg* 2003; 76: 37–40.

11 van der Heijden GJMG, Nathoe HM, Jansen EWL et al. Meta-analysis on the effect of off-pump coronary bypass surgery. *Eur J Cardiothorac Surg* 2004; 26: 81–4.

12 Bolon MK, Morlote M, Weber SG et al. Glycopeptides are no more effective than beta-lactam agents for prevention of surgical site infection after cardiac surgery: a meta-analysis. *Clin Infect Dis* 2004; 38: 1357–63.

13 Liu SS, Block BM, Wu CL. Effects of perioperative central neuraxial analgesia on outcome after coronary artery bypass surgery: a meta-analysis. *Anesthesiology* 2004; 101: 153–61.

14 Bothe W, Olschewski M, Beyersdorf F et al. Glucose-insulin-potassium in cardiac surgery: a meta-analysis. *Ann Thorac Surg* 2004; 78: 1650–7.

15 Cina CS, Abouzahr L, Arena GO et al. Cerebrospinal fluid drainage to prevent paraplegia during thoracic and thoracoabdominal aortic aneurysm surgery: a systematic review and meta-analysis. *J Vasc Surg* 2004; 40: 36–44.

16 Khan SN, Stansby G. Cerebrospinal fluid drainage for thoracic and thoracoabdominal aortic aneurysm surgery. *The Cochrane Database of Syst Rev*, Issue 4, 2003. Art. No. CD003635. DOI: 10.1002/14651858.CD003635.pub2.

17 Rees K, Beranek-Stanley M, Burke M et al. Hypothermia to reduce neurological damage following coronary artery bypass surgery. *The Cochrane Database of Syst Rev* 2001, Issue 1. Art. No. CD002138. DOI: 10.1002/14651858.

18 Himpe D. Colloids versus crystalloids as priming solutions for cardiopulmonary bypass: a meta-analysis of prospective, randomised clinical trials. *Acta Anaesthesiol Belg* 2003; 54: 207–15.

19 Wilkes MM, Navickis RJ, Sibbald WJ. Albumin versus hydroxyethyl starch in cardio-pulmonary bypass surgery: a meta-analysis of postoperative bleeding. *Ann Thorac Surg* 2001; 72: 527–33.

20 Laupacis A, Fergusson D and For the International Study of Peri-operative Transfusion. Erythropoietin to minimize perioperative blood transfusion: a systematic review of random-ized trials. *Transfus Med* 1998; 8: 309–17.

21 Casbard AC, Williamson LM, Murphy MF et al. The role of prophylactic fresh frozen plasma in decreasing blood loss and correcting coagulopathy in cardiac surgery. A systematic review. *Anaesthesia* 2004; 59: 550–8.

22 Fergusson D, Glass KC, Hutton B et al. Randomized controlled trials of aprotinin in cardiac surgery: could clinical equipoise have stopped the bleeding? *Clin Trial* 2005; 2: 218–29.

23 Sedrakyan A, Treasure T, Elefteriades JA. Effect of aprotinin on clinical outcomes in coronary artery bypass graft surgery: a systematic review and meta-analysis of randomized clinical trials. *J Thorac Cardiovasc Surg* 2004; 128: 442–8.

24 Henry DA, Moxey AJ, Carless PA et al. Anti-fibrinolytic use for minimising perioperative allogeneic blood transfusion. *The Cochrane Database of Syst Rev*, Issue 4, 1999. Art. No. CD001886. DOI: 10.1002/14651858.CD001886.

25 Carless PA, Henry DA, Moxey AJ et al. Desmopressin for minimising perioperative allogeneic blood transfusion. *The Cochrane Database of Syst Rev*, Issue 1, 2004. Art. No. CD001884. DOI: 10.1002/14651858.CD001884.pub2.

26 Carless PA, Henry DA, Moxey AJ et al. Cell salvage for minimising perioperative allogeneic blood transfusion. *The Cochrane Database of Syst Rev*, Issue 4, 2003. Art. No. CD001888. DOI: 10.1002/14651858.CD001888.

27 Hawkes CA, Dhileepan S, Foxcroft D. Early extubation for adult cardiac surgical patients. *The Cochrane Database of Syst Rev*, Issue 4, 2003. Art. No. CD003587. DOI: 10.1002/14651858.CD003587.

28 Wallen M, Morrison A, Gillies D et al. Mediastinal chest drain clearance for cardiac surgery. *The Cochrane Database of Syst Rev*, Issue 2, 2002. Art. No. CD003042.pub2. DOI: 10.1002/14651858.CD003042.pub2.

29 Overend TJ, Anderson CM, Lucy SD et al. The effect of incentive spirometry on postoperative pulmonary complications: a systematic review. *Chest* 2001; 120: 971–8.

30 Crystal E, Connolly SJ, Sleik K et al. Interventions on prevention of postoperative atrial fib-rillation in patients undergoing heart surgery: a meta-analysis. *Circulation* 2002; 106: 75–80.

31 Zimmer J, Pezzullo J, Choucair W et al. Meta-analysis of antiarrhythmic therapy in the preven-tion of postoperative atrial fibrillation and the effect on hospital length of stay, costs, cerebro-vascular accidents, and mortality in patients undergoing cardiac surgery. *Am J Cardiol* 2003; 91: 1137–40.

32 Athanasiou T, Aziz O, Mangoush O et al. Do off-pump techniques reduce the incidence of postoperative atrial fibrillation in elderly patients undergoing coronary artery bypass graft-ing? *Ann Thorac Surg* 2004b; 77: 1567–74.

33 Shiga T, Wajima Z, Inoue T et al. Magnesium prophylaxis for arrhythmias after cardiac sur-gery: a meta-analysis of randomized controlled trials. *Am J Med* 2004; 117: 325–33.

34 Alghamdi AA, Al-Radi OO, Latter DA. Intravenous magnesium for prevention of atrial fibrillation after coronary artery bypass surgery: a systematic review and meta-analysis. *J Card Surg* 2005; 20: 293–9.

35 Miller S, Crystal E, Garfinkle M et al. Effects of magnesium on atrial fibrillation after cardiac surgery: a meta-analysis. *Heart* 2005; 91: 618–23.

36 Daoud EG, Snow R, Hummel JD et al. Temporary atrial epicardial pacing as prophylaxis against atrial fibrillation after heart surgery: a meta-analysis. *J Cardiovasc Electrophysiol* 2003; 14: 127–32.

37 Crystal E, Garfinkle MS, Connolly SS et al. Interventions for preventing post-operative atrial fibrillation in patients undergoing heart surgery. *The Cochrane Database of Syst Rev*, Issue 4, 2004. Art. No. CD003611.pub2. DOI: 10.1002/14651858.CD003611.pub2.

24

Postoperative pain therapy

Timothy Canty[1] and Jane Ballantyne[2]

[1]Arnold Pain Management Center, Beth Israel Deaconess Medical Center, Boston, USA
[2]Massachusetts General Hospital Department of Anesthesiology, Boston, USA

Opioid analgesics have long been the mainstay of postoperative pain management. Although effective, their usefulness is offset by opioid-related side effects such as nausea and vomiting, sedation, and bowel and bladder dysmotility, all of which can delay the return to normal physiologic functioning after surgery. In this chapter we review alternative and adjunctive modes of delivering postoperative analgesia and summarise what is known about efficacy and outcome. Current evidence demonstrates convincingly that epidural analgesia, patient-controlled analgesia (PCA), and adjuncts (non-steroidal anti-inflammatory drugs (NSAIDs), acetaminophen, and gabapentin) improve postoperative analgesia and patient satisfaction. Each of these modalities (except PCA) show a measurable opioid-sparing effect, but the reduction of opioid intake although theoretically beneficial, has not consistently been shown to improve outcome and recovery. Epidural analgesia does offer a number of distinct benefits that hasten recovery. Its use has not however been shown to reduce mortality. It is unclear at this point whether pre-emptive interventions can affect postoperative outcome, but the evidence is increasingly supporting this approach for certain treatments (epidural analgesia, local anaesthetics, NSAIDs, and gabapentin). The current trend in postoperative analgesia is a movement towards a multimodal approach of treating pain throughout the perioperative period.

In the last two decades efforts have been made to promote evidence-based guidelines for postoperative pain management [1]. Opioid analgesics administered by injection or by mouth have long been the mainstay of postoperative pain control. Although the effectiveness of this approach cannot be contested, it is clear that opioid-related side effects such as postoperative nausea and vomiting (PONV), sedation, and bowel and bladder immobility contribute to the delay in recovery and return to normal function that is sought in our current paradigm for postoperative management. Much of the evidence in the literature compares newer modalities and opioid adjuncts with standard opioid management, with an emphasis on whether or

Key words: Postoperative analgesia, pre-emptive analgesia, epidural analgesia, PCA, multimodal analgesia, gabapentin, NSAIDs.

not postoperative morbidity and mortality could be affected and opioid intake decreased. Our focus in this chapter is to present the evidence for the commonly utilised analgesic modalities as they pertain to postoperative outcome in light of our overall goal of rapid return to normal physiologic function after surgery and the increasing movement towards a multimodal approach to analgesia.

Evidence in support of epidural analgesia

Epidural analgesia can be accomplished by infusing a variety of drugs (typically low dose local anaesthetics and opioids) into the epidural space. With direct application of opioids to spinal receptors, overall lower doses are needed so that the central and systemic effects of sedation and bowel immobility are minimised. Conceptually, the provision of epidural analgesia is an attractive means of minimising opioid requirement while providing excellent analgesia, thereby promoting recovery after surgery. Does the evidence support the superior analgesic efficacy of epidural analgesia compared to systemic opioids, and its ability to promote recovery after surgery with improved outcomes? A summary of the current literature on the beneficial effects of epidural analgesia is presented in Table 24.1.

Randomised trials and meta-analyses overwhelmingly support the superior analgesic efficacy of epidural analgesia compared with "conventional analgesia" and PCA administered opioids [1,9]. Early smaller randomised controlled trials [2,26] (RCTs) even concluded that mortality associated with high-risk patients undergoing major operations could be reduced with epidural analgesia, but the validity of these studies has been called into question [27]. Since the initial promising studies suggesting a mortality benefit, larger well-designed RCTs and meta-analyses have not shown the same improved mortality from epidural analgesia compared with standard opioid analgesia [3–6]. Other than an improvement in pulmonary function [3,4], and an additional improvement in rates of myocardial infarction, stroke, and death in patients undergoing abdominal aortic surgery [3], the large studies suggest that there is no benefit in terms of major morbidity and mortality. A recent meta-analysis also finds no benefit to combined epidural–general anaesthesia (prolonged as epidural analgesia) versus general anaesthesia with standard postoperative analgesia in terms of mortality (odds ratio (OR): 0.86; confidence interval (CI): 0.54–1.37) [18]. The evidence currently suggests, therefore, that epidural analgesia is effective in terms of analgesia, but fails to influence major morbidity or mortality after extensive surgery.

One of the deficiencies of the contributing studies, which may have led to an absence of demonstrated benefit, was the variability in epidural management. Many used primarily opioid rather than local anaesthetic mixtures, which presumably would more completely block the sympathetic and humoral response to surgical stress. Level of catheter placement certainly must be congruent with the dermatomes

Table 24.1 Summary of evidence supporting the benefits of epidural analgesia

Combined epidural/general anaesthesia with postoperative epidural analgesia

Outcome	Positive findings	Key references	Negative findings	Key references
Mortality	One small study shows improved mortality in high-risk patients.	[2][b]	Large studies do not find a difference.	[3–5][a], [6][c,d]
Postoperative pain	Continuous epidural infusions provide superior analgesia postoperatively in selected patients.	[4][a], [1][c], [7][b], [8][b], [5][a], [9][c], [6][c,d] [10][a]		
Ileus and bowel mobility	In patients undergoing intraabdominal procedures, the use of intra- and postoperative epidural analgesia (especially thoracic) has been associated with decrease in ileus resulting in shorter hospital stay. Epidural local anaesthetic alone may have a superior effect on the bowel compared with combined local anaesthetic and opioid, but both are effective.	[11][b], [12][b], [13][d]		
Cardiac events	A meta-analysis finds a reduced rate of myocardial infarction with the use of epidural anaesthesia/analgesia. Other studies show improved cardiac outcome, especially after cardiac and aortic surgery.	[3][a], [14][c], [2][b], [15][b]	In some patient populations, no improvement in cardiac outcome is shown.	[3][a], [4][a], [16][b], [17][b], [7][b], [5][a]
Pulmonary function	Postoperative epidural analgesia has been associated with a lower incidence of postoperative pulmonary complications when compared to systemic analgesia.	[3][a], [4][a], [18][c], [19][c], [15][b]		
	In intensive care unit patients, intra- and postoperative epidural analgesia has been convincingly shown to be associated with earlier extubation compared with intra- and postoperative systemic analgesia.	[3][a], [4][a], [20][b], [21][b], [15][b], [7][b], [5][a]		
Activity levels and mobility	Epidural anaesthesia/analgesia has been associated with increased activity and improved mobility in the immediate and the long-term postoperative period. In one study, epidural analgesia also had an impact on health-related quality of life after surgery.	[22][b], [8][b], [23][b], [24][b]	Time to first ambulation and other outcomes do not appear to be reduced by epidural anaesthesia/analgesia.	[25][b], [6][c,d]

Selected key references are presented that support the benefits of regional anaesthesia. Papers are identified as: large ($n > 800$) [a]multicentre RCT, [b]RCT, [c]meta-analysis and [d]review. Modified from table in Journal of Clinical Anesthesia. 17(5), Ballantyne JC. Kupelnick B. McPeek B. Lau J. *Does the evidence support the use of spinal and epidural for surgery?* 382–91, © 2005 Elsevier Inc with permisson form Elsevier.

affected for a particular surgery with thoracic placement being preferred for thoracic or upper abdominal procedures [14,18]. The duration of epidural analgesia in the postoperative period has not been standardised in many trials, but evidence suggests that epidural analgesia continued for at least 24–48 h postoperatively may be beneficial [14,28,29].

Remember, though, that our goal is to provide analgesia that promotes rapid recovery as part of the overall goal of postoperative management which is to restore normal physiological function as rapidly as possible in order to avoid adverse outcomes associated with prolonged immobilisation and hospital stay. Epidural analgesia has been shown to promote early mobilisation and reduce rehabilitation time, particularly after joint surgery [22,23,30]. In addition, it has been shown to reduce pulmonary morbidity [3,4,15,19]; reduce time to extubation of the trachea after major thoracic and vascular procedures [3,4,7,15,20,21]; reduce cardiac ischemia and dysrhythmia in high-risk patients [7,14]; and reduce postoperative ileus thereby reducing hospital stay [8,12,13]. A meta-analysis by Beattie et al. [14] finds a reduction in myocardial infarction associated with the use of postoperative epidural analgesia (OR: 0.56; CI: 0.30–1.03).

In summary, the superior analgesic efficacy of epidural analgesia compared to "conventional analgesia" seems absolutely clear, and benefits in terms of minor morbidity and length of hospital stay (by contributing to an accelerated return to normal physiological function) have also been demonstrated. It remains unclear whether epidural analgesia has a role in reducing major morbidity and mortality.

Evidence in support of PCA

Although patients and nurses seem to prefer PCA to conventional analgesia, the questions we must ask are: does PCA result in better analgesia, lower opioid requirements, superior patient satisfaction with treatment, fewer side effects and better surgical outcome? Two meta-analyses of PCA versus "conventional analgesia" have been published, one in 1993 [31], the second more recently in 2001 [32]. Fifteen trials (787 patients) are included in the first analysis, 32 (2072 patients) in the second. The first meta-analysis was able to show convincingly that patients prefer PCA to conventional analgesia, and that PCA has slightly better analgesic efficacy. The mean difference in satisfaction is 42% ($P = 0.02$), while the mean difference in pain score on a scale of 0–100 is 5.6 ($P = 0.006$). However, there is no difference in opioid usage, side effects or length of hospital stay. The initial opioid selection does not appear to affect efficacy or side effects, but certain opioids may be better tolerated in some individuals [33]. Despite the passing of almost 10 years, and the addition of 12 trials (1000 patients) to the first meta-analysis, the results of the second analysis differ very little from those of the first. Patients' preference for PCA is confirmed, as is slightly better analgesic efficacy. This seems reason enough that PCA analgesia has been established as the standard of care for routine management of moderate to severe postoperative pain when epidural analgesia is not appropriate.

Evidence in support of NSAIDs as adjuncts

Multiple studies, and meta-analyses, confirm an average 30–50% opioid-sparing effect of NSAIDs [34–39]. Whether this reduction in opioid dose with NSAIDs translates into improved recovery and morbidity is not so apparent. The most recent meta-analysis of 22 RCTs by Marret et al. affirmed a reduction in PONV and sedation by 30% and 29%, respectively, but effects on urinary retention and respiratory complications were inconclusive. Individual studies demonstrated reduced incidence and degree of respiratory depression [34,35,40,41], but improvements in pulmonary function (less opioid induced suppression of cough, and of hypoxic and hypercapnic responses), have not been convincingly shown [36]. A limited number of studies demonstrate accelerated recovery in association with less nausea and sedation, improved mobility and earlier return of bowel function [42,43] but others fail to show any benefit in terms of recovery [34,35,44,45]. Since an important goal of postoperative pain management is to minimise opioid side effects, NSAIDs must be preferable to systemic opioids when supplementary analgesia is needed and one study has shown improvements in recovery time after total knee replacement in combination with epidural analgesia [46].

The issue of NSAID safety in patients undergoing major surgery is important since these drugs are being used with the explicit aim of improving the safety of another class of drugs, the opioids. The adverse effects of NSAIDs that cause the greatest concern are bleeding, particularly from the gastrointestinal (GI) tract and renal toxicity. In a multicentre RCT with 11 245 patients a low occurrence of serious side effects was found with appropriately administered ketorolac, diclofenac, and ketoprofen after elective major surgery (0.17% mortality, 1.04% surgical site bleeding, 0.09% acute renal failure, GI bleeding 0.04%, overall 1.38%) [47]. The route of administration in this study (intravenous versus oral) did not affect complication rate. Caution is noted since adverse events do seem to increase with higher doses, prolonged therapy >5 days, and the elderly population [48]. In a systematic review, although the incidence of gastric irritation was low, pooled data showed that risk does pertain even with single-dose regimens [49]. With the introduction of NSAIDs that selectively block inducible cyclo-oxygenase-2 (COX-2), a new therapeutic option has emerged with the promise of decreased gastric irritation and no anti-platelet effects and therefore no increase in the bleeding complications observed with non-selective NSAIDs [28,50]. Enthusiasm about the benefits of COX-2 inhibitors has been tempered by the recent association with cardiovascular complications with their long-term use. This concern now extends to the demonstrated deleterious effects of NSAIDs in general on cardiac function and blood pressure, especially in susceptible patients [51]. The exact relevance of perioperative short-term usage in surgical patients is unknown at this time.

The NSAIDs also have a deleterious effect on the kidneys when used chronically, and when used perioperatively [35]. Dysfunctional kidneys are at greater risk than healthy kidneys. Particular risk pertains to the elderly, patients undergoing extensive surgery with episodes of hypotension and/or hypovolemia, and patients receiving nephrotoxic drugs [52–54]. Surgeons, particularly orthopaedic surgeons, are also concerned about the retrospective and animal model evidence that non-selective NSAIDs suppress bone remodelling perhaps leading to fracture nonunion [55,56]. It is unclear at present whether this inhibition occurs through COX-1 or COX-2 inhibition, or through an alternative, yet unidentified pathway [57,58]. In the only prospective randomised study in humans, there was no increased risk of nonunion with the administration of the COX-2 inhibitor Celecoxib for 5 postoperative days after spinal fusion, raising the hypothesis that treatment duration and COX selectivity may have a crucial role in bone healing [59]. At this time it seems many surgeons still prefer to avoid all NSAIDs when new bone growth is important (e.g. fracture surgery, non-cemented joint surgery, bone fusion surgery), but this perception may change if further studies support the safety of perioperative COX-2 inhibitors.

Issues surrounding the timing of NSAID dosing in relation to surgery are not straightforward. Whether or not there is a pre-emptive effect is debatable, and will be addressed in a later section of this chapter. In studies that specifically examine the issue of timing of doses related to their effects, the benefit of NSAIDs was not seen until 4 h or more after initial doses (even intravenous doses), and effectiveness continued to improve even after this. In some studies, the effectiveness, particularly opioid sparing, could not be demonstrated until 4 or 5 h after surgery, which may explain the relatively low analgesic efficacy observed in the early postoperative period [34]. In practice, the timing of NSAID dosing tends to be based on safety rather than on efficacy. Preoperative administration may offer better postoperative efficacy after short, benign procedures, and is likely to be safe. On the other hand, there is no clear evidence that early dosing in the case of major surgery is beneficial, and from the safety standpoint, it is better to avoid NSAIDs until after surgery when the full extent of surgery and bleeding is known.

Evidence in support of acetaminophen and gabapentin as adjuncts

Acetaminophen, although only weakly analgesic when given alone, has synergistic effects with opioids for mild pain. But what about its use for postoperative analgesia after major surgery? A meta-analysis of 7 RCTs observed a 20% morphine PCA-sparing effect, but no difference in morphine-related adverse effects or patient satisfaction was evident [60]. In the USA, only oral forms of acetaminophen are available, but recently an intravenous formulation of paracetamol has been introduced in Europe, which may have added utility during the perioperative period. Caution is advised in patients at risk for liver damage and daily doses should be kept below 4 g. The generally favourable side effect profile of acetaminophen, and its ability to decrease opioid requirements, suggests that it should be included in postoperative pain regimens.

Gabapentin was originally designed as a gamma-aminobutyric acid (GABA) analogue for use as an anti-convulsant. Its anti-convulsant properties were unremarkable, but gabapentin was found to have a substantial ability to modulate and relieve neuropathic pain presumably through its effects on calcium channels in the dorsal horn of the spinal cord [61,62]. Recently, several studies have documented the effectiveness of gabapentin for perioperative analgesic use [63–70]. All eight small RCTs in the literature showed an opioid-sparing effect with typical doses of 1200 mg orally given as a single dose 1–2 h prior to surgery. Dizziness and sedation are the most common dose limiting side effects when gabapentin is used to treat chronic pain. Two trials measured a small increase in dizziness and sedation with gabapentin, whereas no difference in the incidence of side effects could be shown in the other six studies. Thus gabapentin appears to be a safe analgesic adjunct with documented reductions in opioid consumption when used in the perioperative period. More studies will be required to determine if this opioid-sparing effect translates into improved outcome, analgesia, or patient satisfaction. Future studies may also address the potential for reductions in the incidence of chronic pain with pre-emptive dosing of gabapentin.

Pre-emptive analgesia

Does the timing of medication administration affect postoperative pain? Much controversy has surrounded this topic since it was originally demonstrated in animal models that by blocking stimuli prior to a noxious insult, central sensitization could effectively be reduced or abolished [71]. Clinically defined, pre-emptive analgesia is any anti-nociceptive therapy that prevents the establishment of altered central processing of afferent input, which amplifies postoperative pain [72]. Practically, the clinical model used to demonstrate pre-emptive analgesia has largely consisted of comparing a treatment (epidural, NSAIDs, opioids, local infiltration, and N-methyl-D-aspartate (NMDA) antagonists) applied prior to surgical incision with the same treatment administered after surgical stimuli, and comparing short-term outcomes such as postoperative visual analogue scale (VAS) scores and opioid consumption as well as chronic postoperative pain. Earlier successful experimental models led to clinical trials with mixed results. These were summarised in a systematic review by Moiniche et al. [73]: no benefit could be demonstrated through the pre-emptive administration of epidural analgesia, systemic opioids, NSAIDs, NMDA antagonists, and local infiltration.

Despite this overall disappointing result, Ong et al. performed another meta-analysis in 2005, which included 10 newly published RCTs [74]. They used a slightly different approach for analysing VAS differences, and used the exclusion criteria proposed by The Cochrane Collaboration. This resulted in the inclusion of 66 out of 102 RCTs (Moiniche included 80 of 93 possible RCTs). With added trials and a different data analysis, they were able to turn around the negative result of Moiniche et al., and showed a significant pre-emptive effect with some interventions. Pre-emptive epidural analgesia reduced VAS scores by 25% (CI of 10–41%, P value is 0.002) and total analgesic consumption by 58% (CI of 42–74%, P value is $<10^{-8}$). Pre-emptive NSAID administration and wound infiltration diminished opioid consumption by 48% (CI of 31–65%, $P < 0.001$) and 44% (CI of 23–65%, $P < 0.001$), respectively, although they did not improve VAS scores. Pre-emptive opioid and NMDA antagonist administration failed to show any positive effect in this study [74]. There was in fact a trend for pre-emptive opioid administration to cause increased VAS scores in the postoperative period, which may support the growing body of evidence of opioid induced acute tolerance and hyperalgesia through central mechanisms [75–77].

Although the literature is unclear at this point, the suggestion by recent studies and a meta-analysis that some pre-emptively administered interventions may improve postoperative pain seems reasonable. If not contraindicated (NSAID bleeding risk with major surgeries) it seems appropriate to administer NSAIDs/COX-2s, epidural analgesia or local infiltration prior to incision. As concluded by Moiniche, future studies should focus on assessing the impact of "protective analgesia" aimed at the prevention of pain hypersensitivity through intensive and prolonged, multimodal analgesic interventions which may protect more completely against central sensitisation [73]. With this multimodal approach of combining dense perioperative epidural analgesia with NSAIDs and other adjuncts, a greater ability to block physiologically detrimental cascades induced by surgery may be demonstrated.

Practice points

- Patient preference for PCA is overwhelming supported by trials, but analgesia and surgical outcome are not affected.
- Epidural analgesia provides superior analgesia and additional circumscribed benefits, yet there is no overall improvement in mortality.
- NSAIDs and acetaminophen should be combined with systemic opioid analgesic regimens unless contraindicated because of their 20–50% opioid-sparing effects.
- NSAIDs should be avoided or used with caution in the elderly and in those patients at high risk for GI toxicity, renal toxicity, bleeding, or poor bony fusion.

- COX-2 inhibitors are as efficacious as non-selective NSAIDs without the increased risk of bleeding. They also have less impact on bony healing and therefore could be used for short-term orthopaedic perioperative pain.
- Gabapentin (400–1600 mg daily) preoperatively and perioperatively reduces opioid consumption with a low incidence of mild side effects. It may also reduce chronic pain in high-risk procedures, but future studies are needed to provide evidence of this effect.
- Pre-emptive interventions (NSAIDs, neural blockade and wound infiltration) may be effective in reducing postoperative pain.

Summary

The focus of postoperative pain trials has been on assessing new modes of analgesia with particular regard both to their analgesic efficacy and to their ability to improve surgical outcome. Knowing that opioid side effects can delay recovery, the studies also assess the ability of the new treatments to reduce opioid usage. The opioid-sparing effects of epidural analgesia and adjunctive NSAIDs, acetaminophen, and gabapentin are confirmed. It is not clear, however, whether opioid-sparing per se actually improves recovery, and the evidence from the literature is equivocal on this issue. It is also unclear about the existence of additional benefits with pre-emptively administered treatments. Epidural analgesia offers a number of distinct benefits and appears to hasten recovery (largely because of its favourable effects on the bowel). However, although improvements in morbidity have been demonstrated, analysis of current trials suggests that epidural analgesia offers no benefit in terms of major morbidity and mortality.

Current evidence demonstrates convincingly that epidurals, PCA, and adjuncts (NSAIDs, acetaminophen, and gabapentin) improve postoperative analgesia. Epidural analgesia, but not PCA, has the additional benefit of sometimes promoting rapid recovery after surgery, although an effect on major morbidity or mortality has not been demonstrated. In the case of PCA, improvements in pain relief are slight compared to nurse administered opioids, but patients clearly prefer PCA. Epidurals and PCA are recommended for their demonstrated ability to provide good analgesia, improve patient satisfaction and, in the case of epidurals, hasten recovery. However, the need for rational decision-making at an institutional level is respected. Since it has not been possible yet to demonstrate improvements in major morbidity and mortality in association with epidurals (or PCA), the question of whether to offer these advanced pain treatments often turns on cost and feasibility. The use of adjunctive NSAIDs, acetaminophen, and gabapentin to supplement opioid therapy also has demonstrated benefit in terms of improved analgesia and opioid sparing, although the ability of these adjuncts to improve surgical outcome has not been substantiated.

Trials have tended to segregate treatments, and have not assessed pain treatments as part of a multimodal approach, or in terms of their integration into accelerated recovery programmes, and a movement for future progress will be assessing multiple interventions in conjunction [78]. Uncertainty about the benefits of various modes of analgesia will remain until we can be clearer about the importance of pain control to the overall goal of restoring normal physiological function as rapidly as possible.

REFERENCES

1 Ballantyne JC, Ulmer JF, Mahrenholz D. Acute Pain Management, ACHPR Guideline Technical Report. US Department of Health and Human Services, Agency for Health Care Policy and Research; 1995.

2 Yeager MP, Glass DD, Neff RK, Brinck-Johnsen T. Epidural anesthesia and analgesia in high-risk surgical patients. *Anesthesiology* 1987; 66: 729–36.

3 Park WY, Thompson J, Lee K. Effect of epidural anesthesia and analgesia on perioperative outcome. A randomized, controlled Veterans Affairs Cooperative Study. *Ann Surg* 2001; 234: 560–71.

4 Rigg J, Jamrozik K, Myles P, Silbert B, Peyton P, Parsons R et al. Epidural anaesthesia and analgesia and outcome of major surgery: a randomised trial. *Lancet* 2002; 359(9314): 1276–82.

5 Peyton PJ, Myles PS, Silbert BS, Rigg JA, Jamrozik K, Parsons R. Perioperative epidural analgesia and outcome after major abdominal surgery in high-risk patients. *Anesth Analg* 2003; 96: 548.

6 Choi PT, Bhandari M, Scott J, Douketis J. Epidural analgesia for pain relief following hip or knee replacement. *The Cochrane Database Syst Rev* 2003, Issue 3. Art. No.: CD003071. DOI: 10.1002/14651858.

7 Boylan JF, Katz J, Kavanagh BP, Klinck JR, Cheng DCH, DeMajo WC et al. Epidural bupivacaine-morphine analgesia versus patient-controlled analgesia following abdominal aortic surgery. Analgesic, respiratory, and myocardial effects. *Anesthesiology* 1998; 89: 585–93.

8 Carli F, Trudel JL, Belliveau P. The effect of intraoperative thoracic epidural anesthesia and postoperative analgesia on bowel function after colorectal surgery: a prospective, randomized trial. *Diseases of the Colon and Rectum* 2001; 44: 1083–9.

9 Block BM, Liu SS, Rowlingson AJ, Cowan AR, Cowan JA, Wu CL. Efficacy of postoperative epidural analgesia: a meta-analysis. *JAMA* 2003; 290: 2455–63.

10 Flisberg P, Rudin A, Linner R, Lundberg CJ. Pain relief and safety after major surgery. A prospective study of epidural and intravenous analgesia in 2696 patients. *Acta Anaesth Scand* 2003; 47: 457–65.

11 Jørgensen H, Wetterslev J, Møiniche S, Dahl JB. Epidural local anaesthetics versus opioid-based analgesic regimens on postoperative gastrointestinal paralysis, PONV and pain after abdominal surgery. *The Cochrane Database Syst Rev* 2001, Issue 1. Art. No.: CD001893. DOI: 10.1002/14651858.

12 Stevens RA, Mikat-Stevens M, Flanigan R, Water WB. Does the choice of anesthetic technique affect the recovery of bowel function after radical prostatectomy. *Urology* 1998; 52: 213–18.

13 Steinbrook RA. Epidural anesthesia and gastrointestinal motility. *Anesth Analg* 1998; 86: 837–44.

14 Beattie W, Badner N, Choi P. Epidural analgesia reduced postoperative myocardial infarction: a meta-analysis. *Anesth Analg* 2001; 93: 853–8.

15 Scott NB, Turfrey DJ, Ray DAA, Nzewi O, Sutcliffe NP, Lal AB et al. A prospective randomized study of the potential benefits of thoracic epidural anesthesia and analgesia in patients undergoing coronary artery bypass grafting. *Anesth Analg* 2001; 93: 528–35.

16 Davies MJ, Silbert BS, Mooney PJ, Dysart RH, Meads AC. Combined epidural and general anaesthesia versus general anaesthesia for abdominal aortic surgery: a prospective randomised trial. *Anaesth Intens Care* 1993; 21: 790–4.

17 Garnett RL, MacIntyre A, Lindsay P, Barber GG, Cole CW, Hajjar G et al. Perioperative ischaemia in aortic surgery: combined epidural/general anaesthesia and epidural analgesia vs general anaesthesia and IV analgesia. *Can J Anaesth* 1996; 43: 769–77.

18 Rodgers A, Walker WS, McKee A, Kehlet H, van Zundert A, Sage D et al. Reduction of postoperative mortality and morbidity with epidural or spinal anaesthesia: results from overview of randomised trials. *BMJ* 2000; 321: 1493–7.

19 Ballantyne JC, Carr DB, DeFerranti S, Suarez T, Lau J, Chalmers TC et al. The comparative effects of postoperative analgesic therapies on pulmonary outcome: cumulative meta-analyses of randomized, controlled trials. *Anesth Analg* 1998; 86: 598–612.

20 Norris EJ, Beattie C, Perler BA, Martinez EA, Meinert CL, Anderson GF et al. Double-masked randomized trial comparing alternate combinations of intraoperative anesthesia and postoperative analgesia in abdominal aortic surgery. *Anesthesiology* 2001; 95: 1054–67.

21 Priestley MC, Cope L, Halliwell R, Gibson P, Chard RB, Skinner M et al. Thoracic epidural anesthesia for cardiac surgery: the effects on tracheal intubation time and length of hospital stay. *Anesth Analg* 2002; 94: 275–82.

22 Gottschalk A, Smith DS, Jobes DR, Kennedy SK, Lally SE, Noble VE et al. Preemptive epidural analgesia and recovery from radical prostatectomy. A randomized controlled trial. *JAMA* 1998; 279: 1076–82.

23 Singleyn FJ, Deyaert M, Joris D, Pendiville E, Gouverneur JM. Effects of intravenous patient-controlled analgesia with morphine, continuous epidural analgesia, and continuous three-in-one block on postoperative pain and knee rehabilitation after unilateral total knee arthroplasty. *Anesth Analg* 1998; 87: 88–92.

24 Capdevila X, Barthelet Y, Biboulet P, Ryckwaert Y, Rubenovitch J, Athis F. Effects of perioperative analgesic technique on the surgical outcome and duration of rehabilitation after major knee surgery. *Anesthesiology* 1999; 91: 8–15.

25 Moiniche S, Hjortso NC, Hansen BL, Dahl JB, Rosenberg J, Gebuhr P et al. The effect of balanced analgesia on early convalescence after major orthopaedic surgery. *Acta Anaesth Scand* 1994; 38: 328–35.

26 Tuman KJ, McCarthy RJ, March RJ et al. Effects of epidural anesthesia and analgesia on coagulation and outcome after major vascular surgery. *Anesth Analg* 1991; 73: 696–704.

27 McPeek B. Inference, generalizability and a major change in anesthetic practice. *Anesthesiology* 1987; 66: 723–4.

28 Joshi GP. Multimodal analgesia techniques and postoperative rehabilitation. *Anesthesiol Clin North Am* 2005; 23: 185–202.

29 Badner NH, Knill RL, Brown JE, Novick TV, Gelb AW. Myocardial infarction after noncardiac surgery. *Anesthesiology* 1998; 88: 572–8.

30 Williams-Russo P, Sharrock NE, Haas SB, Insall J, Windsor RE, Laskin RS et al. Randomized trial of epidural versus general anesthesia: outcomes after primary total knee replacement. *Clin Orthopaed Rel Res* 1996; 331: 199–208.

31 Ballantyne JC, Carr DB, Chalmers TC, Dear KBG, Angelillo IF, Mosteller F. Postoperative patient-controlled analgesia: meta-analyses of initial randomized control trials. *J Clin Anesth* 1993; 5: 182–93.

32 Walder B, Schafer M, Henzi I, Tramer MR. Efficacy and safety of patient-controlled opioid analgesia for acute postoperative pain: a quantitative systematic review. *Acta Anaesth Scand* 2001; 45: 795–804.

33 Woodhouse A, Ward ME, Mather LE. Intra-subject variability in post-operative patient-controlled analgesia (PCA): is the patient equally satisfied with morphine, pethidine and fentanyl? *Pain* 1999; 80: 545–53.

34 Moote C. Efficacy of nonsteroidal anti-inflammatory drugs in the management of post-operative pain. *Drugs* 1992; 44(Suppl 5): 14–30.

35 Ballantyne JC. Use of nonsteroidal anti-inflammatory drugs for acute pain management. *Probl Anesth* 1998; 10: 23–36.

36 Kehlet H, Rung GW, Callesen T. Postoperative opioid analgesia: time for a reconsideration? *J Clin Anesth* 1996; 8: 441–5.

37 Ballantyne JC, Chalmers TC, Dear KBG, Mosteller F, Carr DB. Qualitative analysis of drug interventions: adult postoperative and trauma patients. In: *Acute Pain Management: Guideline Technical Report*. Agency of Health Care Policy and Research (US Department of Health and Human Services), 1995; 28–106.

38 Marret E, Kurdi O, Zufferey P, Bonnet F. Effects of nonsteroidal antiinflammatory drugs on patient-controlled analgesia morphine side effects: meta-analysis of randomized controlled trials. *Anesthesiology* 2005; 102: 1249–60.

39 Kehlet H. Postoperative opioid sparing to hasten recovery: what are the issues? *Anesthesiology* 2005; 102: 1083–5.

40 Gillies GW, Kenny GN, Bullingham RE, McArdle CS. The morphine sparing effect of ketorolac tromethamine. A study of a new, parenteral non-steroidal anti-inflammatory agent after abdominal surgery. *Anaesthesia* 1987; 42: 727–31.

41 Hodsman NB, Burns J, Blyth A, Kenny GN, McArdle CS, Rotman H. The morphine sparing effects of diclofenac sodium following abdominal surgery. *Anaesthesia* 1987; 42: 1005–8.

42 Reasbeck PG, Rice ML, Reasbeck JC. Double-blind controlled trial of indomethacin as an adjunct to narcotic analgesia after major abdominal surgery. *Lancet* 1982; 2: 115–8.

43 Grass JA, Sakima NT, Valley M, Fischer K, Jackson C, Walsh P et al. Assessment of ketorolac as an adjuvant to fentanyl patient-controlled epidural analgesia after radical retropubic prostatectomy. *Anesthesiology* 1993; 78: 642–8.

44 Thind P, Sigsgaard T. The analgesic effect of indomethacin in the early postoperative period following abdominal surgery; a double-blind controlled study. *Acta Chir Scand* 1988; 154: 9–12.

45 Higgins MS, Givogre JL, Marco AP, Blumenthal PD, Furman WR. Recovery from outpatient laparoscopic tubal ligation is not improved by preoperative administration of ketorolac or ibuprofen. *Anesth Analgesia* 1994; 79: 274–80.

46 Buvanendran A, Kroin JS, Tuman KJ, Lubenow TR, Elmofty D, Moric M et al. Effects of perioperative administration of a selective cyclooxygenase 2 inhibitor on pain management and recovery of function after knee replacement: a randomized controlled trial. *JAMA* 2003; 290: 2411–18.

47 Forrest JB, Camu F, Greer IA, Kehlet H, Abdalla M, Bonnet F et al. Ketorolac, diclofenac, and ketoprofen are equally safe for pain relief after major surgery. *Br J Anaesth* 2002; 88: 227–33.

48 Macario A, Lipman AG. Ketorolac in the era of cyclo-oxygenase-2 selective nonsteroidal anti-inflammatory drugs: a systematic review of efficacy, side effects, and regulatory issues. *Pain Med* 2001; 2: 336–51.

49 Ready LB, Edwards WT. *Management of Acute Pain: A Practical Guide.* Seattle: International Association for the Study of Pain Press; 1992

50 Romsing J, Moiniche S. A systematic review of COX-2 inhibitors compared with traditional NSAIDs, or different COX-2 inhibitors for post-operative pain. *Acta Anaesth Scand* 2004; 48: 525–46.

51 Hillis WS. Areas of emerging interest in analgesic cardiovascular complications. *Am J Therapeut* 2002; 9: 259–69.

52 Mather LE. Do the pharmacodynamics of the nonsteroidal anti-inflammatory drugs suggest a role in the management of postoperative pain? *Drugs* 1992; 44(Suppl 5): 1–13.

53 Nuutinen LS, Aitinen JO, Salomaki TE. A risk-benefit appraisal of injectable NSAIDs in the management of postoperative pain. *Drug Safety* 1993; 9: 380–93.

54 Souter AJ, Fredman B, White PF. Controversies in the perioperative use of nonsterodial anti-inflammatory drugs. *Anesth Analg* 1994; 79: 1178–90.

55 Glassman SD, Rose SM, Dimar JR, Puno RM, Campbell MJ, Johnson JR. The effect of post-operative nonsteroidal anti-inflammatory drug administration on spinal fusion. *Spine* 1998; 23: 834–8.

56 Long J, Lewis S, Kuklo T, Zhu Y, Riew KD. The effect of cyclooxygenase-2 inhibitors on spinal fusion. *J Bone Joint Surg* 2002; 84-A: 1763–8.

57 McGlew IC, Angliss DB, Gee GJ, Rutherford A, Wood AT. A comparison of rectal indomethacin with placebo for pain relief following spinal surgery. *Anaesth Intens Care* 1991; 19: 40–5.

58 Goodman S, Ma T, Trindade M, Ikenone T, Matsuura I, Wong N et al. COX-2 selective NSAID decreases bone ingrowth in vivo. *J Orthopaed Res* 2002; 20: 1164–9.

59 Reuben SS, Ekman EF. The effect of cyclooxygenase-2 inhibition on analgesia and spinal fusion. *J Bone Joint Surg* 2005; 87: 536–42.

60 Remy C, Marret E, Bonnet F. Effects of acetaminophen on morphine side-effects and consumption after major surgery: meta-analysis of randomized controlled trials. *Br J Anaesth* 2005; 94: 505–13.

61 Habib AS, Gan TJ. Role of analgesic adjuncts in postoperative pain management. *Anesthesiol Clin North Am* 2005; 23: 85–107.

62 Gee NS, Brown JP, Dissanayake VU, Offord J, Thurlow R, Woodruff GN. The novel anti-convulsant drug, gabapentin (Neurontin), binds to the alpha2delta subunit of a calcium channel. *J Biol Chem* 1996; 271: 5768–76.

63 Dirks J, Fredensborg BB, Christensen D, Fomsgaard JS, Flyger H, Dahl JB. A randomized study of the effects of single-dose gabapentin versus placebo on postoperative pain and morphine consumption after mastectomy. *Anesthesiology* 2002; 97: 560–4.

64 Dierking G, Duedahl T, Rasmussen ML, Fomsgaard JS, Moiniche S, Romsing J et al. Effects of gabapentin on postoperative morphine consumption and pain after abdominal hysterectomy: a randomized, double-blind trial. *Acta Anaesth Scand* 2004; 48: 322–7.

65 Fassoulaki A, Patris K, Sarantopoulos C, Hogan Q. The analgesic effect of gabapentin and mexiletine after breast surgery for cancer. *Anesth Analg* 2002; 95: 985–91.

66 Pandey CK, Priye S, Singh S, Singh U, Singh RB, Singh PK. Preemptive use of gabapentin significantly decreases postoperative pain and rescue analgesic requirements in laparoscopic cholecystectomy. *Can J Anaesth* 2004; 51: 358–63.

67 Turan A, Memis D, Karamanlioglu B, Yagiz R, Pamukcu Z, Yavuz E. The analgesic effects of gabapentin in monitored anesthesia care for ear-nose-throat surgery. *Anesth Analg* 2004; 99: 375–8.

68 Rorarius MG, Mennander S, Suominen P, Rintala S, Puura A, Pirhonen R et al. Gabapentin for the prevention of postoperative pain after vaginal hysterectomy. *Pain* 2004; 110: 175–81.

69 Turan A, Karamanlioglu B, Memis D, Hamamcioglu MK, Tukenmer B, Pamukcu Z et al. Analgesic effects of gabapentin after spinal surgery. *Anesthesiology* 2004; 100: 935–8.

70 Turan A, Karamanlioglu B, Memis D, Usar P, Pamukcu Z, Ture M. The analgesic effects of gabapentin after total abdominal hysterectomy. *Anesth Analg* 2004; 98: 1370–3.

71 Woolf CJ. Evidence for a central component of post-injury pain hypersensitivity. *Nature* 1983; 306: 686–8.

72 Kissin I. Preemptive analgesia. *Anesthesiology* 2000; 93: 1138–43.

73 Moiniche S, Kehlet H, Dahl JB. A qualitative and quantitative systematic review of preemptive analgesia for postoperative pain relief: the role of timing of analgesia. *Anesthesiology* 2002; 96: 725–41.

74 Ong CK, Lirk P, Seymour RA, Jenkins BJ. The efficacy of preemptive analgesia for acute postoperative pain management: a meta-analysis. *Anesth Analg* 2005; 100: 757–73.

75 Vinik HR, Kissin I. Rapid development of tolerance to analgesia during remifentanil infusion in humans. *Anesth Analg* 1998; 86: 1307–11.

76 Guignard B, Bossard AE, Coste C, Sessler DI, Lebrault C, Alfonsi P et al. Acute opioid tolerance: intraoperative remifentanil increases postoperative pain and morphine requirement. *Anesthesiology* 2000; 93: 409–17.

77 Mao J. Opioid-induced abnormal pain sensitivity: implications in clinical opioid therapy. *Pain* 2002; 100: 213–7.

78 Kehlet H. A multi-modal approach to control postoperative pathophysiology and rehabilitation. *Br J Anaesth* 1997; 78: 606–17.

25

Critical care medicine

Harald Herkner[1] and Christof Havel[2]

[1]Editor Cochrane Anaesthesia Review Group, Specialist Internal Medicine, Intensive Care Medicine, Cochrane Anaesthesia Group; Department of Emergency Medicine, Vienna General Hospital/Medical University of Vienna, Austria
[2]Department of Emergency Medicine, Vienna General Hospital/Medical University of Vienna, Austria

This chapter will deal with a selection of topics, which are currently of practical and scientific importance. We discuss *respiratory support* including indication and conditions requiring respiratory support, examine the choice of artificial airway (tracheal tube, mask, tracheostoma). We present practical examples of ventilation strategies: lung-protective ventilation for acute respiratory distress syndrome (ARDS) and non-invasive ventilation for obstructive lung disease (OLD). Weaning from respiratory support will end this part.

Antibiotic therapy can be used as prophylactic therapy or to treat manifest sepsis. The current concept of initial empirical antimicrobial therapy and de-escalating strategy will be described. The part dealing with *nutrition* contains the steps necessary in practice: estimating the required energy, deciding kind of nutrient and route of administration, and management of problems. We will demonstrate that evidence regarding *Vasopressors* is sparse and give some practical information for treating cardiac arrest and septic shock.

Antithrombotic therapy goes beyond heparin alone. We exemplify this for deep vein thrombosis and sepsis.

Respiratory support

Indication for respiratory support

Some vague guidance is available to decide whether respiratory support should be provided to the individual patient. Nonetheless it is important to mention here that – on top of the available evidence – patient centredness, ethical considerations, and critical assessment of the actual situation are necessary to appropriately supply this core element of intensive care medicine. Respiratory support can effectively sustain

Key words: Lung-protective ventilation, non-invasive ventilation, ARDS, intensive insulin therapy, sepsis, heparin, activated protein C, initial empirical antimicrobial therapy, early enteral nutrition, vasopressors, shock.

vital functions, but it is not a harmless intervention. Some patients are too healthy to benefit and are exposed to excess risk if respiratory support is provided; some may well benefit; and others may be too sick so that respiratory support is a desperate deed only to cover physicians' feelings of helplessness.

Several conditions typically lead to the initiation of respiratory support in adult patients. These conditions may be related to the lung itself, like the acute exacerbation of obstructive lung diseases (OLD), acute congestive heart failure, and acute respiratory distress syndrome (ARDS). Non-pulmonary conditions that make respiratory support necessary include neuromuscular diseases, intoxications, diseases of the chest wall, and other conditions where patients have compromised airway protection or inefficient respiratory drive. Respiratory support in patients with ARDS and OLD is common clinical standard with differing levels of evidence to support its benefit. For neuromuscular and chest wall diseases the current evidence about the therapeutic benefit of mechanical ventilation is weak, but it consistently suggests alleviation of the symptoms of chronic hypoventilation and prolongation of survival [1]. Another Cochrane Review is currently performed to examine the efficacy of mechanical ventilation (tracheostomy and non-invasive ventilation) in improving survival in ALS [2].

Conditions requiring respiratory support

Respiratory support strategies vary to a great extent between the extremes OLD and ARDS. Bronchospasm and overinflation of the lungs is the major problem in OLD (hypercapnic failure), whereas a hampered diffusion via the pulmonary membranes is found in ARDS (hypoxic failure). It is therefore important to keep these two conditions strictly apart because therapeutic strategies are contradictory (Box 25.1).

Choosing the artificial airway

Tracheal intubation

Several strategies and devices have been developed to facilitate respiratory support. The classical approach is the tracheal intubation, which is considered the gold standard for airway protection. The early placement of an endotracheal tube is justified to limit the work of breathing, protect the threatened airway, or prevent respiratory arrest. All forms of controlled and assisted ventilation can be applied via a tracheal tube (Box 25.2).

Clinical judgement must be used when making decisions. Many patients have acute or chronic conditions, therefore values normal for the individual patients should be considered, as well as trends in the acute course.

There are, however, no randomised trials evaluating endotracheal intubation in patients with sepsis and acute lung injury (ALI) [8]. Whether oral or nasal endotracheal intubation should be preferred remains undetermined [9].

Box 25.1. Definitions of typical diseases requiring respiratory support

Definitions of OLD

COPD [3]
"Chronic obstructive pulmonary disease (COPD) is a disease state characterised by airflow limitation that is not fully reversible. The airflow limitation is usually both progressive and associated with an abnormal inflammatory response of the lungs to noxious particles or gases". (Stages I–IV)

Acute exacerbation of COPD [3]
"Increased breathlessness, the main symptom of an exacerbation, is often accompanied by wheezing and chest tightness, increased cough and sputum, change of the colour and/or tenacity of sputum, and fever. Exacerbations may also be accompanied by a number of non-specific complaints, such as malaise, insomnia, sleepiness, fatigue, depression, and confusion. A decrease in exercise tolerance, fever, and/or new radiological anomalies suggestive of pulmonary disease may herald a COPD exacerbation. An increase in sputum volume and purulence points to a bacterial cause, as does a prior history of chronic sputum production".

Asthma [4]
"Asthma is a chronic inflammatory disorder of the airways in which many cells and cellular elements play a role. The chronic inflammation causes an associated increase in airway hyperresponsiveness that leads to recurrent episodes of wheezing, breathlessness, chest tightness, and coughing, particularly at night or in the early morning. These episodes are usually associated with widespread but variable airflow obstruction that is often reversible either spontaneously or with treatment".

A Definition of ARDS
Currently the American–European Consensus Conference definition is most frequently used [5].
For the clinical diagnosis of ARDS it requires:
1 Acute onset
2 Evidence on chest radiographs of airspace changes in all 4 quadrants
3 No clinical evidence of left atrial hypertension or pulmonary artery wedge pressure <18 mmHg (if measured)
4 Ratio of PO_2 to inspired fraction of oxygen (FiO_2) of <200
If the other criteria are fulfilled but the ratio of PO_2 to FiO_2 is <300, the condition is referred to as ALI.
  It may result from pulmonary conditions (mainly pneumonia or aspiration) or extrapulmonal conditions (mainly sepsis or shock) [6]. Noteworthy, in severely ill patients, clinical criteria and pathological findings for ARDS are not closely linked [7].

Box 25.2. Common indications for institution of mechanical ventilation

Indications may include:

• Apnea with respiratory arrest

ARDS

• Tachypnea

• Use of accessory respiratory muscles

• Refractory hypoxaemia on high levels of inspired FiO_2

• Compromised cardiac performance

• Life-threatening metabolic acidosis

• Altered mental status.

Acute exacerbations of OLD

• Clinical deterioration – respiratory muscle fatigue, coma, hypotension, tachypnea or bradypnea

• Persistent hypoxaemia, marked hypercapnia or acidosis

Neuromuscular diseases

• Decreased inspiratory pressure

• Markedly reduced vital capacity

Importantly, long-term tracheal intubation is related to a number of potential complications like increased risk of mucosal damage, ventilator associated pneumonia, and prolonged intensive care unit (ICU) stay [9]. In about 15–20% cases, withdrawal from artificial ventilation may be a strenuous process [10].

Non-invasive devices

Due to drawbacks of tracheal intubation other strategies were developed, which may be summarised as non-invasive airway management. The devices which are merely used in intensive care medicine are face masks and helmets [11].

Non-invasive devices are effective tools for respiratory support, but they need good skills in handling. New developments in the shape of masks could overcome some discomfort and local complications that limited these therapies. Air leakage at higher ventilation pressure is another major problem with mask ventilation. Finding a well fitting mask requires an assortment of different masks at hand. In addition specialised software is available for many ventilators to quantify leakage and allow for it. Nonetheless it is necessary that both nurses and physicians are familiar with details of equipment. Professionalism and confidence are important for a good patient – carer relationship, which is a key for the success of non-invasive respiratory support. Several modes of ventilation can be applied via non-invasive devices. Commonly used forms are continuous positive airway pressure (CPAP), pressure support ventilations (PSV), volume support ventilations, and biphasic positive airway pressure (BiPAP) (Box 25.3).

> **Box 25.3. Relative contraindications for non-invasive ventilation (see Hillberg and Johnson [12], Copyright © 1997 Massachusetts Medical Society. All rights reserved adapted with permission 2006).**
> - Failure of prior attempts at non-invasive ventilation
> - Haemodynamic instability
> - High risk of aspiration
> - Impaired mental status
> - Inability to use face mask
> - Life-threatening refractory hypoxaemia (PaO$_2$ < 60 mmHg at FiO$_2$ 1.0)

The domain of non-invasive ventilation is the treatment of acute exacerbation of COPD, but it may also be used in cardiogenic lung oedema, in ARDS/ALI, and as a weaning tool. Data from good quality randomised controlled trials (RCTs) show benefit of non-invasive ventilation as first line intervention as an adjunct therapy to usual medical care in all suitable patients for the management of acute exacerbation of COPD. Non-invasive ventilation should be considered early in the course of respiratory failure [13,14]. The application of non-invasive positive pressure ventilation (NIPPV) in patients suffering from status asthmaticus, despite some interesting and very promising preliminary results, still remains unclear [15].

It appears reasonable that NIPPV is also beneficial in acute cardiogenic pulmonary oedema, but there remain a number of controversies [16]. Currently a Cochrane Review is underway to investigate whether there is sufficient evidence to generally recommend this strategy [17].

Tracheostoma

Another option of airway interface is the intubation via a tracheostoma. For patients who cannot be weaned and when non-invasive methods cannot be used the translaryngeal tube should be replaced by a tracheostoma tube. Earlier placement of a tracheostoma in critically ill patients does not alter mortality but reduces duration of artificial ventilation and length of ICU stay and should therefore be considered [18].

Percutaneous techniques are available as well as a surgical approach to perform tracheotomy. There are currently only a limited number of small studies prospectively evaluating percutaneous techniques and surgical tracheostoma. A meta-analysis of these studies suggests potential advantages of percutaneous techniques compared to surgical tracheotomy, including ease of performance, and lower incidence of peristomal bleeding and postoperative infection [19].

Humidifiers

Respiratory support can lead to lacking humidification of ventilated air, resulting in a number of potentially severe complications [20]. Humidification is therefore essential in respiratory support. There are different systems in use although currently heat and moisture exchangers are regarded superior to heat humidifiers in order to prevent ventilator-associated pneumonia [9]. In non-invasive ventilation humidification may not be so important, because the humidifying capacity of the upper airway is sustained. Nonetheless it is more agreeable for many patients to inhale moist air instead of dry air. An exception comes about if helmets are used for respiratory support, because moist air leads to discomforting condensations in the helmet.

Respiratory support in ARDS/ALI: lung-protective ventilation

A major achievement in intensive care medicine was the implementation of lung-protective ventilation strategy for ARDS/ALI. It aims at (1) limited airway pressure and tidal volume to reduce barotrauma and volutrauma, and (2) medium to high levels of positive end-expiration pressure (PEEP) to avoid collapse of the alveoli.

Low tidal volume ventilation and permissive hypercapnia: accepting a rise in the arterial partial pressure of carbon dioxide.

It was proposed that low tidal volume ($6 \, mL \, kg^{-1}$ body weight) and limited ventilation pressure ($<30 \, cmH_2O$) would be able to avoid distension, barotrauma, volutrauma and it measurably reduced inflammation. But lowering the tidal volume is potentially not harmless, because it may be accompanied by rise in $PaCO_2$ and decrease of pH. The clinical consequences of severe hypercapnia and acidosis include increased intracranial pressure, depressed myocardial contractility, pulmonary hypertension, and depressed renal blood flow [21]. Weighing up the potential benefits of low tidal ventilation and harms of permissive hypercapnia was the issue of recent research. A Cochrane Review demonstrates a generally beneficial effect of lower tidal ventilation, but this result is not unequivocal. Mortality at day 28 was significantly reduced by lung-protective ventilation in all eligible trials, whereas beneficial effect on long-term mortality was uncertain. The comparison between low and conventional tidal volume was not significantly different if a plateau pressure $\leq 31 \, cmH_2O$ in control group was used. The reviewers' concluded that intensivists should choose which technique is most appropriate for each individual patient. Lower tidal volume ventilation may be preferable when lung recovery is a priority [22]. Lung protective ventilation is contraindicated if hypercapnia has potentially deleterious effects, like in patients with increased intracranial pressure.

Open lung ventilation (moderate to high PEEP)

A number of factors including failure of surfactant may lead to collapsing of alveoli and atelectasis in ARDS/ALI. Shear stress along the lung tissue at re-opening is the consequence. Moderate to high levels of PEEP are used to facilitate bronchoalveolar

Table 25.1. Adjustment of PEEP according to required FiO2 in patients with ARDS/ALI (Copyright © 2004 Massachusetts Medical Society. All rights reserved. Adapted with permission 2006) [24]

FiO_2	0.3	0.4	0.4	0.5	0.5	0.6	0.7	0.7	0.7	0.8	0.9	0.9	0.9	1.0
PEEP (cmH_2O)	5	5	8	8	10	10	10	12	14	14	14	16	18	18–24

patency to avoid deleterious effects of repeated opening and collapsing of the airways. Thereby PEEP may also minimise the need for high oxygen concentrations, and hence reduces oxygen toxicity. In contrast, too high PEEP may lack additional recruitment and increase the risk of lung damage, therefore the lowest necessary PEEP level should be chosen [23].

Two strategies to adjust PEEP levels are commonly used:

1 PEEP according to FiO_2: PEEP levels are derivated from the current FiO_2 requirement. To avoid oxygen toxicity FiO_2 should be regularly adapted and used as low as possible to fulfil oxygenation goals (PaO_2 55–80 mmHg, SpO_2 88–95%) (Table 25.1).
2 PEEP according to lung compliance: This procedure involves identification of the lower deflection point in the pressure–volume curves. This method deserves some expertise (Table 25.2). A ventilation strategy for patients with ARDS is presented in Table 25.2.

High-frequency ventilation

High-frequency ventilation is often used to treat patients with ARDS/ALI but there is not enough evidence to conclude whether high-frequency ventilation reduces mortality or long-term morbidity in patients with ALI or ARDS [25].

Prone positioning

Some studies have shown that a majority of patients with ALI/ARDS respond to the prone position with improved oxygenation and lower incidences in ventilator associated pneumonia. On the other hand prone positioning may have potentially life-threatening complications, including accidental dislodgement or obstruction of the endotracheal tube and central venous catheters. The success of improved oxygenation did not directly translate into improvement in mortality rates [26,27].

According to a recent review prone positioning is of uncertain value but could be considered in severely diseased patients who are not at high risk for adverse positional changes and who are in facilities with adequate experience [8]. Another systematic review which had some methodological limitations arrived at a similar conclusion [28]. In summary prone position cannot be recommended a routine procedure to date.

Table 25.2. A ventilation strategy for patients with ARDS as suggested by the ARDS network group (Copyright © 2004 Massachusetts Medical Society. All rights reserved. Adapted with permission 2006) [24]

Inclusion criteria	Exclusion criteria
Patients who were intubated	Younger than 13 years of age
Sudden decrease in the ratio of PaO_2 to $FiO_2 \leqslant 300$	Pregnant
	Increased intracranial pressure
Recent appearance of bilateral pulmonary infiltrates consistent with the presence of oedema	Severe neuromuscular disease
	Sickle cell disease
	Severe chronic respiratory disease
No clinical evidence of left atrial hypertension (pulmonary-capillary wedge pressure of $\leqslant 18$ mmHg, if measured).	A body weight >1 kg cm^{-1} of height
	Burns over $> 40\%$ of their body-surface area
	Severe chronic liver disease
	Vasculitis with diffuse alveolar haemorrhage had received a bone marrow or lung transplant

Ventilator mode Volume assist/control
Tidal volume 6 mL kg^{-1} predicted body weight
PEEP According to FiO_2 (see Table 25.1)
Plateau pressure goal $\leqslant 30$ cmH$_2$O
Ventilator rate and pH goal 6–35 min adjusted to achieve pH $\geqslant 7.30$ if possible
I:E time 1:1–1:3
Oxygenation goal PaO_2 55–80 mmHg, SpO_2 88–95%

Weaning attempt by means of pressure support when acceptable oxygenation (at PEEP $\leqslant 8$ cmH$_2$O and $FiO_2 \leqslant 0.4$) [24].

Respiratory support in OLD

The common problem in OLD is a hypercapnic respiratory failure due to bronchial obstruction and a hampered expiration. Dynamic hyperinflation is a consequence of bronchial obstruction, which increases airways resistance, and causes intrinsic positive end-expiratory pressure (auto-PEEP) and potentially barotrauma. This auto-PEEP can be measured by an end-expiratory hold manoeuvre. Respirator settings can be guided by auto-PEEP, oxygenation goals and $PaCO_2$. Respirator settings should yield to allow for longer expiration, which can be achieved by lower respiratory rates, and manoeuvres to gain inspiration:expiration time (*I:E*) in favour of longer expiration. In controlled modes and BiPAP *I:E* can be easily adjusted, but in assisted modes it may be more complicated and requires more detailed knowledge of the ventilator type in use. A way to influence *I:E* in assisted modes is to change termination criteria or shape of inspiratory flow.

Alveolar hyperinflation can also be allayed by using adequate levels of applied PEEP. Levels of applied PEEP can be estimated from the measured auto-PEEP. Levels

Table 25.3. Example of initial respirator settings for acute OLD with non-invasive device

Mode	CPAP/PSV
PEEP	6–8 cmH$_2$O
Pressure support	10 cmH$_2$O
FiO$_2$	To achieve PaO$_2$ 55–80 mmHg, SpO$_2$ 88–95%, but as low as possible to avoid oxygen-induced hypercapnia

Table 25.4. Example of initial respirator settings for acute OLD with a tracheal tube

Ventilator mode	Assist/control ventilation
Tidal volume	10 mL kg^{-1} predicted body weight*
PEEP	start at 8 cmH$_2$O*
Ventilator rate	10 min*
I:E	1:2–1:4*
FiO$_2$	Oxygenation goal: PaO$_2$ 55–80 mmHg, SpO$_2$ 88–95%

* Adjust to PaCO$_2$ and intrinsic PEEP.

of PEEP may be set lower with non-invasive devices, because the unprotected glottis produces some natural PEEP, and lower pressure protects against mask leakage.

Additionally to PEEP, assisted or controlled ventilation is often necessary in more severe cases of acute OLD. PEEP and assisted/controlled ventilation reduce work of breathing, which is often a crucial factor in patients with OLD (Tables 25.3 and 25.4).

Weaning from respiratory support

In many patients weaning from respiratory support is not a big deal at all, but a considerable number of patients are difficult to wean. Withdrawal from artificial ventilation may become a strenuous process [10]. More importantly long-term tracheal intubation is related to a number of potential complications [9] and should be terminated as soon as possible.

There is good evidence, that in clinically stable intubated patients who are arousable, without high ventilation, PEEP, or FiO$_2$ requirements, daily spontaneous breathing trials or weaning protocols reduce the duration of mechanical ventilation [8]. Daily interruption of sedation, may avoid excessive accumulation of sedative drugs and may avoid prolonged mechanical ventilation [29].

Compared to intuitive approaches, explicit weaning protocols have consistently performed as well or better [30] (Box 25.4).

> **Box 25.4. A proposed screening protocol; the process is divided into two parts: (1) a screen to determine suitability for weaning and (2) a defined period of spontaneous breathing (Copyright Lippincott Williams & Wilkins reprinted with permission)**
>
> • Consider weaning if
>   1 Original illness resolving; no new illness
>   2 Off vasopressors and continuous sedatives
>   3 Cough during suctioning
>   4 $PaO_2/FiO_2 > 200$
>   5 PEEP $\leqslant 5\,cmH_2O$
>   6 Minute ventilation $<15\,L\,min$
>   7 Frequency/tidal volume (F/TV) ratio $\leqslant 105$ during 2 min spontaneous breathing test
> • Spontaneous breathing trial (T-piece, CPAP (5–$10\,cmH_2O$) or pressure support)
> Achieving a consistent plateau without criteria for weaning failure*, and cough adequate to clear excretions, and able to protect airway:
> – if all apply: extubate
> – if any no: continue mechanical ventilation
> *Weaning failure if respiratory rate >35, O_2 saturation <90, pulse >140 (or change $\geqslant 20\%$), systolic blood pressure >180 or $<90\,mmHg$, agitation, diaphoresis, or anxiety, F/TV ratio >105. Any of the above criteria at any time during the trial represents a weaning failure.
>
> Example of a weaning protocol for patients with ARSD/ALI [8].

Successful completion of a spontaneous breathing trial for either 30 or 120 min led to a $>80\%$ chance of discontinuation of mechanical ventilation [31].

Modes for weaning

Three modes for weaning from mechanical ventilation have been compared in a systematic review (good quality but restricted to English language): T-piece, synchronised intermittent mandatory ventilation (SIMV), or pressure support ventilation (PSV) [32]. Participants from mixed medical-surgical populations and chest trauma patients required a gradual weaning process from the ventilator (either requiring prolonged initial ventilation of $>72\,h$ or a failed trial of spontaneous breathing after $>24\,h$ of ventilation). None of the weaning technique was superior (T-piece, PSV, or SIMV) in the difficult-to-wean patient. However, SIMV may result in a longer weaning time than either T-piece or PSV. Whether PSV is particularly superior for weaning in COPD patients is currently examined in a Cochrane Review [33].

Non-invasive positive pressure ventilation (NIPPV) for weaning

There is good evidence that the use of NIPPV to facilitate weaning in mechanically ventilated patients with predominantly COPD is associated with promising evidence of clinical benefit. Compared to weaning strategies involving invasive positive pressure ventilation the NIPPV strategy decreased mortality, the incidence of ventilator associated pneumonia, and hospital length of stay [34].

Antibiotic therapy

Bacterial, viral, and fungal infections remain a common challenge for intensivists, and treatment of sepsis is one of the focuses in intensive care medicine. Antimicrobial treatment is therefore of great importance, but good evidence is still missing for a number of critical questions. The aim of this chapter is to give a short overview of the principals of antimicrobial therapy.

An increasing number of antibacterial, antifungal, and antiviral agents are available which enables effective empiric and specific therapy. However, to keep antimicrobial resistance low and to maximise efficacy, detailed knowledge of the likely pathogens in the hospital and community is essential for intensivists [35]. Regularly updated protocols/standards should therefore be used.

Prophylactic antibiotics

Prophylactic antibiotics are suggested for intensive care patients for a long time, because infections are an important cause of mortality in intensive care medicine. After many controversies a large Cochrane Review (36 trials involving 6922 patients) could demonstrate that a combination of topical and systemic antibiotics reduces mortality and infections. The use of topical antibiotics alone reduces infections but does not influence survival [36]. Which combination of antibiotics is preferable remains open and may be an issue of local circumstances.

Community acquired pneumonia

Community acquired pneumonia is caused by pathogens which are usually referred to as "typical" and "atypical". In a Cochrane Review no benefit of survival or clinical efficacy was shown to initial empirical atypical coverage in hospitalised patients with community acquired pneumonia. This conclusion relates mostly to the comparison of quinolone monotherapy to non-atypical monotherapy [37].

Severe sepsis and septic shock

Initial empirical antimicrobial therapy

According to common sense, as early as severe sepsis or septic shock is recognised appropriate cultures should be obtained. Intravenous antibiotic therapy should be started early [38]. To achieve that, a system for rapid administration of a rationally chosen drug when sepsis or septic shock is suspected should be established [35].

The choice of appropriate initial empiric therapy is a key factor for outcome [39,40]. Appropriateness of empirical therapy is determined by the likely pathogens (guided by the susceptibility patterns of microorganisms in the community and in the hospital), by the potential to penetrate into the presumed source of sepsis and by the patient's history (including prior prescriptions and intolerances). Initial selection of an empirical antimicrobial regimen warrants broad-spectrum therapy until the causative organism and its antibiotic susceptibilities are defined.

De-escalating strategy

Once the causative pathogens are identified, broad-spectrum treatment should be narrowed appropriately and shorter courses of antimicrobial therapy to prevent emergence of antibiotic-resistant bacteria [41,42].

Nutrition

Appropriate nutrition is an integral part of critical care. It is made up of (1) estimating the required energy, (2) choosing the route of nutrition, (3) defining the kind of nutrients, and (4) managing problems.

Estimating the required energy

Basal metabolism (BM) (kcal day^{-1}) can be estimated by 25 times body weight (kg). A better estimate can be derived from the Harris–Benedict equation [43] (Box 25.5).

Currently the best method is indirect calorimetry, although this method is limited if $FiO_2 > 0.5$ [45].

These values of required energy can be adapted for specific conditions: For fever the energy requirement is multiplied by 1.1 for every degree Celsius above 38°C. For stress a factor of 1.2–1.6 is used, depending on its intensity.

Route of nutrient administration

There is an enormous body of literature regarding the route of nutrient administration, including 17 systematic reviews currently. Accordingly, enteral nutrition – if

---

Box 25.5. Estimating energy: BM (Harris–Benedict equation)

BM (men) (kcal/24 h) = 66 + (13.7 kg bw) + (5 cm height) − (6.7 years of age)

BM (women) (kcal/24 h) = 65.5 + (9.6 kg bw) + (1.85 cm height) − (4.7 years of age)

To allow for the thermic effect of ingestion the value of BM must be increased by the factor 1.2. [44]. "bw" denotes presumed body weight.

given within the first 24 h after admission – is equal to parenteral nutrition in terms of mortality. Enteral nutrition is superior to parenteral nutrition in terms of infectious complications, length of hospital stay and lower costs [46–48]. This applies to surgical patients, to medical critically ill patients including those with acute pancreatitis [49] and head injured patients [50]. Therefore enteral nutrition should be established within 24 h as first line management, unless contraindicated (shock, intestinal ischaemia, or intestinal obstruction). Otherwise parenteral nutrition should be supplied. Potential drawbacks of enteral nutrition are increased rates of diarrhoea and vomiting, but less rates of hyperglycaemia compared to parenteral nutrition.

Kind of nutrient

Depending on the route of administration several commercially available formulas are available. Usually they contain 1 kcal mL^{-1}. Some nutrients contain additional amino acids or are enriched with additives. For many of these a beneficial effect in terms of reduced infections was demonstrated, although there is no evidence for reduced mortality [51,52]. A number of useful software solutions exist for the prescription of parenteral and enteral nutrition, but it may also be calculated by hand [44].

Management of problems with nutritional support

Many patients develop diarrhoea during their course of enteral nutrition. Enteral nutrition is usually administered in 12 h intervals. If diarrhoea appears the more physiological way of bolus administration may help. Though nutrients may potentially produce diarrhoea, sorbitol-containing drugs, or Clostridium difficile should be considered causal, too.

Regurgitation may be another problem of enteral nutrition. Laying the patient in a 45° upright position may attenuate the problem. Jejunal tubes may be applied instead of usual gastric feeding. However, there is reasonable evidence that postpyloric tubes do not influence mortality but delay feeding when used as primary strategy [53]. Erythromycin (70 mg intravenously) may also be used to enhance gastric emptying [54]. Currently there is no good evidence to support the use of metoclopramide to enhance the migration of naso-enteral tubes [55].

Tight control of blood glucose is particularly important in patients with parenteral feeding, because hyperglycaemia is a frequent problem. Furthermore there is some evidence that tight glucose control using an intensive insulin protocol reduces mortality in critically ill patients (most of them postoperative). Target glucose values were 80–110 mg dL^{-1} [56]. A Cochrane Review is currently underway to further investigate this topic [57].

Vasopressors

Vasopressors may be used in many circumstances in medicine, administered either systemically or topically. This chapter will concentrate on the two indications, which are common in intensive care medicine: cardiac arrest and septic shock.

Cardiac arrest

The drug of choice in adult cardiac arrest is adrenaline. It is given in repetitive doses of 1 mg intravenously or 2 mg (diluted in 10 mL saline) via a tracheal tube [58]. Adrenaline has been used in resuscitation for more than 100 years [59], but the evidence is still sparse. Moreover, it may have deleterious side effects after restoration of spontaneous circulation. A retrospective study indicates that increasing cumulative doses of epinephrine are independently associated with unfavourable neurological outcome [60]. Vasopressin was introduced as an alternative to adrenalin recently [58]. In an RCT in out-of-hospital cardiac arrest 40 IU vasopressin or 1 mg of epinephrine was compared, each followed by additional treatment with epinephrine if required. The effects of vasopressin were similar to those of epinephrine in the management of ventricular fibrillation and pulseless electrical activity. Only in a subgroup with asystole vasopressin was superior to epinephrine. Vasopressin followed by epinephrine could be more effective than epinephrine alone in the treatment of refractory cardiac arrest [61].

Septic shock

Circulatory shock is usually defined as circulatory failure, where the organ perfusion does not meet oxygen demands. Noteworthy there is no simple parameter to measure organ perfusion, therefore all variables like blood pressure, serum lactate or central venous oxygen saturation require clinical appraisal, too. First line therapy of shock is fluid resuscitation [62]. Whether crystalloids or colloids should be used remains unclear [63]. Currently albumin cannot be recommended for fluid resuscitation in patients with shock [64].

When an appropriate fluid challenge fails to restore adequate organ perfusion or if hypotension is too profound during fluid resuscitation, vasopressors should be started, best via a central venous line [38]. However, evidence from RCTs about vasopressors in shock is sparse and generally limited to septic shock [65]. The vasopressors of choice in septic shock are noradrenaline or dopamine [65].

There is good evidence that low-dose dopamine should not be used for renal protection as part of the treatment of severe sepsis [66].

Low doses of vasopressin may be considered in patients with shock refractory to fluids and other vasopressors, although no outcome data on this are available [65]. Vasopressin should be used with caution in patients with cardiac dysfunction, and

Table 25.5. Commonly used vasopressors to treat circulatory shock. Always adapt dose to the changing individual requirements (from [44,67,68] and suppliers' information)

Vasopressor	Usual dose	Comments
Noradrenaline	$0.01–3\ \mu g\,kg^{-1}min^{-1}$	α agonist; more potent than dopamine, may induce ischaemia
Dopamine	$1.5–20\ \mu g\,kg^{-1}min^{-1}$	Dose-depending δ, β, α agonist; increase in 10–30 min intervals according to effect; increases cardiac output but may induce tachycardia
Vasopressin	$0.01–0.04$ units min^{-1}	Direct vasoconstriction, no outcome data yet; not for patients with reduced cardiac output; may cause myocardial infarction
Adrenaline	$0.01–0.1\ \mu g\,kg^{-1}min^{-1}$	α and β agonist; first line in anaphylaxis; not primarily for septic shock; may induce tachycardia, impair splanchnic perfusion

higher doses may promote myocardial ischaemia, significant decreases in cardiac output, and cardiac arrest (Table 25.5).

Antithrombotics

Deep vein thrombosis

Prophylaxis of deep vein thrombosis

Up to 80% of critically ill patients have deep vein thrombosis with a great heterogeneity between several patient groups [69]. To prevent deep venous thrombosis critically ill patients should receive low-dose unfractionated heparin or low molecular weight heparin. If heparin is contraindicated graduated compression stockings or intermittent compression device are recommended except for those who have peripheral vascular disease [38].

Initial treatment of venous thromboembolism

For the initial treatment of venous thromboembolism low molecular weight heparin is more effective than unfractionated heparin. Low molecular weight heparin significantly reduces the occurrence of major haemorrhage and overall mortality [70]. In the intensive care setting a twice-daily application of low molecular weight heparin is preferable [71].

Attention must be paid to heparin-induced thrombocytopaenia (HIT), which is a serious complication of heparin therapy that has a high rate of morbidity and mortality. Particularly in patients with impaired renal function low molecular weight heparin should be adapted to anti-Xa activity. For unfractionated heparin regular measurements of a partial thromboplastin time (PTT) are mandatory.

Sepsis

In severe sepsis, coagulation abnormalities often develop following endothelial damage or organ dysfunction. Recent research activities yield at controlling these abnormalities with recombinant endogenous and exogenous anticoagulants.

Heparin

Heparin is an old [72] and inexpensive anticoagulant, which is commonly used to prevent deep venous thrombosis or catheter occlusion also in patients with sepsis. There is an ongoing debate about clinical benefits of heparin in severe sepsis [73,74], but good evidence from rigorous studies is still missing.

Protein C

In high-risk patients with sepsis-induced multiple organ failure, septic shock, or sepsis-induced ARDS activated protein C is recommended if the APACHE II score is 25 or more and if no contraindications are present [38,75]. Activated protein C should not be given to patients with severe sepsis who are at low risk for death (APACHE score <25 or single organ failure), because of increased risk of serious bleeding complications and the absence of a beneficial treatment effect [76].

Other anticoagulants: currently not recommended

Tifacogin (recombinant tissue factor pathway inhibitor) is currently not recommended in patients with severe sepsis and high international normalised ratio (INR). In a large phase III study tifacogin had no effect on mortality but was associated with an increased risk of bleeding, irrespective of baseline INR [77].

Early high-dose *antithrombin III* therapy does not reduce mortality in adult patients with severe sepsis and septic shock. Antithrombin III was associated with an increased risk of haemorrhage when administered with heparin [78].

Practice points

What we know: Beneficial interventions in critical care include: non-invasive ventilation early for exacerbated COPD and for weaning; weaning protocols for mechanically ventilated patients; early broad protocol guided empiric antibiotic therapy in sepsis followed by a de-escalating strategy; early enteral in favour of parenteral nutrition; tight glucose control with intensive insulin therapy; thrombosis prophylaxis in patients with severe sepsis. A futile intervention is low-dose dopamine for renal failure in septic shock.

What is undetermined: Interventions which may be beneficial include: lung-protective ventilation in ARDS; non-invasive ventilation for asthma, cardiac lung oedema or ARDS; method to find best PEEP; high-frequency ventilation in ARDS; prone positioning in severe ARDS; enriched nutrients; activated protein C in severe sepsis; vasopressin in cardiac arrest; vasopressors for septic shock.

What we don't know: indication for mechanical ventilation, which ventilation mode is preferable in non-invasive or mechanical ventilation or for weaning; adrenaline for resuscitation; which antibiotic for empiric therapy in sepsis; valid indicators of shock; vasopressors for shock other than septic shock; heparin as antithrombotic in sepsis.

Conclusion

Current intensive care medicine includes some key interventions which are merely related to the therapy of severe sepsis and septic shock, although the spectrum of intensive care is rather wide. Non-invasive ventilation for acute exacerbation of COPD, lung protective ventilation for ARDS, tight glucose control using intensive insulin therapy, activated protein C for severely ill patients with sepsis, early empiric followed by de-escalation antibiotic therapy in sepsis and early enteral nutrition are among the most cited ones. Numerous concepts and details for customary interventions like the use of vasopressors for shock or heparin in sepsis are lacking sufficient evidence. Research in intensive care is hampered by heterogeneity and relatively low patient numbers in particular departments, which requires usually more complicated multi-centre studies. Moreover ethical restrictions are a continuing problem when research is performed in unconscious patients who are unable to provide informed consent.

REFERENCES

1 Annane D, Chevrolet JC, Chevret S, Raphaël JC. Nocturnal mechanical ventilation for chronic hypoventilation in patients with neuromuscular and chest wall disorders. *The Cochrane Database of Syst Rev* 2000, Issue 1. Art. No.: CD001941. DOI: 10.1002/14651858.

2 Leigh PN, Annane D, Jewitt K, Mustfa N. Mechanical ventilation for amyotrophic lateral sclerosis/motor neuron disease. (Protocol) *The Cochrane Database of Syst Rev* 2003, Issue 4. Art. No.: CD004427. DOI: 10.1002/14651858.

3 GOLD (The Global Initiative for Chronic Obstructive Lung Disease). Pocket Guide to COPD Diagnosis, Management, and Prevention. Retrieved November 01, 2005 from WWW. http://www.goldcopd.org/GuidelineItem.asp?intId=1116

4 GINA (The Global Initiative for Asthma). A Pocket Guide for Physicians and Nurses. Retrieved November 01, 2005 from WWW. http://www.ginasthma.org/Guidelineitem.asp??l1=2&l2=1&intId=37

5 Bernard GR, Artigas A, Brigham KL, Carlet J, Falke K, Hudson L, Lamy M, LeGall JR, Morris A, Spragg R. The American-European Consensus Conference on ARDS. Definitions, mechanisms, relevant outcomes, and clinical trial coordination. *Am J Respir Crit Care Med* 1994; 149: 818–24.

6 Ware LB, Matthay MA. Medical progress: the acute respiratory distress syndrome. *New Engl J Med* 2000; 342: 1334–49.

7 Esteban A, Fernandez-Segoviano P, Frutos-Vivar F, Aramburu JA, Najera L, Ferguson ND, Alia I, Gordo F, Rios F. Comparison of clinical criteria for the acute respiratory distress syndrome with autopsy findings. *Ann Intern Med* 2004; 141(6): 440–5.

8 Sevransky JE, Levy MM, Marini JJ. Mechanical ventilation in sepsis-induced acute lung injury/acute respiratory distress syndrome: an evidence-based review. *Crit Care Med* 2004; 32(Suppl): S548–53.

9 Cook D, De Jonghe B, Brochard L, Brun-Buisson C. Influence of airway management on ventilator-associated pneumonia: evidence from randomized trials. *JAMA* 1998; 279(10): 781–7.

10 Tahvanainen JM, Salmenpera. Extubation criteria after weaning from intermittent mandatory ventilation and continuous positive airway pressure. *Crit Care Med* 1983; 11: 702–79.

11 Antonelli M, Conti G, Pelosi P, Gregoretti C, Pennisi MA, Costa R, Severgnini P, Chiaranda M, Proietti R. New treatment of acute hypoxemic respiratory failure: noninvasive pressure support ventilation delivered by helmet – a pilot controlled trial. *Crit Care Med* 2002; 30(3): 602–8.

12 Hillberg RE, Johnson DC. Noninvasive ventilation. *New Engl J Med* 1997; 337: 1746–52.

13 Ram FSF, Picot J, Lightowler J, Wedzicha JA. Non-invasive positive pressure ventilation for treatment of respiratory failure due to exacerbations of chronic obstructive pulmonary disease. *The Cochrane Database of Syst Rev* 2004, Issue 3. Art. No.: CD004104. DOI: 10.1002/14651858.

14 Peter JV, Moran JL, Phillips-Hughes J, Warn D. Noninvasive ventilation in acute respiratory failure: a meta-analysis update. *Crit Care Med* 2002; 30(3): 555–62.

15 Ram FSF, Wellington SR, Rowe B, Wedzicha JA. Non-invasive positive pressure ventilation for treatment of respiratory failure due to severe acute exacerbations of asthma. *The Cochrane Database of Syst Rev* 2005, Issue 3. Art. No.: CD004360. DOI: 10.1002/14651858.

16 Nadar S, Prasad N, Taylor RS, Lip GY. Positive pressure ventilation in the management of acute and chronic cardiac failure: a systematic review and meta-analysis. *Int J Cardiol* 2005; 99(2): 171–85.

17 Vital FMR, Sen A, Atallah AN, Ladeira MTT, Soares BGDO, Burns KEA, Hawkes C. Non-invasive positive pressure ventilation (CPAP or BiPAP) in cardiogenic pulmonary oedema. (Protocol) *The Cochrane Database of Syst Rev* 2005, Issue 3. Art. No.: CD005351. DOI: 10.1002/14651858.

18 Griffiths J, Barber VS, Morgan L, Young JD. Systematic review and meta-analysis of studies of the timing of tracheostomy in adult patients undergoing artificial ventilation. *BMJ* 2005; 330(7502): 1243.

19 Freeman BD, Isabella K, Lin N, Buchman TG. A meta-analysis of prospective trials comparing percutaneous and surgical tracheostomy in critically ill patients. *Chest* 2000; 118(5): 1412–18.

20 Kelly M, Gillies D, Lockwood C, Todd D. Heated humidification versus heat and moisture exchangers for ventilated adults and children. (Protocol) *The Cochrane Database of Syst Rev* 2004, Issue 1. Art. No.: CD004711. DOI: 10.1002/14651858.

21 Feihl F, Perret C. Permissive hypercapnia: how permissive should we be? *Am J Respir Crit Care Med* 1994; 150: 1722–37.

22 Petrucci N, Iacovelli W. Ventilation with lower tidal volumes versus traditional tidal volumes in adults for acute lung injury and acute respiratory distress syndrome. *The Cochrane Database of Syst Rev* 2004, Issue 2. Art. No.: CD003844. DOI: 10.1002/14651858.

23 Grasso S, Fanelli V, Cafarelli A, Anaclerio R, Amabile M, Ancona G, Fiore T. (2005) Effects of high versus low positive end-expiratory pressures in acute respiratory distress syndrome. *Am J Respir Crit Care Med*. May 1; 171(9): 1002–8

24 Brower RG, Lanken PN, MacIntyre N, Matthay MA, Morris A, Ancukiewicz M, Schoenfeld D, Thompson BT, The National Heart, Lung, and Blood Institute ARDS Clinical Trials Network Higher versus lower positive end-expiratory pressures in patients with the acute respiratory distress syndrome. *New Engl J Med* 2004; 351: 327–36.

25 Wunsch H, Mapstone J. High-frequency ventilation versus conventional ventilation for treatment of acute lung injury and acute respiratory distress syndrome. *The Cochrane Database of Syst Rev* 2004, Issue 1. Art. No.: CD004085. DOI: 10.1002/14651858.pub2.

26 Gattinoni L, Tognoni G, Pesenti A, Taccone P, Mascheroni D, Labarta V, Malacrida R, Di Giulio P, Fumagalli R, Pelosi P, Brazzi L, Latini R, Prone-Supine Study Group. Effect of prone positioning on the survival of patients with acute respiratory failure. *New Engl J Med* 2001; 345: 568–73.

27 Guerin C, Gaillard S, Lemasson S, Ayzac L, Girard R, Beuret P, Palmier B, Le QV, Sirodot M, Rosselli S, Cadiergue V, Sainty JM, Barbe P, Combourieu E, Debatty D, Rouffineau J, Ezingeard E, Millet O, Guelon D, Rodriguez L, Martin O, Renault A, Sibille JP, Kaidomar M. Effects of systematic prone positioning in hypoxemic acute respiratory failure: a randomized controlled trial. *JAMA* 2004; 292(19): 2379–87.

28 Curley MA. Prone positioning of patients with acute respiratory distress syndrome: a systematic review. *Am J Crit Care* 1999; 8(6): 397–405.

29 Kress JP, O'Connor MF, Hall JB. Daily interruption of sedative infusions in critically ill patients undergoing mechanical ventilation. *New Engl J Med* 2000; 342: 1471–7.

30 Cook D, Meade M, Guyatt G, Griffith G, Booker L. Criteria for weaning from mechanical ventilation. *Evid Rep Technol Assess* (Summary) 2000; (23): 1–4.

31 Esteban A, Alia I, Tobin MJ, Gil A, Gordo F, Vallverdu I, Blanch L, Bonet A, Vazquez A, de Pablo R, Torres A, de La Cal MA, Macias S. Effect of spontaneous breathing trial duration on outcome of attempts to discontinue mechanical ventilation. *Am J Respir Crit Care Med* 1999; 159: 512–18.

32 Butler R, Keenan SP, Inman KJ, Sibbald WJ, Block G. Is there a preferred technique for weaning the difficult-to-wean patient: a systematic review of the literature. *Crit Care Med* 1999; 27(11): 2331–6.

33 Pant S. Pressure support ventilation following acute ventilatory failure in chronic obstructive pulmonary disease. (Protocol) *The Cochrane Database of Syst Rev* 2002, Issue 1. Art. No.: CD003529. DOI: 10.1002/14651858.

34 Burns KEA, Adhikari NKJ, Meade MO. Noninvasive positive pressure ventilation as a weaning strategy for intubated adults with respiratory failure. *The Cochrane Database of Syst Rev* 2003, Issue 4. Art. No.: CD004127. DOI: 10.1002/14651858.

35 Bochud PY, Bonten M, Marchetti O, Calandra T. Antimicrobial therapy for patients with severe sepsis and septic shock: an evidence-based review. *Crit Care Med.* 2004; 32(Suppl 11): S495–512.

36 Liberati A, D'Amico R, Pifferi, Torri V, Brazzi L. Antibiotic prophylaxis to reduce respiratory tract infections and mortality in adults receiving intensive care. *The Cochrane Database of Syst Rev* 2004, Issue 1. Art. No.: CD000022. DOI: 10.1002/14651858.

37 Shefet D, Robenshtok E, Paul M, Leibovici L. Empiric antibiotic coverage of atypical pathogens for community acquired pneumonia in hospitalized adults. *The Cochrane Database of Syst Rev* 2005, Issue 2. Art. No.: CD004418. DOI: 10.1002/14651858.pub2.

38 Dellinger RP, Carlet JM, Masur H, Gerlach H, Calandra T, Cohen J, Gea-Banacloche J, Keh D, Marshall JC, Parker MM, Ramsay G, Zimmerman JL, Vincent JL, Levy MM, Surviving Sepsis Campaign Management Guidelines Committee. Surviving Sepsis Campaign guidelines for management of severe sepsis and septic shock. *Crit Care Med* 2004; 32(3): 858–73.

39 Leibovici L, Shraga I, Drucker M, Konigsberger H, Samra Z, Pitlik SD. The benefit of appropriate empirical antibiotic treatment in patients with bloodstream infection. *J Intern Med* 1998; 244: 379–86.

40 Ibrahim EH, Sherman G, Ward S, Fraser VJ, Kollef MH. The influence of inadequate antimicrobial treatment of bloodstream infections on patient outcomes in the ICU setting. *Chest* 2000; 118: 146–55.

41 Singh N, Rogers P, Atwood CW, Wagener MM, Yu VL. Short-course empiric antibiotic therapy for patients with pulmonary infiltrates in the intensive care unit. *Am J Respir Crit Care Med* 2000; 162: 505–11.

42 Hoffken G, Niederman MS. Nosocomial pneumonia: the importance of a de-escalating strategy for antibiotic treatment of pneumonia in the ICU. *Chest* 2002; 122: 2183–96.

43 Harris JA, Benedict FG. A biometric study of basal metabolism in man. Washington, DC: Carnegie Institute of Washington, Publication 279, 1919.

44 Marino PL. *The ICU Book.* Philadelphia, PA: Lippincott Williams & Wilkins, 1998.

45 McClave SA, Snider HL. Use of indirect calorimetry in clinical nutrition. *Nutr Clin Pract* 1992; 7: 207–21.

46 Peter JV, Moran JL, Phillips-Hughes J. A meta analysis treatment outcomes of early enteral versus early parenteral nutrition in hospitalized patients. *Crit Care Med* 2005; 33(1): 213–20.

47 Simpson F, Doig GS. Parenteral vs. enteral nutrition in the critically ill patient: a meta-analysis of trials using the intention to treat principle. *Intens Care Med* 2005; 31(1): 12–23.

48 Gramlich L, Kichian K, Pinilla J, Rodych NJ, Dhaliwal R, Heyland DK. Does enteral nutrition compared to parenteral nutrition result in better outcomes in critically ill adult patients? A systematic review of the literature. *Nutrition* 2004; 20(10): 843–8.

49 Marik PE, Zaloga GP. Meta-analysis of parenteral nutrition versus enteral nutrition in patients with acute pancreatitis. *BMJ* 2004; 328(7453): 1407.

50 Yanagawa T, Bunn F, Roberts I, Wentz R, Pierro A. Nutritional support for head-injured patients. *The Cochrane Database of Syst Rev* 2002, Issue 3. Art. No.: CD001530. DOI: 10.1002/14651858.

51 Montejo JC, Zarazaga A, Lopez-Martinez J, Urrutia G, Roque M, Blesa AL, Celaya S, Conejero R, Galban C, Garcia de Lorenzo A, Grau T, Mesejo A, Ortiz-Leyba C, Planas M, Ordonez J, Jimenez FJ. Spanish Society of Intensive Care Medicine and Coronary Units. Immunonutrition in the intensive care unit. A systematic review and consensus statement. *Clin Nutr* 2003; 22(3): 221–33.

52 Heyland DK, Novak F, Drover JW, Jain M, Su X, Suchner U. Should immunonutrition become routine in critically ill patients? A systematic review of the evidence. *JAMA* 2001; 286(8): 944–53.

53 Marik PE, Zaloga GP. Gastric versus post-pyloric feeding: a systematic review. *Crit Care* 2003; 7(3): R46–51.

54 Ritz MA, Chapman MJ, Fraser RJ, Finnis ME, Butler RN, Cmielewski P, Davidson GP, Rea D. Erythromycin dose of 70 mg accelerates gastric emptying as effectively as 200 mg in the critically ill. *Intens Care Med* 2005; 31(7): 949–54.

55 Silva CCR, Saconato H, Atallah AN. Metoclopramide for migration of naso-enteral tube. *The Cochrane Database of Syst Rev* 2002, Issue 4. Art. No.: CD003353. DOI: 10.1002/14651858.

56 van den Berghe G, Wouters P, Weekers F, Verwaest C, Bruyninckx F, Schetz M, Vlasselaers D, Ferdinande P, Lauwers P, Bouillon R. Intensive insulin therapy in the critically ill patients. *New Engl J Med* 2001; 345(19): 1359–67.

57 Henderson WR, Chittock D, Dhingra V, Doyle-Waters M, Fitzgerald M, Ronco J. Intensive insulin therapy and strict glucose control for critically ill patients. (Protocol) *The Cochrane Database of Syst Rev* 2005, Issue 3. Art. No.: CD005366. DOI: 10.1002/14651858.

58 ECC Guidelines Part 1: Introduction to the international guidelines 2000 for CPR and ECC: a consensus on science. *Circulation* 2000; 102 (Suppl I-1).

59 Gottlieb R. (1896–97) Ueber die Wirkung der Nebennieren Extracte auf Herz und Blutdruck. *Arch Exp Path Pharmakol* 38: 99–112.

60 Behringer W, Kittler H, Sterz F, Domanovits H, Schoerkhuber W, Holzer M, Mullner M, Laggner AN. Cumulative epinephrine dose during cardiopulmonary resuscitation and neurologic outcome. *Ann Intern Med* 1998; 129(6): 450–6.

61 Wenzel V, Krismer AC, Arntz HR, Sitter H, Stadlbauer KH, Lindner KH, European Resuscitation Council Vasopressor during Cardiopulmonary Resuscitation Study Group. A comparison of vasopressin and epinephrine for out-of-hospital cardiopulmonary resuscitation. *New Engl J Med* 2004; 350(2): 105–13.

62 Weil MH, Nishjima H. Cardiac output in bacterial shock. *Am J Med* 1978; 64: 920–2.

63 Choi PT, Yip G, Quinonez LG, Cook DJ. Crystalloids vs. colloids in fluid resuscitation: a systematic review. *Crit Care Med.* 1999; 27(1): 200–10.

64 The Albumin Reviewers (Alderson P, Bunn F, Li Wan Po A, Li L, Roberts I, Schierhout G.) Human albumin solution for resuscitation and volume expansion in critically ill patients. *The Cochrane Database of Syst Rev* 2004, Issue 4. Art. No.: CD001208. DOI: 10.1002/14651858.pub2.

65 Müllner M, Urbanek B, Havel C, Losert H, Waechter F, Gamper G. Vasopressors for shock. *The Cochrane Database of Syst Rev* 2004, Issue 3. Art. No.: CD003709. DOI: 10.1002/14651858.

66 Kellum J, Decker J. Use of dopamine in acute renal failure: A meta-analysis. *Crit Care Med* 2001; 29: 1526–31.

67 Beale RJ, Hollenberg SM, Vincent JL, Parrillo JE. Vasopressor and inotropic support in septic shock: an evidence-based review. *Crit Care Med* 2004; 32: S455–65.

68 Malay MB, Ashton JL, Dahl K, Savage EB, Burchell SA, Ashton Jr RC, Sciacca RR, Oliver JA, Landry DW. Heterogeneity of the vasoconstrictor effect of vasopressin in septic shock. *Crit Care Med* 2004; 32(6): 1327–31.

69 Attia J, Ray JG, Cook DJ, Douketis J, Ginsberg JS, Geerts WH Deep vein thrombosis and its prevention in critically ill adults. *Arch Intern Med* 2001; 161(10): 1268–79.

70 van Dongen CJJ, van den Belt AGM, Prins MH, Lensing AWA. Fixed dose subcutaneous low molecular weight heparins versus adjusted dose unfractionated heparin for venous thromboembolism. *The Cochrane Database of Syst Rev* 2004, Issue 4. Art. No.: CD001100. DOI: 10.1002/14651858.

71 van Dongen CJ, Mac Gillavry MR, Prins MH. Once versus twice daily LMWH for the initial treatment of venous thromboembolism. *The Cochrane Database of Syst Rev* 2005, Issue 3. Art. No.: CD003074. DOI: 10.1002/14651858.pub2.

72 Corrigan JJ. Heparin therapy in bacterial septicemia. *J Pediatr* 1977; 91: 695–700.

73 Davidson BL, Geerts WH, Lensing AWA. Low-dose heparin for severe sepsis. *New Engl J Med* 2002; 347: 1036–7.

74 Opal SM. Unintended bias, clinical trial results, and the heparin post hoc crossover fallacy. *Crit Care Med* 2004; 32(3): 874–5.

75 Bernard GR, Vincent JL, Laterre PF, LaRosa SP, Dhainaut JF, Lopez-Rodriguez A, Steingrub JS, Garber GE, Helterbrand JD, Ely EW, Fisher Jr CJ, Recombinant human protein C Worldwide Evaluation in Severe Sepsis (PROWESS) study group. Efficacy and safety of recombinant human activated protein C for severe sepsis. *New Engl J Med* 2001; 344: 699–70.

76. Abraham E, Laterre PF, Garg R, Levy H, Talwar D, Trzaskoma BL, Rea-Neto A, Roissant R, Perrotin D, Sablotzki A, Arkins N, Utterback BG, Macias WL. Drotrecogin alfa (activated) for adults with severe sepsis and a low risk of death. *New Eng J Med* 2005; 353: 1332–41.

77. Abraham E, Reinhart K, Opal S, Demeyer I, Doig C, Rodriguez AL, Beale R, Svoboda P, Laterre PF, Simon S, Light B, Spapen H, Stone J, Seibert A, Peckelsen C, De Deyne C, Postier R, Pettila V, Artigas A, Percell SR, Shu V, Zwingelstein C, Tobias J, Poole L, Stolzenbach JC, Creasey AA, OPTIMIST Trial Study Group. Efficacy and safety of tifacogin (recombinant tissue factor pathway inhibitor) in severe sepsis: a randomized controlled trial. *JAMA* 2003; 290: 238–47.

78 Warren BL, Eid A, Singer P, Pillay SS, Carl P, Novak I, Chalupa P, Atherstone A, Penzes I, Kubler A, Knaub S, Keinecke HO, Heinrichs H, Schindel F, Juers M, Bone RC, Opal SM, KyberSept Trial Study Group. High-dose antithrombin III in severe sepsis: a randomized controlled trial. *JAMA* 2001; 286: 1869–78.

26

Emergency medicine: cardiac arrest management, severe burns, near-drowning and multiple trauma

Stephen Priestley[1] and Michael Ragg[2]

[1]Emergency Medicine, Sunshine Hospital, St Albans, Melbourne, Australia
[2]Emergency Medicine, Geelong Hospital, Geelong, Australia

This chapter explores four important practical topics in emergency medicine. The management of cardiac arrest, drowning, burns and multiple trauma all require specific knowledge and skills in order to achieve best outcomes. We have provided an overview of the general principles of management of these four clinical scenarios and identified a number of specific questions regarding novel or emerging therapies. In attempting to answer these questions we reviewed the evidence and further identified what is known and what requires further study. Whilst there is some good-quality evidence to support practice in the areas of cardiac arrest, traumatic brain injury and some aspects of fluid resuscitation in trauma, there is little evidence to guide clinicians in the choice of burns dressings, management of near drowning and differing strategies in trauma fluid resuscitation. Opportunities for further research are highlighted.

Cardiac arrest management

The patient in cardiac arrest is the most important time-critical emergency that the anaesthetist will face. The earliest possible initiation of basic and advanced life support offers the best chance of patient survival.

In 1997 the International Liaison Committee On Resuscitation (ILCOR) published *The Universal ALS Algorithm*. The updated version is shown in Figure 26.1. It was designed to be simple, concise and easy to memorise.

In 2000, The American Heart Association (AHA) in collaboration with the ILCOR developed and published the *International Guidelines 2000 for CPR* (Guidelines 2000 for cardiopulmonary resuscitation and emergency cardiovascular care: a consensus

Key words: Cardiac arrest, near-drowning, burns, multiple trauma, traumatic brain injury, fluid resuscitation.

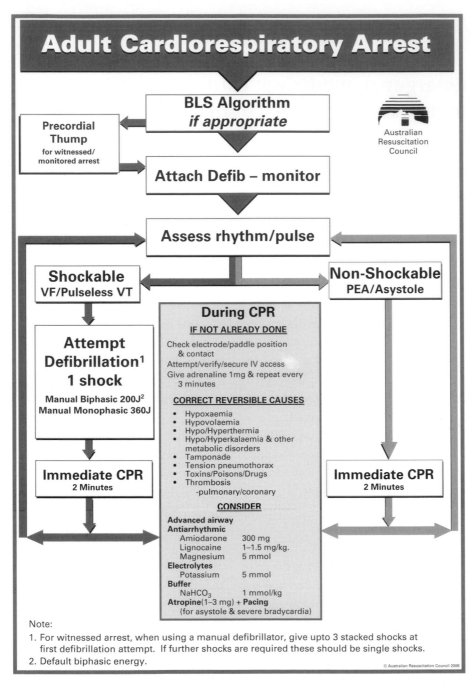

Adult Cardiorespiratory Arrest

BLS Algorithm *if appropriate*

Precordial Thump
for witnessed/ monitored arrest

Attach Defib – monitor

Assess rhythm/pulse

Shockable
VF/Pulseless VT

Non-Shockable
PEA/Asystole

Attempt Defibrillation[1]
1 shock

Manual Biphasic 200J[2]
Manual Monophasic 360J

During CPR

IF NOT ALREADY DONE

Check electrode/paddle position & contact
Attempt/verify/secure IV access
Give adrenaline 1mg & repeat every 3 minutes

CORRECT REVERSIBLE CAUSES

- Hypoxaemia
- Hypovolaemia
- Hypo/Hyperthermia
- Hypo/Hyperkalaemia & other metabolic disorders
- Tamponade
- Tension pneumothorax
- Toxins/Poisons/Drugs
- Thrombosis
   -pulmonary/coronary

CONSIDER

Advanced airway
Antiarrhythmic
  Amiodarone   300 mg
  Lignocaine   1–1.5 mg/kg.
  Magnesium 5 mmol
Electrolytes
  Potassium   5 mmol
Buffer
  $NaHCO_3$ 1 mmol/kg
Atropine(1–3 mg) + **Pacing**
  (for asystole & severe bradycardia)

Immediate CPR
2 Minutes

Immediate CPR
2 Minutes

Australian Resuscitation Council

Note:
1. For witnessed arrest, when using a manual defibrillator, give upto 3 stacked shocks at first defibrillation attempt. If further shocks are required these should be single shocks.
2. Default biphasic energy.

© Australian Resuscitation Council 2006

Figure 26.1   ALS Universal algorithm figure reproduced with permission of the Australian Resuscitation Council

on science. *Circulation* 102 (Suppl 8): II-1384). These guidelines were evidence based and serve as a very useful adjunct to the Universal ALS Algorithm.

More recently, there has been much interest in the use of the drugs: vasopressin and amiodarone in adult cardiac arrest patients; biphasic waveforms for defibrillation of ventricular fibrillation (VF) and pulseless ventricular tachycardia (VT) and finally, the role of therapeutic hypothermia in post-cardiac arrest coma in adults.

In this section on cardiac arrest management, we will seek to answer the following questions:

1 What is the role of vasopressin in cardiac arrest in adults?
2 What is the role of amiodarone in cardiac arrest in adults?
3 How does biphasic defibrillation compare to monophasic defibrillation in patients with VF or pulseless VT?
4 What is the role of therapeutic hypothermia in post cardiac arrest coma in adults?

What is the role of vasopressin in cardiac arrest in adults?

Although adrenaline has been used in cardiac arrest management for many years, there has been recent interest in the use of vasopressin in adult cardiac arrest. A number of prospective, randomised studies have looked at this and recently a systematic review and meta-analysis has been published [1]. It looked at 1519 patients from five randomised controlled trials. All trials studied patients with cardiac arrest who underwent CPR in or out of hospital. In all studies, the control group received intravenous adrenaline and the experimental group received intravenous vasopressin.

The results of this systematic review and meta-analysis showed no significant differences between the two groups in any of the following:

Parameter	Risk ratio	95% Confidence interval
Return of spontaneous circulation	0.81	0.58–1.12
Death before hospital admit	0.72	0.38–1.39
Death within 24 h	0.74	0.38–1.43
Death before hospital discharge	0.96	0.87–1.05
Combination of number of deaths + neurologically impaired survivors	1.00	0.94–1.07

The largest study had 1186 patients [2] which is 78% of the total patient number. In this study, subgroup analysis showed a benefit in both survival to hospital admission and survival to hospital discharge in the subgroup of patients with asystole who received vasopressin. This has not been validated prospectively and should be interpreted with caution until such prospective data is available.

There are two studies currently recruiting patients looking specifically at whether the addition of vasopressin to adrenaline improves survival of cardiac arrests [3,4].

What is the role of amiodarone in adults with cardiac arrest?

Historically, lignocaine has been the initial antiarrhythmic drug recommended for VF or pulseless VT. More recently the question has been asked: is amiodarone better than lignocaine in treating adult patients with VF or pulseless VT? The Cochrane Heart Group is looking at the use of intravenous amiodarone for the treatment of VT and VF, however it is still in the protocol stage [5].

There have been two prospective, randomised, placebo control, double-blinded studies looking at the use of intravenous amiodarone in adult cardiac arrest. Dorian et al. [6] compared amiodarone with lignocaine in 347 patients with out-of-hospital VF. The primary endpoint was the proportion of patients who survived to hospital admission. After treatment with amiodarone, 22.8% of 180 patients survived to hospital admission versus 12% of 167 patients treated with lignocaine ($P = 0.009$; odds ratio (OR): 2.17; 95% confidence interval (CI): 1.21–3.83). There were however no significant differences between groups in rates of survival to hospital discharge (5% in amiodarone group versus 3% in lidocaine group).

Kudenchuk et al. [7] compared amiodarone to placebo in 504 adults with pre-hospital VF or pulseless VT. Once again, the 246 subjects who received amiodarone were more likely to survive to hospital admission when compared with placebo (44% versus 34%; $P = 0.03$; OR: 1.6; 95% CI: 1.1–2.4), however there was no difference to hospital discharge.

In summary, the only benefit shown from these two well-constructed studies was survival to hospital admission, not to neurologically intact discharge. The latter requires further study. Nonetheless, AHA and ILCOR state that amiodarone is an acceptable alternative to lidocaine in this group of patients [8].

How does biphasic defibrillation compare to monophasic defibrillation in VF and pulseless VT in adults?

There has been growing interest in the use of biphasic, impedance-compensating waveforms for defibrillation. The use of less current leads to less cardiac damage.

In adults with VF or pulseless VT, are biphasic waveforms more effective than monophasic waveforms in achieving successful defibrillation?

No systematic reviews are available to help answer this question. Several prospective, randomised studies have been performed. The most recent of these looked at 123 Dutch cardiac arrest patients in VF [9]. In this study looking at out-of-hospital patients, the primary endpoint was removal of VF after the first shock. The secondary endpoint was termination of VF at 5 s. VF was the initial rhythm in 120 patients, 51 of these received biphasic defibrillation and 69 received monophasic shocks.

In terms of the primary endpoint, biphasic defibrillation was more successful than monophasic in removing VF after one shock (69% versus 45%; $P = 0.01$; OR: 4.01; 95% CI: 1.01–10.0). However, there was no difference between the groups in terms of return of spontaneous circulation (ROSC) (61% biphasic versus 65% monophasic), survival to hospital admission (40% versus 48%) or survival to hospital discharge (14% versus 19%).

The next largest prospective, randomised study, the Optimal Response to Cardiac Arrest (ORCA) study compared biphasic and two types of monophasic shocks in 115 pre-hospital cardiac arrest victims [10]. Biphasic defibrillation was associated with significantly higher rates of defibrillation after the first shock; ROSC and survival to hospital admission. However, there was no difference in survival to hospital discharge.

In summary, it would appear that biphasic shocks are more likely to revert VF and pulseless VT, however there is no proven advantage in neurologically intact survival to hospital discharge.

What is the role of therapeutic hypothermia therapy in post cardiac arrest coma in adults?

The Advanced Life Support Task Force of the ILCOR [11] made the following recommendations in October 2002:

- Unconscious adult patients with spontaneous circulation after out-of-hospital cardiac arrest should be cooled to 32–34°C for 12–24 h when the initial rhythm was VF.
- Such cooling may also be beneficial for other rhythms or in-hospital cardiac arrest. There have been two sentinel prospective, randomised, controlled trials identified [12,13]. More recently, a systematic review and individual patient meta-analysis by a collaborative group including the principal authors of the above two studies has been published [14]. It identified three randomised trials. The total number of patients in this systematic review was 385. Analyses were conducted on an intention-to-treat basis. The major conclusions were that patients treated with hypothermia had a higher likelihood of discharge in good neurological condition (risk ratio (RR): 1.68; 95% CI: 1.29–2.07). In addition, being alive at 6 months with good neurological function was more likely in the hypothermia group (RR: 1.44; 95% CI: 1.11–1.76). Table 26.1 gives the data from this systematic review.

Concerns have been raised about how selected the patients were in both trials and that treating clinicians were not blinded. In the European study only 8% of patients assessed for eligibility were enrolled (257 of 3551). In the Australian study, four participating hospitals over 33 months enrolled only 77 patients.

Table 26.1. Long- and short-term neurological recovery (Figure modified from the original supplied by Michael Holzer. Copyright Lippincott Williams & Wilkins reprinted with permission)

Trial	Hypothermia (%)	Normothermia (%)	RR (95% CI)	P-value
Alive at hospital discharge with favourable neurological recovery				
HACA [41][c]	72/136 (53%)	50/137 (36%)	1.51 (1.14 to 1.89)[a]	0.006[a]
Bernard [42]	21/43 (49%)	9/34 (26%)	1.75 (0.99 to 2.43)[a]	0.052[a]
Idrissi [49]	3/16 (19%)	0/17 (0%)	7.41 (0.83 to ∞)[b]	0.15[b]
Summary estimate			1.68 (1.29 to 2.07)	
Alive at 6 months with favourable neurological recovery				
HACA [41]	71/136 (52%)	50/137 (36%)	1.44 (1.11 to 1.76)[a]	0.009[a]

CI: confidence interval.

[a] Random effects models, centre random.

[b] Fisher's exact test and exact confidence limits (StatXact), the point estimate was calculated by adding 0.5 to each cell.

[c] Two patients were transferred under sedoanalgesia to non-participating hospitals; neurological outcome could not be assessed; it is known that these two patients survived until 6 months.

Further studies are required to determine long-term prognostic data and how best to cool patients and for how long.

Practice points
- At present there is no clear difference between adrenaline and vasopressin for adults with cardiac arrest.
- Amiodarone is an acceptable alternative to lignocaine for VF and pulseless VT.
- Biphasic defibrillation is at least as effective as monophasic defibrillation in the adult cardiac arrest patient.
- Hypothermia therapy (32–34°C for 12–24 h) in the patient with post-cardiac arrest coma is now recommended.
- How best to cool patients and for exactly how long is not known.

Research agenda
- In relation to vasopressin, two questions need to be answered:
- In patients with asystole, does vasopressin confer any benefit over adrenaline in cardiac arrest?
- Is the combination of vasopressin and adrenaline more effective than adrenaline alone in cardiac arrest?
- Though amiodarone appears to be more effective than lignocaine in patients with VF or pulseless VT in terms of survival to hospital admission, further research needs to look specifically at the more important outcome of survival to hospital discharge.
- In relation to therapeutic hypothermia, future research needs to address how best to cool patients and for how long.

REFERENCES

1 Aung KA, Htay T. Vasopressin for Cardiac Arrest. A systematic review and meta-analysis. *Arch Intern Med* 2005; 165: 17–24.

2 Wenzel V, Krismer AC, Arntz HR et al. A comparison of vasopressin and epinephrine for out-of-hospital cardiopulmonary resuscitation. *New Eng J Med* 2004; 350: 105–13.

3 ClinicalTrials.gov Identifier: NCT00127907.

4 University of Pittsburgh News Bureau. Public Forum 16 March 2004.

5 Lunxian T, Hu X, Qing H. Intravenous amiodarone for treatment of ventricular fibrillation and ventricular tachycardia [Protocol]. *The Cochrane Database of Systematic Reviews* 2003, Issue 2. Art No.: CD 004195. DOI: 10.1002/14651858.CD004195.

6 Dorian P, Cass D, Schwartz B et al. Amiodarone as compared with lidocaine for shock-resistant ventricular fibrillation. *New Eng J Med* 2002; 346(12): 884–90.

7 Kudenchuk PJ, Cobb LA, Copass MK et al. Amiodarone for resuscitation after out-of-hospital cardiac arrest due to ventricular fibrillation. *New Eng J Med* 1999; 341(12): 871–8.

8 AHA with ILCOR (International Liaison Committee on Resuscitation). Guidelines 2000. *Circulation* 2000; 102: 112–28.

9 van Alem AP, Chapman FW, Lank P. A prospective, randomised and blinded comparison of first shock success of monophasic and biphasic waveforms in out-of-hospital cardiac arrest. *Resuscitation* 2003; 58(1): 17–24.

10 Martens PR, Russell JK, Wolcke B et al. Optimal response to cardiac arrest study: defibrillation waveform effects. *Resuscitation* 2001; 49(3): 233–43.

11 Nolan JP, Morley PT, Vanden Hoek TL et al. Therapeutic Hypothermia After Cardiac Arrest: An Advisory Statement by the Advanced Life Support Task Force of the International Liaison Committee on Resuscitation. *Circulation* 2003; 108: 118–21.

12 Bernard SA, Gray TW, Buist MD et al. Treatment of comatose survivors of out-of-hospital cardiac arrest with induced hypothermia. *New Eng J Med* 2002; 346(8): 557–64.

13 Holzer MD et al. Mild therapeutic hypothermia to improve the neurologic outcome after cardiac arrest. *New Eng J Med* 2002; 346(8): 549–56.

14 Holzer MD, Bernard SA, Hachimi-Idrissi S et al. Hypothermia for neuroprotection after cardiac arrest: systematic review and individual patient data meta-analysis. *Crit Care Med* 2005; 33(2): 414–18.

Severe burns in adults

Severe burns continue to cause significant morbidity and mortality despite advances in burns management. Airway burns account for most deaths. Patients with severe burns are best managed in specialised centres.

The principles of the initial management of the patient with severe burns can be summarised as below:

1 Stopping the burning process by application of cold water. Prolonged exposure to cool water however should be avoided to prevent hypothermia.

2   Assessing and stabilising the airway as part of primary survey. This may involve early intubation before airway oedema develops. 100% oxygen should be given to all patients, particularly if carbon monoxide exposure is likely.

3   Assessment of burn surface area (BSA) followed by application of a clean, preferably sterile dressing to burned skin. Plastic cling wrap is also useful as a non-adherent temporary dressing.

4   Fluid resuscitation if BSA >15%. Most formulae use 3–4 mL kg^{-1}% burn over 24 h. Such formulae are a guide only and haemodynamic status and urine output should be used to determine fluid requirements. Isotonic salt solutions (e.g. 0.9% saline, Hartmann's solution) are generally used in the first 24 h.

5   Intravenous analgesia.

6   Insertion of urinary catheter and nasogastric tube.

7   Early escharotomy may be required for circumferential burns where the circulation is compromised.

8   Attention to tetanus prophylaxis.

9   Disposition to a specialised burns unit.

10 Chemical burns are treated like thermal burns once decontamination and administration of specific antidotes has occurred.

In this section we look specifically at the evidence for fluid resuscitation in the severely burned patient as well as evidence to guide clinicians in deciding which type of dressing to apply.

Which fluid is best in severe burns in adults?

The fluid management of the patient with severe burns remains controversial. Several Cochrane Reviews have looked at fluid management in the non-defined critically ill patient [15–17]. The conclusion from all of these reviews was that in the subset of these critically ill patients with severe burns, there was no difference in mortality between colloids and crystalloids [15], hypertonic versus isotonic crystalloids [16] and with the use of human albumin solution [17].

In terms of what rate fluids should be given, various formulae exist for fluid resuscitation. Most standard regimes use between 3 and 4 mL kg^{-1}% burn of crystalloid in the first 24 h. A single randomised study of 50 patients with burns to >20% BSA compared a control group receiving 4 mL kg^{-1}% burn over the first 24 h to the study group where fluids were determined by invasive haemodynamic monitoring [18]. The authors concluded that the control group were significantly hypovolaemic during the first 48 h and that haemodynamic monitoring was associated with a significant increase in fluid administration. The small study population limits the author's conclusion however.

All other studies found in relation to fluid resuscitation in severe burns were retrospective in nature.

There has been recent interest in the clinical syndrome of abdominal compartment syndrome in the severe burns patient. Raised intra-abdominal pressure (IAP) correlates with large volumes of fluid. A recently published randomised study compared IAPs in burns patients receiving crystalloids or colloids [19]. Only 31 patients who had >25% BSA burns with inhalational injury or >40% with no respiratory tract involvement were studied. Patients who received colloids had significantly lower IAPs than the crystalloid group and the colloid group remained below the threshold for complications of intra-abdominal hypertension. Once again, however, the sample size was very small.

To conclude, in relation to both the type and volume of fluid for severe burns patients, there appears to very little high-level evidence looking specifically at burns patients. Resuscitation formulae serve only as guidelines.

Which initial dressing is best in severe burns in adults?

Severely burned patients are particularly at risk of infection as bacteria proliferate rapidly in burn wounds and the patient's immune system is impaired. Various dressings and topical agents have been used in the initial management of the patient with severe burns. Examples include simple sterile dressings, silver sulfadiazine (SSD) cream and plastic cling wrap. Though many small studies exist in both human and animal models, there is currently no high level evidence to guide such management. There is currently a Cochrane Protocol for a systematic review underway looking at the evidence for dressings and topical agents in burn wounds [20]. It will try to specifically answer the following questions:

1 Is there any difference in the effectiveness and side-effects of different dressings?
2 Is there any difference in the effectiveness and side-effects of dressings and topical agents?
3 Is there any difference in the effectiveness and side-effects of different topical agents?

There has also been interest in the use of hyperbaric oxygen therapy (HBOT) to treat severe burns. A Cochrane Systematic Review did not find sufficient evidence to support or refute the effectiveness of HBOT in the treatment of thermal burns.

Practice points
- Very little high level evidence exists for determining both the type and volume of fluid for severe burns patients. Resuscitation formulae such as the Parkland formula serve only as guidelines. There appears to be no differences between colloids, crystalloids, hypertonic solutions and human albumin in terms of mortality.
- Similarly, there is very little high level evidence pertaining to initial dressing types or topical agents in the severely burned victim.

Research agenda
- Prospective study looking at various dressings and topical agents in severely burned patients.

REFERENCES

15 Roberts I, Alderson P, Bunn F, Chinnock P, Ker K, Schierhout G. Colloids versus crystalloids for fluid resuscitation in critically ill patients. *The Cochrane Database Syst Rev* 2004, Issue 4: Art. No.: CD000567. DOI: 10.1002/14651858.

16 Bunn F, Roberts I, Tasker R et al. Hypertonic versus near isotonic crystalloid for fluid resuscitation in critically ill patients. *The Cochrane Database Syst Rev* 2004, Issue 3: CD002045.

17 Roberts I, Alderson P, Bunn F et al. Human albumin solution for resuscitation and volume expansion in critically ill patients. *The Cochrane Database Syst Rev* 2004, Issue 4: CD001208.

18 Holm C, Mayr M, Tegeler J et al. A clinical randomized study on the effects of invasive monitoring on burn shock resuscitation. *Burns* 2004; 30(8): 798–807.

19 O'Mara MS, Slater H, Goldfarb I et al. A prospective, randomized evaluation of intra-abdominal pressures with crystalloid and colloid resuscitation in burn patients. *J Trauma* 2005; 58: 1011–18.

20 Campbell F, Seers K. Dressing and topical agents for burns [Protocol]. *The Cochrane Database of Systematic Reviews* 2000, Issue 2. Art No.: CD002106. DOI: 10.1002/14651858.

Near-drowning in adults

There is much confusion surrounding terminology relating to drowning and near-drowning. The most common definitions are as follows:

(a) Drowning is defined as death by asphyxia due to submersion in a liquid medium.

(b) Near-drowning is defined as immediate survival after asphyxia due to submersion. This includes those patients that later die from complications such as adult respiratory distress syndrome and hypoxic encephalopathy.

The term "secondary drowning" is no longer used as this simply relates to delayed lung complications.

The principles of initial treatment of the near-drowning victim is summarised as follows:

1 Earliest possible initiation of cardiopulmonary resuscitation at the scene.

2 Cervical spine protection if there is any possibility of trauma (e.g. diving accident).

3 Endotracheal intubation in the hypoxic, unconscious patient with IPPV/PEEP.

4 Continuous positive airways pressure (CPAP) in the hypoxic but conscious and cooperative patient.

5 Intravenous fluids to maintain normovolaemia.

From an evidence based perspective, there is very little high level evidence looking at near-drowning. There were no systematic reviews nor good-quality prospective studies. We have summarised the available evidence for corticosteroids, antibiotics and therapeutic hypothermia below.

What are the roles of other therapies in adult victims of near-drowning?

(a) *Steroids in the management of near-drowning*:

There have been no prospective randomised placebo-controlled trials looking at the role of corticosteroids in near-drowning however there has been a single prospective study in 10 patients [21]. Based on the current poor evidence, victims of near-drowning should not be given steroids.

(b) *Prophylactic antibiotics in the management of near-drowning*:

All studies found looking at this question were retrospective case reports. No prospective studies were identified nor systematic reviews found. Based on these four retrospective studies of a total of approximately 350 patients, there was no evidence of benefit when prophylactic antibiotics were given to near-drowning victims [22–25].

(c) *Therapeutic hypothermia in the management of near-drowning*:

The World Congress on Drowning in 2002 recommended that victims of near-drowning who remained comatosed after restoration of adequate spontaneous circulation should be treated with controlled hypothermia as a neuroprotective therapy [26]. ILCOR have also suggested that therapeutic hypothermia may be beneficial for near-drowning victims [27]. There are no prospective studies, however looking specifically at this group of patients.

Practice points

1 In adult victims of near-drowning, therapeutic hypothermia may have a neuro-protective role based on expert opinion only. There is no evidence of benefit from prophylactic corticosteroids or antibiotics.

2 The most useful prognostic predictors of favourable outcome include:
  – less than 5 min submersion time
  – CPR instituted within 10 min
  – first spontaneous breath within 30 min of rescue
  – return of spontaneous circulation prior to hospital arrival.

Research agenda

• Newer treatment modalities such as nitric oxide and exogenous surfactant therapy require further study.

REFERENCES

21 Sladen A, Zauder HL. Methylprednisolone therapy for pulmonary edema following near drowning. *JAMA* 1971; 215: 1793–5.

22 Modell JH, Graves SA, Ketover A. Clinical course of 91 consecutive near-drowning victims. *Chest* 1976; 70(2): 231–8.

23 Corbin DO, Fraser HS. A review of 98 cases of near-drowning at the Queen Elizabeth Hospital, Barbados. *West Ind Med J* 1981; 30(1): 22–9.

24 Oakes DD, Sherck JP, Maloney JR et al. Prognosis and management of victims of near-drowning. *J Trauma* 1982; 22(7): 544–9.

25 van Berkel M, Bierens JJ, Lie RL et al. Pulmonary oedema, pneumonia and mortality in submersion victims: a retrospective study in 125 patients. *Int Care Med* 1996; 22(2): 101–7.

26 Bierens JJ, Knape JT, Gelissen HP. Drowning. *Curr Opin Crit Care* 2002; 8: 578–86.

27 Nolan JP, Morley PT, Hoek TL et al. Advanced life support task force of the International Liaison Committee on Resuscitation. *Resuscitation* 2003; 57: 231–3.

Multiple trauma in adults

Overview of initial emergency department management

In accordance with the principles of advanced trauma life support, injured patients are treated in a fashion that establishes priorities based on their presenting vital signs, mental status and mechanism of injury. The priorities in the treatment of trauma patients are similar to those in any other life-threatening condition – securing the airway, maintaining ventilation, controlling haemorrhage and treating shock are first priorities because of their crucial importance for survival.

In the emergency department (ED) it is preferable to utilise a predetermined response or trauma team with defined roles so that multiple therapeutic and diagnostic procedures can be performed simultaneously. In this model a team leader assesses the patient, orders and interprets diagnostic studies, and prioritises diagnostic and therapeutic concerns using the team to manage particular aspects of care. The team leader helps the team focus on the injuries that are immediately life-threatening and formulates the plan for the evaluation of less threatening injuries in sequence.

A structured approach to the initial management of the multiply injured patient allows initial assessment, prioritisation of care and resuscitative treatment to proceed in an orderly fashion.

The most widely adopted approach is that of Advanced Trauma Life Support Guidelines from the American College of Surgeons [28]. This approach includes sequential assessment and management in a series of steps with the goal of identifying and treating immediately life-threatening conditions followed by specific interventions and laboratory and radiology testing and a final thorough examination prior to the provision of definitive care for all injuries.

The primary survey identifies the acute life-threatening problems that must be managed immediately. The secondary survey identifies the remaining major injuries and sets priorities for definitive management.

Primary survey

Primary survey comprises a rapid assessment of ABCDE with immediate management of life-threatening conditions:

1 **Airway** maintenance with cervical spine immobilisation
2 **Breathing**
3 **Circulation** and haemorrhage control
4 **Disability**/neurological assessment
5 **Exposure** – where the patients is completely undressed ensuring no serious injuries requiring immediate care are missed.

Depending upon findings during the primary survey, initial portable radiographs and indicated procedures such as bladder catheterisation and insertion of a gastric tube should be performed immediately and not be delayed for the secondary survey.

Relatively routine emergent radiographs in bluntly injured patients are the lateral cervical spine, chest and pelvis.

Secondary survey

The secondary survey is a complete re-assessment of the patient and injuries. A more complete and traditional history and physical exam is performed. Multiple sources (friends, relatives, law enforcement and emergency services personnel) often are required to obtain a complete history. Much can be learned from the mechanism of injury.

Throughout this portion of the evaluation, the patient's vital signs of pulse rate, blood pressure (BP), respiratory rate, and effort and conscious state should be continuously observed along pulse oximetry and potentially end-tidal CO_2 monitoring. If at any time during the secondary survey the patient's clinical status deteriorates, the treating team should return to the elements of the primary survey.

Once the secondary survey is completed, more specific imaging and diagnostic may be performed allowing a full assessment of all injuries and planning for definitive care.

Current issues and controversies in the emergency care of multiple trauma patients

In this section we present a brief overview of evidence relating to a number of specific interventions and controversies in the management of the multiple trauma patients.

These include:

- Fluid resuscitation – timing, amount and type of intravenous fluid for initial resuscitation of adult multiple trauma patients.
- Use of blood substitutes in trauma.
- Interventions in acute traumatic brain injury (TBI) – use of hypothermia, mannitol, steroids, hyperventilation and calcium channel blockers.
- Endpoints and monitoring in trauma resuscitation.

Fluid resuscitation in trauma

When and how quickly?

For the past four decades, the standard approach to the trauma victim who presents hypotensive from presumed haemorrhage has focused on early aggressive resuscitation with large volumes of crystalloid, and blood products as deemed appropriate [28].

The goal of this treatment is to restore intravascular volume and vital signs back to normal as quickly as possible to maintain vital organ perfusion. This has been the approach regardless of whether the victim is bleeding from a readily controllable source such as an extremity, or from an inaccessible injury within the chest or abdomen. The rationale for this approach is derived from controlled haemorrhage studies in animals in the 1950s and 1960s in which isotonic fluid resuscitation was a life saving treatment of severe hypotension due to haemorrhage. Untreated animals died or suffered irreversible organ damage whilst those animals who received fluids to restore perfusion to vital organs generally survived [29].

The recommendations for and practice of aggressive fluid replacement to restore vital signs to normal values in all forms of trauma continues to be questioned with a number of authorities and studies suggesting that there is a role for limited volume or delayed fluid resuscitation in some clinical circumstances. In particular investigators are questioning fluid replacement regimes in patients with uncontrolled ongoing haemorrhage such as might be seen in a severe penetrating wound of the torso [30].

More recent animal studies have used an uncontrolled haemorrhage animal model to better represent the patient rapidly exsanguinating from a major vessel injury. These studies have demonstrated results opposite to the classic controlled haemorrhage studies – aggressive fluid resuscitation may be harmful, resulting in increased haemorrhage volume and increased short term mortality [31–33].

In 1994, Bickell et al. published a randomised trial comparing immediate with delayed fluid resuscitation of 598 hypotensive patients over 15 years of age with penetrating torso injuries [34]. All patients had systolic blood pressure (SBP) less than or equal to 90 mmHg at the initial on scene assessment and were randomised to one of two groups – the immediate resuscitation group in which intravascular fluid resuscitation was given before surgical intervention or the delayed resuscitation group in which intravascular fluid resuscitation was delayed until operative intervention. The overall rate of survival to hospital discharge was higher in the delayed resuscitation group than the immediate resuscitation group (70% versus 62%; $P = 0.04$) despite adjustment for other variables such as pre-hospital scene to hospital times. Notwithstanding a number of methodological flaws this large study strongly suggested a more favourable outcome with delayed fluid resuscitation in this selected group of patients and hypothesised that fluids given before surgical control of bleeding lead to either accentuation of ongoing haemorrhage or hydraulic disruption of an effective thrombus, followed by a fatal secondary haemorrhage. In addition, they raised the possibility that intravenous infusions of crystalloid may promote haemorrhage by diluting clotting factors and by lowering blood viscosity.

The study authors concluded that their findings challenged the notion that aggressive fluid resuscitation was beneficial in all groups of trauma patients and made the important point that it is not the value of fluid resuscitation that should be debated, but rather the volume, timing and extent of that resuscitation for certain patients.

A second clinical trial evaluating in-hospital mortality in haemorrhagic shock randomised 110 patients to one of two fluid resuscitation protocols: target SBP > 100 mmHg or target SBP of 70 mmHg. Fluid therapy was titrated to this endpoint until definitive haemostasis was achieved by either operative intervention or clinical and radiological confirmation of no ongoing haemorrhage [35]. This study included patients with haemorrhagic shock secondary to penetrating and blunt injury. In this study, the eventual difference in mean BP between the two groups was 114 mmHg versus 100 mmHg ($p < 0.04$) rather than the intended larger difference as described in the methodology. Infused fluid volumes were not reported. There was no significant differences in mortality between the low and normal BP resuscitation protocols though it can be argued that a SBP of 100 mmHg does not constitute hypotensive resuscitation.

In 2003 a systematic review assessed the effects of early versus delayed, and larger versus smaller volume of fluid administration in trauma patients with bleeding [36]. Although this review identified over 4000 reports only six met the review's inclusion criteria – three studying the effect of early versus delayed fluid administration and three studying larger versus smaller volumes of intravenous fluids. Despite all six trials reporting mortality data it was not possible to perform a meta-analysis because of their heterogeneity in terms of patient types and fluids used. In summary, the authors concluded that they found no evidence for or against the use of early or larger volume intravenous fluid administration in uncontrolled haemorrhage.

The best fluid resuscitation strategy in trauma has not yet been definitively established. Whilst there is a considerable amount of animal data suggesting that hypotensive or limited resuscitation may be preferable to the current standard of care, there is still a relative paucity of clinical outcome based studies comparing different fluid resuscitation regimes in selected groups of patients and as a consequence trauma resuscitation protocols have changed little in the last 10 years.

Large, well-concealed, randomised controlled trials are required to delineate the optimum fluid resuscitation strategy in our heterogenous trauma population. It appears clear that one standard regime will not fit all cases – it is most likely that differing regimes will be required to manage blunt injuries compared with penetrating injuries and mild versus severe circulatory compromise. The presence of head injury and the relationship of cerebral perfusion pressure with mean arterial pressure will be another factor requiring consideration when choosing between limited or delayed fluid resuscitation regimes.

Which fluid is best in trauma resuscitation?

There are a large number of studies, systematic reviews and meta-analyses examining the question of the most appropriate fluid choice in patients requiring fluid resuscitation. In particular, the choice of crystalloid versus colloid in fluid resuscitation has been debated over many years and this subject has been presented in detail in an earlier chapter of this book.

In relation to trauma fluid resuscitation there is considerable interest in the use of hypertonic crystalloids as these fluids are considered to have a greater ability to expand blood volume and improve BP, and can be administered as a relatively small volume infusion in a short period of time. Additionally, their administration may be associated with less interstitial oedema formation when compared with isotonic crystalloid solutions. The use of hypertonic solutions in hypotensive patients with head injury is being increasingly advocated [37–40].

Reductions in intracranial pressure (ICP) may be achieved by establishing an osmotic gradient across the blood–brain barrier that draws water from the brain tissue into the vascular space. Hypertonic solutions, therefore, have the potential to restore BP rapidly, but without increasing ICP.

A meta-analysis of patients with severe TBI from randomised trials of hypertonic saline (HTS) combined with dextran colloid solution for pre-hospital trauma resuscitation reported an 11% absolute increase in survival compared with standard resuscitation fluids [41].

Cooper et al. published a double-blind randomised controlled trial of 229 patients with TBI who were comatose (Glasgow Coma Score <9) and hypotensive (SBP < 100 mmHg). Patients were randomly assigned to receive a rapid infusion of either 250 mL of 7.5% saline or 250 mL Ringers lactate solution in addition to conventional intravenous fluids and resuscitation protocols administered by paramedics [42].

The proportion of patients surviving to hospital discharge was similar in both groups ($n = 63$ [55%] for the HTS group and $n = 57$ [50%] for controls; $P = 0.32$). The proportion of patients surviving at 6 months was $n = 62$ (55%) in the HTS group and $n = 53$ (47%) in the control group ($P = 0.23$; RR: 1.17; 95% CI: 0.9–1.5).

In this well-designed study comparing hypertonic and isotonic fluid resuscitation there were no significant differences between the groups with respect to the primary study endpoint – the extended Glasgow Outcome Score – or other measures of functional neurological status at either 3 or 6 months after injury.

In 2004, 14 trials underwent a meta-analysis in an effort to determine whether hypertonic crystalloid decreased mortality in patients with hypovolaemia secondary to trauma, burns or surgery [43].

The trials compared hypertonic with isotonic and near isotonic solutions and the principal outcome was mortality from all causes and disability as measured by the Glasgow Outcome Scale. In the 14 trials reported in the meta-analysis, patients with burns were included in three ($n = 72$), patients undergoing surgery in five ($n = 230$) and trauma patients in six ($n = 654$).

Due to the clinical heterogeneity of the different patient groups it was felt to be inappropriate to pool them; therefore, only the results for the subgroups are given. The pooled relative risk for death in trauma patients was 0.84 (95% CI: 0.69–1.04), for patients with burns 1.49 (95% CI: 0.56–3.95) and for patients undergoing surgery 0.51 (95% CI: 0.09–2.73). Only one trial gave data on disability and the relative risk for a poor outcome was 1.00 (95% CI: 0.82–1.22).

This review did not provide enough data to be able to say whether hypertonic crystalloid is better than isotonic crystalloid for the resuscitation of patients with trauma or burns, or those undergoing surgery. However, the confidence intervals are wide and do not exclude clinically significant differences between hypertonic and isotonic crystalloid.

In critically ill patients with hypovolaemia, burns or hypoalbuminaemia systematic reviews in 1998, and 2004 have reported colloid resuscitation and albumin therapy to be associated with increased mortality [44,45].

Another systematic review looking at crystalloids versus colloids in fluid resuscitation on mortality and pulmonary oedema in a wide group of patient types found no apparent differences in these outcomes between the two groups [46]. The strength of the findings was limited by the amount of data studied as there was not enough data to generate sufficient power to detect significant differences. Additionally, this review reported a subgroup analysis of trauma patients which suggested that crystalloid resuscitation was associated with a lower mortality than colloid resuscitation. Again, no firm conclusions should be drawn from such a finding – further study in trauma patients is strongly recommended to confirm or refute a beneficial effect of crystalloid fluid resuscitation over colloid.

During November 2001 and June 2003 the Saline versus Albumin Fluid Evaluation (SAFE) study randomised 6997 intensive care unit (ICU) patients to receive either 4% albumin or normal saline for intravascular fluid resuscitation over a 28-day period [47]. In this heterogenous group there was no significant difference in 28-day all-cause mortality between the two groups. The group reported a subgroup analyses of 1186 trauma patients with and without head injury and found an increased risk of death amongst the albumin group compared with the saline group of 1.36. This increased risk of death derived from a greater number of patients with head injury who died in the albumin group (59/241 = 24.5%) compared with the saline group (38/251 = 15.1%). When the trauma group was analysed without patients with head injury there was no difference between the groups in mortality. The authors cautioned against placing too much emphasis on the reported higher risk of death in the trauma group treated with albumin compared with saline. This was a subgroup analysis only and the finding may have arisen by chance as this subgroup was not adequately powered to establish a significant difference.

Practice points
- Intravenous fluid resuscitation is a key component in the management of multiple trauma.
- Optimum fluid resuscitation strategies for differing groups of patients have not yet been defined.
- In penetrating trauma, over aggressive fluid resuscitation aiming for normal vital signs prior to operative control of haemorrhage may be associated with worsened outcomes. In these cases, it is prudent to consider smaller volumes of fluid resuscitation and maintenance of vital organ perfusion.
- There is no proven difference in outcomes of trauma patients resuscitated with colloid fluids versus crystalloid fluids. Given this lack of difference, crystalloid fluid resuscitation may be preferred on the basis of availability and cost.
- Hypertonic saline and hypertonic saline with colloid is increasingly recommended for initial resuscitation of patients with hypotension and trauma, particularly those with head injuries.

Research agenda

Large well-designed outcome studies are needed of differing fluid resuscitation strategies in trauma.

In particular, differing types of trauma – blunt, penetrating and patients with associated head injury compared with no head injury should be studied separately as it is likely that optimal strategies will be different for each of these groups.

Important variables to consider include:

- Type of fluid, crystalloid versus colloid, hypertonic versus isotonic.
- Endpoints of resuscitation (e.g. target BP or measurement of perfusion).
- Timing of resuscitation, early versus delayed.
- Total time to definitive care.

Blood substitutes in trauma

There is an increasing focus on the utility and safety of blood substitutes in the resuscitation of haemorrhagic shock secondary to trauma and in perioperative transfusion therapy. A successful blood substitute is one that can temporarily replace the principal functions of transfused blood: volume expansion and oxygen delivery. Disadvantages of blood transfusion include risk of disease transmission, incompatibility reactions, immunomodulation combined with a diminishing supply of donated blood and storage time limitations.

Though blood substitutes have been under development for many years, problems with unacceptable side-effects including nephrotoxicity, abdominal pain and hepatic dysfunction has made progress slow. Two general classes of blood substitutes are under development – perfluorocarbon (PFC) emulsions and modified haemoglobin (Hb) solutions. PFCs are synthetic fluorinated hydrocarbons that increase dissolved oxygen in the fluid phase and thus rely on a high FiO_2 to achieve maximal oxygen carrying capacity. Modified Hbs are derived from either human or bovine red blood cells or can be genetically engineered. These Hb based oxygen carriers are cross-linked and modified in a variety of ways to minimise side-effects whilst optimising the oxygen carrying and dissociation properties to mimic red blood cells as far as possible [48].

Whilst the majority of trials so far have been testing the safety and utility of blood substitutes in different clinical settings, a single randomised trial of 44 trauma patients compared Polyheme® (Northfield Laboratories Inc, Evanston, IL) with red cells as initial blood replacement after trauma and during emergent operations [49].

The study reported no serious or unexpected adverse events related to the Polyheme® and no difference in total [Hb] between the two groups. The experimental group also received significantly lower numbers of red blood cell units through the first 24 h (10.4 ± 4.2 units in control group versus 6.8 ± 3.9 units in the Polyheme group; $P < 0.05$) but there was no significant reduction in total red blood cell units given by the end of day 3. This study illustrated the ability of a modified Hb to maintain circulating Hb at a therapeutic level safely in the setting of urgent haemorrhage. The results of this trial are promising though too small to properly evaluate clinically relevant benefit or harm as there is no mortality or outcome data reported. Large randomised controlled trials are certainly required to delineate the place of these red cell alternatives in trauma resuscitation. A Cochrane Review examining the evidence for the use of blood substitutes as a means of avoiding allogeneic blood transfusions is underway at the present time [50].

Stabilisation of circulation in multiple trauma/haemorrhagic shock

Primary strategies for stabilization of the circulation in the multiple trauma patient include fluid or blood administration and control of bleeding source by operative intervention or pressure/elevation. Additionally, medical anti-shock trousers (MAST) have been used in cases of haemorrhagic shock or hypotension in the pre-hospital or ED setting to stabilise patients until definitive care can be provided. MAST were thought to cause an autotransfusion of blood from the lower extremities and an increase in systemic vascular resistance which, combined with compression of blood vessels would cause movement of blood from the lower body to the brain, heart and lungs. A systematic review of randomised controlled trials was published in 1999 in an effort to quantify the effectiveness and safety of MAST usage in patients following trauma [51]. Two studies met the inclusion criteria (total patients = 1202) and were included in this review [52,53].

In this systematic review the relative risk of death with MAST was 1.13 (95% CI: 0.97–1.32) and there was an increased length of stay in the ICU (weighted mean difference of 1.7 days; 95% CI: 0.33–2.98) and a longer total hospitalisation. This data did not support the routine use of MAST in cases of multiple trauma and suggested there may be a worse outcome with its application. Since this report, the use of MAST in multiple trauma has dramatically lessened. Notwithstanding the author's cautions in drawing conclusions from only two trials, both of which suffered from methodological flaws, their recommendations that further well-designed randomised trials should be conducted to ensure there is no benefit in trauma has not been acted upon so we have no further evidence to support or discount their use in multiple trauma. Having said this, MAST devices are still in use in cases of severe pelvic and lower extremity injuries and can be helpful for immediate mechanical stabilisation at an accident scene. "Pre-hospital" personnel can apply these garments promptly to facilitate transfer to the trauma centre [54].

Practice points
- MAST should not be used routinely in patients with multiple trauma.
- MAST may be useful in the initial care of selected cases of severe pelvic and lower limb trauma to aid in mechanical stabilisation of fractures in the pre-hospital setting.

In patients with multiple trauma, including head injury, does induced hypothermia therapy improve outcome?

Induced hypothermia is defined as the controlled lowering of core temperature for therapeutic reasons and is commonly used intraoperatively in different procedures.

There is evidence from trials and a systematic review that such cooling therapy following cardiac arrest is associated with improved neurological outcome [55–57] and there has been renewed interest in the use of induced hypothermia in reducing secondary brain injury in head injured patients. A meta-analysis of seven randomised clinical trials involving a total of 668 patients found no benefit from induced hypothermia for the treatment of traumatic brain injury (TBI) on Glasgow Outcome Scores or intracranial pressure (ICP) [58]. Nevertheless, because hypothermia is still being used in a number of centres in posttraumatic head injury, the authors concluded that additional studies are justified and urgently needed.

Ca channel blockers in TBI

A Cochrane Review published in 2003 reported that there is insufficient evidence to support the use of calcium channel blockers in an unselected group of patients with traumatic head injury, although a clinically significant benefit cannot be ruled out with the data available [59]. There is some evidence to suggest that nimodipine may be of benefit to a subgroup of patients with traumatic subarachnoid haemorrhage, however the promising results in this subgroup of patients need to be replicated in a larger randomised controlled trial before any firm conclusions about the effectiveness of the drug can be drawn.

Hyperventilation therapy for TBI

Patient's with TBI are frequently managed with varying degrees of hyperventilation to prevent or reduce raised ICP. Hyperventilation reduces raised ICP by causing cerebral vasoconstriction and a reduction in cerebral blood flow. Hyperventilation to a $PaCO_2$ of 20–30 mmHg during the first few days after head injury has been recommended widely. The original rationale for the use of hyperventilation following head injury was first described by Bruce in 1981 [60].

However, more recently, uncertaninty has emerged as to the level of $PaCO_2$ that should be targeted during hyperventilation for head injury, in addition to the optimum timing, duration and indications. Although hyperventilation produces a rapid reduction in ICP, and high or uncontrolled ICP is one of the most common precursors of death or neurological disability in traumatically brain injured patients, there is currently little evidence to suggest that reducing ICP through hyperventilation improves clinically relevant outcomes.

A Cochrane Review was performed to quantify the effect of hyperventilation on death and neurological disability following head injury [61].

Only one suitable randomised controlled study involving 113 patients was found. This study randomised severely head injured patients to receive standard head injury therapy ($n = 41$) versus standard therapy and hyperventilation for 5 days with or without the co-administration of a buffer [THAM]. The intervention in the hyperventilation ($n = 36$) and in the hyperventilation-plus-THAM group ($n = 36$) comprised adjusting the respiratory rate and the volume of the ventilator to keep $PaCO_2$ at 24–28 mmHg. For hyperventilation alone, the RR for death or severe disability was 1.14 (95% CI: 0.82, 1.58). The RR for death or severe disability in the hyperventilation-plus-THAM group, was 0.87 (95% CI: 0.58, 1.28).

Owing to the small study size, all of the effect measures were imprecise. The lack of significant findings of this small randomised controlled trial in severely head injured patients, not all of whom had raised ICP highlight the need for further randomised controlled trials to address the question of the appropriateness of this widely used intervention in order to assess any potential benefit or harm that may result from the use of hyperventilation.

Current recommendations from the Brain Trauma Foundation [62] include avoiding prophylactic hyperventilation to $PaCO_2 < 35$ mmHg during the first 24 hours post injury because of the risk of worsening ischaemia.

Steroids in TBI

A Cochrane Review examined a heterogenous group of 20 studies to determine the effectiveness and safety of corticosteroids in the treatment of acute TBI [63]. This review was first published in 1997 and was updated in 2004 after the publication of a very large and relevant trial which effectively changed the conclusions of the review. The largest trial in this group which studied over 10 000 participants [64] contained 80% of all randomised trials participants, and studied the effect of high-dose intravenous methyl prednisolone on 14 day mortality and complications. The authors reported a risk ratio of death of 1.18 (95% CI: 1.09–1.27) indicating a significant increase in death with steroids and in fact the trial was stopped prematurely. The heterogeneity of the studies included in the Cochrane review precluded the derivation of a pooled risk ratio.

Mannitol in TBI

Mannitol is widely used in the control of raised ICP following brain injury, though there is uncertainty about the best total dosage, the optimum timing of administration and duration over which it maintains effectiveness in reducing brain swelling. A Cochrane Review [65] examined these questions and reported that high-dose mannitol (1.4 g kg^{-1}) may be preferable to conventional-dose mannitol (0.7 g kg^{-1}) in the acute management of comatose patients with severe head injury. Single trials examined in the review suggested that mannitol therapy for raised ICP may have a beneficial effect on mortality when compared to pentobarbital treatment, but may have a detrimental effect on mortality when compared to hypertonic saline. In this review ICP-directed treatment showed a small beneficial effect compared to treatment directed by neurological signs and physiological indicators.

Interestingly, despite mannitol use in severe TBI being widespread there is little evidence to direct clinicians in the optimum regime. The authors noted that there are many unanswered questions regarding the optimal use of mannitol following acute traumatic head injury. The widespread current use of mannitol, and lack of clarity regarding optimal administration, present an ideal opportunity for the conduct of randomised controlled trials.

Current recommendations from the Brain Trauma Foundation [62] recommend mannitol doses of $0.25–1.0\,g\,kg^{-1}$ are effective in controlling raised ICP. During its use care should be taken to maintain euvolaemia and avoid serum osmolarity exceeding $320\,mOsm\,L^{-1}$ which may lead to renal failure.

Practice points
- The management of raised ICP in TBI is an important factor in reducing secondary neurological injury.
- Though widely practiced, currently there is insufficient evidence to guide clinicians in the optimum use of hyperventilation or mannitol in managing raised ICP in the initial resuscitation phase.
- Hyperventilation ($PaCO_2 < 35$) may be associated with worsened cerebral blood flow in the first 24 h after injury and an increased risk of ischaemia and should not be routinely used.
- Current clinical practice includes mannitol use in a dose range of $0.25–1.0\,g\,kg^{-1}$.

Research agenda
- Target $PaCO_2$ in TBI.
- Optimum timing and duration of hyperventilation in TBI. Researchers should investigate whether groups of patients with differing levels of ICP of patterns of brain injury should have differing hyperventilation regimes.
- There are many unanswered questions regarding the optimal use of mannitol following acute traumatic head injury. The widespread current use of mannitol, and lack of clarity regarding optimal administration, present an ideal opportunity for the conduct of high-quality randomised controlled trials.

Endpoints of trauma resuscitation: what is the evidence?

A variety of strategies exist to assess circulatory status in traumatic haemorrhagic shock, including haemodynamic monitoring, tissue perfusion measurement and the use of serum markers of metabolism.

There are a number of significant developments in the evaluation of differing methods of assessing the severity of shock and determining the adequacy of resuscitation in multiple trauma. Attention is being focused on how best to use information obtained from non-invasive and invasive monitoring and laboratory tests to guide therapy and achieve best clinical outcomes. A clinical practice guideline was published in 2004 with the goal of reconciling endpoints of trauma resuscitation with patient outcomes [66].

Shock is defined as circulatory dysfunction causing decreased tissue oxygenation and accumulation of oxygen debt, which can ultimately lead to multi-organ system failure if left untreated. In the multiple trauma victim, shock generally occurs due to hypovolaemia from acute blood loss, making the assessment of haemodynamic status and perfusion a key principle of the primary survey of trauma patients. Ongoing monitoring to screen for continuing haemorrhage and to assess the efficacy of resuscitation is vital in avoiding preventable death and significant morbidity in these patients.

Vital signs, such as blood pressure (BP) and heart rate (HR), are the initial parameters used to assess for possible haemorrhage in trauma patients. The early recognition of shock using vital signs alone may be difficult, even in the presence of significant blood loss, due to the effect of compensatory mechanisms in otherwise healthy patients. Interestingly, after normalisation of these parameters (BP and HR), up to 85% of severely injured trauma victims still have evidence of inadequate tissue oxygenation based on findings demonstrating an ongoing metabolic acidosis or evidence of gastric mucosal ischaemia [67]. This condition has been described as compensated shock. The American College of Surgeons defines four classes of haemorrhagic shock [28].

Class I   Blood loss up to 15% total circulating blood volume
Class II   Blood loss 15–30% total circulating blood volume
Class III   Blood loss 30–40% total circulating blood volume
Class IV   Blood loss 40% and greater of total circulating blood volume

Only Classes III and IV include a decrease in BP, requiring blood loss of greater than 30% of the total blood volume. Patients with this severity of illness also begin to display evidence of multiple organ failure, including alterations in mental status and a decrease in urine output.

Thus, an important goal of trauma assessment is the early recognition of circulatory dysfunction, prior to the development of hypotension and end organ dysfunction. In addition, resuscitation strategies should be designed to optimise tissue perfusion while avoiding complications of overaggressive volume replacement, such as the exacerbation of haemorrhage, pulmonary oedema and undesirable increases in intracranial hypertension following brain injury [68].

Haemodynamic monitoring

The cuff BP is most useful when hypotension is measured in the setting of acute trauma, as this provides evidence for significant blood loss; however, a normal BP can be sustained despite loss of up to 30% of blood volume. Thus, the physician must consider other sources of information rather than relying exclusively on BP recordings to diagnose haemorrhage prior to the development of hypotension. Other clinical assessment tools for blood loss include HR, capillary refill, skin temperature and colour, mental status and urine output [28]. None of these parameters is adequately sensitive or specific to detect early haemorrhage or allow appropriate ongoing assessment as to the effectiveness of resuscitation.

Measurement of systolic and mean arterial pressures by placement of arterial catheters in the radial or femoral arteries are generally more reliable than measurements by non-invasive cuff methods and are frequently employed early in the resuscitation phase.

Thoracic electrical bioimpedance (TEB) is a non-invasive technique for calculating cardiac output (CO) using the known changes in electrical impedance produced by blood flow through the aorta [69].

Studies by Shoemaker et al. in critically ill patients (including trauma patients) have found a high degree of correlation in the measurement of CO between the non-invasive TEB and invasive techniques, such as pulmonary artery catheter thermodilution [69,70].

This promising monitoring technique deserves further study in multiple trauma patients to evaluate its accuracy, practicality and effect on outcomes.

CO can also be estimated utilising arterial pulse contour analysis but its accuracy seems to require initial calibration using thermodilution via a pulmonary artery catheter – an invasive procedure which has limited the use of this technique in the emergency setting [71,72].

Invasive haemodynamic monitoring by the insertion of a catheter into the pulmonary vascular system to obtain measurements of CO and function, blood volume status, peripheral resistance and ventricular end diastolic volumes is commonly used in the operating room and intensive care setting in the management of multiple trauma patients, but less so in the ED management of these patients. The practicalities of inserting and managing pulmonary artery catheters in the ED during the acute resuscitation phase of a multiply injured patient coupled with significant potential for complications and a lack of evidence of the efficacy of this form of monitoring means it is unlikely that this form of monitoring will become common place in EDs [73,74].

Central venous pressure measurement via placement of a catheter placed into the superior vena cava gives an indication of intravascular fluid status which is a useful measure to guide ongoing fluid requirements.

Oxygenation and perfusion

Blood flow and haemodynamic variables alone may not be sufficient for assessing a patient at risk for haemorrhagic shock. Oxygen delivery to tissues may be compromised in the presence of normal CO, mean arterial pressure and cardiac filling pressures due to compensatory mechanisms. Determination of oxygen debt that may be accumulating is critical to appropriately assess the patient, evaluate the effectiveness of resuscitation and prevent onset of multi-organ system failure. Measurements of oxygen delivery (DO_2) and oxygen consumption (VO_2) are used to assess oxygen debt (imbalance between oxygen delivery and oxygen consumption at the cellular level) with ongoing debt being linked with increased morbidity and mortality [68,75].

Despite studies in numbers of critically ill patients there is little specific data on the use of oxygen debt measurement in the early emergency management of multiple trauma patients.

Serum markers of shock include lactate and base deficit (BD). Both measurements reflect tissue acidosis and hypoperfusion and are readily available in many laboratories. Not only is the level of lactate associated with morbidity and mortality the resolution of hyperlactaemia also appears to be predictive of survival – particularly with normalisation of the serum lactate within the first 24 h [76,77]. The increasing availability of bedside lactate analysers is leading to increased evaluation of the clinical applications of serum lactate to guide therapy and disposition decisions.

The BD is derived from blood gas analysis and gives an approximation of the global tissue acidosis, thereby indirectly evaluating tissue perfusion. Multiple studies in trauma patients requiring fluid resuscitation have demonstrated the ability of an initial BD to accurately predict the severity of haemorrhagic shock [78–80].

Disappointingly, despite excellent correlation between both BD and lactate in animal models of haemorrhage, a poor correlation between the two measures was found in one study in 52 consecutive ICU patients [81,82].

Further investigation is required to determine the relative clinical utility of BD and serum lactate in both the acute resuscitation and post-resuscitation phases. Currently there is insufficient evidence to use serum lactate alone as an endpoint to reflect adequacy of resuscitation [66,68].

Measurement of tissue specific oxygenation and perfusion can also be achieved by the use of fibre optic sensors placed through the skin, gastric tonometry to reflect gastrointestinal mucosal perfusion and measures of cerebral oxygen consumption and perfusion, such as jugular venous oxygen saturation and brain tissue oxygen tension. These techniques are generally beyond the scope of the early management of severe trauma but a newer technique for assessing cerebral oxygen metabolism and regional perfusion – near infrared spectroscopy (NIRS) – may have some applicability in management of head injury once its exact clinical applications are better defined [83,84]. This technique uses the differential absorption spectra of Hb, HbO_2 and cytochrome oxidase to assess intracellular hypoxia. The technique is non-invasive, easy to use and provides continuous data, similar to pulse oximetry.

There are multiple strategies to diagnose shock and monitor resuscitation in multiple trauma patients. Some of these techniques, such as pulmonary artery catheterisation and gastric tonometry, are highly invasive and impractical in the acute resuscitation phase. Other less-invasive techniques, such as tissue PO_2, PCO_2, and pH measurements and TEB, are not yet well studied but may eventually offer viable alternatives in the ED and trauma suites. Other strategies that measure cerebral perfusion, such as jugular venous oxygen saturation and NIRS, may offer better guidance to resuscitative efforts in head-injured patients. Finally, serum markers of shock, such as BD and serum lactate, can provide rapid assessment of tissue oxygen debt and the need for additional diagnostics or resuscitative measures.

As the technology for assessing haemorrhagic shock improves, additional research will define the accuracy, clinical application and prognostic value of each technique, particularly those related to the assessment of the microcirculation.

Practice points

- Pulse rate and BP measurements alone are not sufficiently sensitive to detect shock or imminent shock in multiple trauma patients.
- The accurate assessment of shock and the efficacy of resuscitation require information from different measures – CO, cardiac filling pressures, measures of oxygen debt and serum markers of perfusion such as lactate and BD are all helpful in defining the severity of shock and guiding resuscitation.
- Presently, there is no clearly superior single measure for monitoring the efficacy of resuscitation.
- Newer non-invasive techniques of measuring CO (such as TEB monitors) and tissue oxygenation and perfusion are promising and have the potential to be used early in guiding resuscitation.

Research agenda

- Studies looking at the utility and accuracy of newer devices for measuring CO and tissue perfusion in multiple trauma are required.
- Studies relating these measurments to patient outcomes are required.

REFERENCES

28 Krantz BE. *Advanced Trauma Life Support for Doctors*. Chicago, IL: The American College of Surgeons, 1997.
29 Wiggers CJ. *Physiology of Shock*. New York: Commonwealth Fund, 1950, pp. 121–46; Shires T, Coln D, Carrico J, Lightfoot S. Fluid therapy in hemorrhagic shock. *Arch Surg* 1964; 88: 688–93.
30 Stern SA. Low-volume fluid resuscitation for presumed hemorrhagic shock: helpful or harmful? *Curr Opin Crit Care* 2001; 7: 422–30.

31 Bickell WH, Bruttig SP, Millnamow GA et al. The detrimental effects of intravenous crystalloid after aortotomy in swine. *Surgery* 1991; 110(3): 529–36.

32 Kowalenko T, Stern SA, Dronen SC. Improved outcome with hypotensive resuscitation of uncontrolled hemorrhagic shock. *J Trauma* 1992; 33: 349–53.

33 Solomonov E, Hirsh M, Yahiya A et al. The effect of vigorous fluid resuscitation in uncontrolled hemorrhagic shock after massive splenic injury. *Crit Care Med* 2000; 28(3): 749–54.

34 Bickell WH, Wall MJ, Pepe PE et al. Immediate versus delayed fluid resuscitation for hypotensive patients with penetrating torso injuries. *New Eng J Med* 1994; 331: 1105–9.

35 Dutton RP, Mackenzie CF, Scale TM. Hypotensive resuscitation during active hemorrhage: impact on in-hospital mortality. *J Trauma* 2002; 52: 1141–6.

36 Kwan I, Bunn F, Roberts I, on behalf of the WHO Pre-Hospital Trauma Care Steering Committee. Timing and volume of fluid administration for patients with bleeding. *The Cochrane Database of Systematic Reviews* 2003, Issue 3. Art No.: CD002245. DOI: 10.1002/14651858.CD002245.

37 Khanna S, Davis D, Peterson B, Fisher B, Tung H, O'Quigley J, Deutsch R. Use of hypertonic saline in the treatment of severe refractory posttraumatic intracranial hypertension in pediatric traumatic brain injury. *Crit Care Med* 2000; 28(4): 1144–51.

38 Fisher B, Thomas D, Peterson B. Hypertonic saline lowers raised intracranial pressure in children after head trauma. *J Neuro-surg Anesthesiol* 1992; 4(1): 4–10.

39 Gabriel EJ, Ghajar J, Jogada A, Pons PT, Scalea T. *Guidelines for the Pre-Hospital Management of Traumatic Brain Injury*. New York, NY: Brain Trauma Foundation, 2000: pp. 7–49.

40 Kramer GC. Hypertonic resuscitation: physiologic mechanisms and recommendations for trauma care. *J Trauma* 2003; 54: S89–99.

41 Vassar MJ, Fischer RP, O'Brien PE et al. Multicenter Group for the Study of Hypertonic Saline in Trauma Patients. A multicenter trial for resuscitation of injured patients with 7.5% sodium chloride: the effect of added dextran 70. *Arch Surg* 1993; 128: 1003–11.

42 Cooper J, Myles P, McDermott F, Murray L, Laidlaw J, Cooper G et al. Prehospital hypertonic saline resuscitation of patients with hypotension and severe traumatic brain injury. *J Am Med Assoc* 2004; 291(11): 1350–7.

43 Bunn F, Roberts I, Tasker R. Hypertonic versus near isotonic crystalloid for fluid resuscitation in critically ill patients. *The Cochrane Database of Systematic Reviews* 2004, Issue 3. Art No.: CD002045.pub2. DOI: 10.1002/14651858.CD002045.pub2.

44 Cochrane Injuries Group. Albumin reviewers: human albumin administration in critically ill patients: systematic review of randomised controlled trials. *BMJ* 1998; 317: 235–40.

45 The Albumin Reviewers: Alderson P, Bunn F, LiWan Po A, Li L, Roberts I, Schierhout G. Human albumin solution for resuscitation and volume expansion in critically ill patients. *The Cochrane Database of Systematic Reviews* 2004, Issue 4. Art No.: CD001208.pub2. DOI: 10.1002/14651858.CD001208.pub2.

46 Choi PT-L, Yip G, Quinone JG. Crystalloids vs colloids in fluid resuscitation: a systematic review. *Crit Care Med* 1999; 27: 200–10.

47 The SAFE Study Investigators. A comparison of albumin and saline for fluid resuscitation in the intensive care unit. *New Eng J Med* 2004; 350: 2247–56.

48 Arnoldo BD, Minei JP. Potential of hemoglobin-based oxygencarriers in trauma patients. *Curr Opin Crit Care* 2001; 7: 431–6.

49 Gould SA, Moore EE, Hoyt DB, Burch JM, Haenel JB, Garcia J, DeWoskin R, Moss GS. The first randomized trial of human polymerized hemoglobin as a blood substitute in acute trauma and emergent surgery. *J Am Coll Surg* 1998; 187: 113–20.

50 Brunskill SJ, Prowse C, Garrioch M, Gill R, Hebert P, Thompson J, Hyde C, Stanworth S, Roberts D. Blood substitutes for avoiding allogeneic blood transfusion [Protocol]. *The Cochrane database of Systematic Reviews* 2003, Issue 3. Art No.: CD004894. DOI: 10.1002/14651858.CD004894.

51 Dickinson K, Roberts I. Medical anti-shock trousers (pneumatic anti-shock garments) for circulatory support in patients with trauma. *The Cochrane Database of Systematic Reviews* 1999, Issue 4. Art No.: CD001856. DOI: 10.1002/14651858.

52 Chang FC, Harrison PB, Beech RR, Helmer SD. PASG: does it help in the management of traumatic shock? *J Trauma* 1995; 39: 453–7.

53 Mattox KL, Bickell W, Pepe PE, Burch J, Feliciano D. Prospective MAST study in 911 patients. *J Trauma* 1989; 29: 1104–12.

54 Mohanty K, Musso D, Powell JN, Kortbeek JB, Kirkpatrick AW. Emergent management of pelvic ring injuries: an update. *Can J Surg* 2005; 48(1): 49–56.

55 Bernard SA, Gray TW, Buist MD et al. Treatment of comatose survivors of out-of-hospital cardiac arrest with induced hypothermia. *New Eng J Med* 2002; 346(8): 557–64.

56 Holzer MD et al. Mild therapeutic hypothermia to improve the neurologic outcome after cardiac arrest. *New Eng J Med* 2002; 346(8): 549–56.

57 Holzer MD, Bernard SA, Hachimi-Idrissi S et al. Hypothermia for neuroprotection after cardiac arrest: systematic review and individual patient data meta-analysis. *Crit Care Med* 2005; 33(2): 414–18.

58 Harris OA, Colford Jr JM, Good MC, Matz PG. The role of hypothermia in the management of severe brain injury: a meta-analysis. *Arch Neurol* 2002; 59: 1077–83.

59 Langham J, Goldfrad C, Teasdale G, Shaw D, Rowan K. Calcium channel blockers for acute traumatic brain injury. *The Cochrane Database of Systematic Reviews* 2003, Issue 4. Art No.: CD000565. DOI: 10.1002/14651858.CD000565.

60 Bruce DA, Alavi A, Bilanuik L et al. Diffuse cerebral swelling following head injuries in children: the syndrome of malignant brain oedema. *J Neurosurg* 1981; 54: 170–8.

61 Roberts I, Schierhout G. Hyperventilation therapy for acute traumatic brain injury. *The Cochrane Database of Systematic Reviews* 1997, Issue 4. Art No.: CD000566. DOI: 10.1002/14651858.CD000566.

62 http://www2.braintrauma.org/guidelines/downloads/btf_guidelines_management.pdf (accessed 21 November 2005).

63 Alderson P, Roberts I. Corticosteroids for acute traumatic brain injury. *The Cochrane Database of Systematic Reviews* 2005, Issue 1. Art No.: CD000196.pub2. DOI: 10.1002/14651858.CD000196.pub2.

64 CRASH trial collaborators. Effect of intravenous corticosteroids on death within 14 days in 10 008 adults with clinically significant head injury (MRC CRASH trial): randomised placebo-controlled trial. *Lancet* 2004; 364: 1321–8.

65 Wakai A, Roberts I, Schierhout G. Mannitol for acute traumatic brain injury. *The Cochrane Database of Systematic Reviews* 2005, Issue 4. Art No.: CD001049.pub2. DOI: 10.1002/14651858.CD001049.pub2.

66 Tisherman SA, Barie P, Bokhari F, Bonadies J, Daley B, Diebel L, Eachempati SR, Kurek S, Luchette F, Puyana JC, Schreiber M, Simon R. Clinical practice guideline: endpoints of resuscitation. *J Trauma* 2004; 57: 898–912.

67 Scalea TM, Maltz S, Yelon J et al. Resuscitation of multiple trauma and head injury: role of crystalloid fluids and inotropes. *Crit Care Med* 1994; 20: 1610–15; Abou-Khalil B, Scalea TM, Trooskin SZ, Henry SM, Hitchcock R. Hemodynamic responses to shock in young trauma patients: need for invasive monitoring. *Crit Care Med* 1994; 22: 633–9.

68 Wilson M, Davis DP, Coimbra R. Diagnosis and monitoring of hemorrhagic shock during the initial resuscitation of multiple trauma patients: a review. *J Emerg Med* 2003; 24: 413–22.

69 Shoemaker WC, Wo CCJ, Bishop MH et al. Multicenter trial of a new thoracic bioimpedance device for cardiac output estimation. *Crit Care Med* 1994; 22: 1907–12.

70 Shoemaker WC, Thangathurai D, Wo CCJ et al. Intra-operative evaluation of tissue perfusion in high-risk patients by invasive and noninvasive hemodynamic monitoring. *Crit Care Med* 1999; 27: 2147–52.

71 Gratz I, Kraidin J, Jacobi AG et al. Continuous noninvasive cardiac output as estimated from the pulse contour curve. *J Clin Monit* 1992; 8: 16–52.

72 Irlbeck M, Forst H, Briegel J, Holler M, Peter K. Continuous measurement of cardiac output with pulse contour analysis. *Anaesthetist* 1995; 44: 493–500.

73 Vender JS. Resolved: a pulmonary artery catheter should be used in the management of the critically ill patient. Pro. *J Cardiothorac Vasc Anesth* 1998; 12: 9–12.

74 Becker Jr K. Resolved: a pulmonary artery catheter should be used in the management of the critically ill patient. Con. *J Cardiothorac Vasc Anesth* 1998; 12: 13–16.

75 Shoemaker WC, Appel PL, Kram HB. Role of oxygen debt in the development of organ failure sepsis, and death in high-risk surgical patients. *Chest* 1992; 102: 208–15.

76 Manikis P, Jankowski S, Zhang H, Kahn RJ, Vincent JL. Correlation of serial blood lactate levels to organ failure and mortality after trauma. *Am J Emerg Med* 1995; 13: 619–22.

77 Abramson D, Scalea TM, Hitchcock R, Trooskin SZ, Henry SM, Greenspan J. Lactate clearance and survival following injury. *J Trauma* 1993; 35: 584–9.

78 Davis JW, Shackford SR, Mackersie RC, Hoyt DB. Base deficit as a guide to volume resuscitation. *J Trauma* 1988; 28: 1464–7.

79 Davis JW, Mackersie RC, Holbrook TL, Hoyt DB. Base deficit as an indicator of significant abdominal injury. *Ann Emerg Med* 1991; 20: 842–4.

80 Davis JW, Parks SN, Kaups KL, Gladen HE, O'Donnell-Nicol S. Admission base deficit predicts transfusion requirements and risk of complications. *J Trauma* 1996; 41: 769–74.

81 Davis JW. The relationship of base deficit to lactate in porcine hemorrhagic shock and resuscitation. *J Trauma* 1994; 36: 168–72.

82 Mikulaschek A, Henry SM, Donovan R, Scalea TM. Serum lactate is not predicted by anion gap or base excess after trauma resuscitation. *J Trauma* 1996; 40: 218–22.

83 Kirkpatrick PJ, Smielewski P, Czosnyka M, Menon DK, Pickard, JD. Near-infrared spectroscopy use in patients with head injury. *J Neurosurg* 1995; 83: 963–70.

84 Kampfl A, Pflauser B, Denchev D, Jaring HP, Schmutzhard E. Near infrared spectroscopy (NIRS) in patients with severe brain injury and elevated intracranial pressure: a pilot study. *Acta Neurochir* 1997; 70(Suppl): 112–14.

Glossary of terms

Modified glossaries from the Cochrane Anaesthesia Review Group and The Cochrane Collaboration. For a more detailed description, see: http://www.mrw.interscience.wiley.com/cochrane/clabout/articles/ANAESTH/frame.html and http://www.cochrane.org/resources/glossary.htm

A

Absolute risk reduction   The absolute arithmetic difference in rates of bad outcomes between experimental and control participants in a trial, calculated as the experimental event rate (EER) and the control event rate (CER), and accompanied by a 95% confidence interval (CI). Depending on circumstances it can be reduction in risk (death or cardiovascular outcomes, for instance, in trials of statins), or an increase (pain relief, for instance, in trials of analgesics).

Adverse effect   An adverse event for which the causal relation between the drug/intervention and the event is at least a reasonable possibility. The term adverse effect applies to all interventions, while adverse drug reaction (ADR) is used only with drugs. The terms are otherwise used interchangeably, though in the case of drugs an adverse effect tends to be seen from the point of view of the drug and an adverse reaction is seen from the point of view of the patient.

Attrition bias   Systematic differences between comparison groups in withdrawals or exclusions of participants from the results of a study. For example, participants may drop out of a study because of side effects of an intervention, and excluding these participants from the analysis could result in an overestimate of the effectiveness of the intervention, especially when the proportion dropping out varies by treatment group.

B

Bias   Bias is an asystematic error or deviation in results or inferences. In studies of the effects of health care bias can arise from systematic differences in the groups that are compared (selection bias), the care that is provided, or exposure to other factors apart from the intervention of interest (performance bias), withdrawals or exclusions of people entered into the study (attrition bias), or how outcomes are assessed (detection bias). Bias does not necessarily carry an imputation of prejudice, such as the investigators' desire for particular results. This differs from conventional use of the word in which bias refers to a partisan point of view.

Blinding   The process used in epidemiological studies and clinical trials in which the participants, investigators, and/or assessors remain ignorant concerning the treatments which participants are receiving. The aim is to minimise observer bias, in which the assessor, the person making a measurement, has a prior interest or belief that one treatment is better than another, and therefore scores one better than another just because of that.

In a single-blind study it may be the participants who are blind to their allocations, or those who are making measurements of interest, the assessors.

In a double-blind study, at a minimum both participants and assessors are blind to their allocations.

To achieve a double-blind state, it is usual to use matching treatment and control treatments. For instance, the tablets can be made to look the same, or if one treatment uses a single pill once a day, but the other uses three pills at various times, all patients will have to take pills during the day to maintain blinding.

The important thing to remember is that lack of blinding is a potent source of bias, and open studies or single-blind studies are potential problems for interpreting results of trials.

C

Case–control study   A study that compares people with a specific disease or outcome of interest (cases) to people from the same population without that disease or outcome (controls), and which seeks to find associations between the outcome and prior exposure to particular risk factors. This design is particularly useful where the outcome is rare and past exposure can be reliably measured. Case–control studies are usually retrospective, but not always.

CENTRAL (Cochrane Central Register of Controlled Trials, CCRCT)   The Cochrane Collaboration's register of reports of studies that may be relevant for inclusion in Cochrane Reviews. CENTRAL aims to include all relevant reports that have been identified through the work of The Cochrane Collaboration, through the transfer of this information to the US Cochrane Center. It is published in *The Cochrane Library*.

Chi-squared test   A statistical test based on comparison of a test statistic to a chi-squared distribution. Used in Review Manager (RevMan) analyses to test the statistical significance of the heterogeneity statistic.

CINAHL (Cumulative Index to Nursing and Allied Health Literature)   Electronic database covering the major journals in nursing and allied health.

Clinical trial   An experiment to compare the effects of two or more health care interventions. Clinical trial is an umbrella term for a variety of designs of health care trials, including uncontrolled trials, controlled trials, and randomised controlled trials (RCTs).

Clinically significant   A result (e.g. a treatment effect) that is large enough to be of practical importance to patients and health care providers. This is not the same thing as statistically significant. Assessing clinical significance takes into account factors such as the size of a treatment effect, the severity of the condition being treated, the side effects of the treatment, and the cost. For instance, if the estimated effect of a treatment for acne was small but statistically significant, but the treatment was very expensive, and caused many of the treated patients to feel nauseous, this would not be a clinically significant result. Showing that a drug lowered the heart rate by an average of 1-beat per minute would also not be clinically significant.

Cluster randomised trial   A trial in which clusters of individuals (e.g. clinics, families, geographical areas), rather than individuals themselves, are randomised to different arms. In such studies, care should be taken to avoid unit of analysis errors.

Cochrane Collaboration, The   An international organisation that aims to help people make well-informed decisions about health care by preparing, maintaining, and ensuring the accessibility of systematic reviews of the effects of health care interventions.

Cochrane Database of Systematic Reviews   One of the databases in *The Cochrane Library*. It brings together all the currently available Cochrane Reviews and Protocols for Cochrane Reviews. It is updated quarterly, and is available via the Internet and CD-ROM.

Cochrane Handbook for Systematic Reviews of Interventions (previously called Cochrane Reviewers Handbook)   Document containing guidance and advice on how to prepare and maintain Cochrane Reviews. Accessible on the Collaboration web site and in the RevMan software.

Cochrane Library   A collection of databases, published on CD-ROM and the Internet and updated quarterly, containing the *Cochrane Database of Systematic Reviews*, the CCRCT, the Database of Abstracts of Reviews of Effects (DARE), the Cochrane Methodology Register, the Health Technology Assessment (HTA) Database, NHS Economic Evaluation database (NHSEED), and information about The Cochrane Collaboration.

Cochrane Review   Cochrane Reviews are systematic summaries of evidence of the effects of health care interventions. They are intended to help people make practical decisions. For a review to be called a Cochrane Review it must be in CDSR (*Cochrane Database of Systematic Reviews*) or CMR (Cochrane Methodology Register). The specific methods used in a Review are described in the text of the review. Cochrane Reviews are prepared using RevMan software provided by the

Collaboration, and adhere to a structured format that is described in the Cochrane Handbook for Systematic Reviews of Interventions.

Cohort study   An observational study in which a defined group of people (the cohort) is followed over time. The outcomes of people in subsets of this cohort are compared, to examine people who were exposed or not exposed (or exposed at different levels) to a particular intervention or other factor of interest. A prospective cohort study assembles participants and follows them into the future. A retrospective (or historical) cohort study identifies subjects from past records and follows them from the time of those records to the present. Because subjects are not allocated by the investigator to different interventions or other exposures, adjusted analysis is usually required to minimise the influence of other factors (confounders).

Collaborative Review Group (CRG)   CRGs are made up of individuals sharing an interest in a particular health care problem or type of problem. The main purpose of a CRG is to prepare and maintain systematic reviews of the effects of health care interventions within the scope of the CRG. Members participate in the CRG not only by preparing Cochrane Reviews but also by handsearching journals and other activities that help the CRG to fulfil its aim. Each CRG is co-ordinated by an editorial team, responsible for regularly updating and submitting an edited module of Cochrane Reviews and information about the CRG, for publication in *The Cochrane Library*.

Concealment of allocation   The process used to prevent foreknowledge of group assignment in a RCT, which should be seen as distinct from blinding. The allocation process should be impervious to any influence by the individual making the allocation by having the randomisation process administered by someone who is not responsible for recruiting participants; for example, a hospital pharmacy, or a central office. Using methods of assignment such as date of birth and case record numbers (see quasi-random allocation) are open to manipulation.

Adequate methods of allocation concealment include: centralised randomisation schemes; randomisation schemes controlled by a pharmacy; numbered or coded containers in which capsules from identical-looking, numbered bottles are administered sequentially; on-site computer systems, where allocations are in a locked unreadable file; and sequentially numbered opaque, sealed envelopes.

Confidence interval (CI)   A measure of the uncertainty around the main finding of a statistical analysis. Estimates of unknown quantities, such as the odds ratio (OR) comparing an experimental intervention with a control, are usually presented as a point estimate and a 95% CI. This means that if someone were to keep repeating a study in other samples from the same population, 95% of the CIs from those studies would contain the true value of the unknown quantity. Alternatives to 95%, such as 90% and 99% CIs, are sometimes used. Wider intervals indicate lower precision; narrow intervals, greater precision. (Also called CI.)

Confounder A factor that is associated with both an intervention (or exposure) and the outcome of interest. For example, if people in the experimental group of a controlled trial are younger than those in the control group, it will be difficult to decide whether a lower risk of death in one group is due to the intervention or the difference in ages. Age is then said to be a confounder, or a confounding variable. Randomisation is used to minimise imbalances in confounding variables between experimental and control groups. Confounding is a major concern in non-randomised studies. See also adjusted analyses.

Controlled (clinical) trial (CCT) This is an indexing term used in MEDLINE and CENTRAL. Within CENTRAL it refers to trials using quasi-randomisation, or trials where double blinding was used but randomisation was not mentioned.

Controlled trial A clinical trial that has a control group. Such trials are not necessarily randomised.

Correlation Linear association between two variables, measured by a correlation coefficient. A correlation coefficient can range from -1 for perfect negative correlation, to $+1$ for perfect positive correlation (with perfect meaning that all the points lie on a straight line). A correlation coefficient of 0 means that there is no linear relationship between the variables.

Critical appraisal The process of assessing and interpreting evidence by systematically considering its validity, results, and relevance.

Cross-over trial A type of clinical trial comparing two or more interventions in which the participants, upon completion of the course of one treatment, are switched to another. For example, for a comparison of treatments A and B, the participants are randomly allocated to receive them in either the order A, B or the order B, A. Particularly appropriate for study of treatment options for relatively stable health problems. The time during which the first interventions are taken is known as the first period, with the second intervention being taken during the second period. See also carry over, and period effect.

D

Database of Abstracts of Reviews of Effects (DARE) A collection of structured abstracts and bibliographic references of systematic reviews of the effects of health care interventions produced by the NHS Centre for Reviews and Dissemination in York, UK. One of the databases in *The Cochrane Library*.

Dependent variable   The outcome or response that results from changes to an independent variable. In a clinical trial, the outcome (over which the investigator has no direct control) is the dependent variable, and the treatment arm is the independent variable. The dependent variable is traditionally plotted on the vertical axis on graphs. (Also called outcome variable.)

Descriptive study   A study that describes characteristics of a sample of individuals. Unlike an experimental study, the investigators do not actively intervene to test a hypothesis, but merely describe the health status or characteristics of a sample from a defined population.

Detection bias   Systematic difference between comparison groups in how outcomes are ascertained, diagnosed, or verified. (Also called ascertainment bias.)

Dichotomous data   Data that can take one of two possible values, such as dead/alive, smoker/non-smoker, present/not present. (Also called binary data.) Sometimes continuous data or ordinal data are simplified into dichotomous data (e.g. age in years could become <75 years or ≥75 years).

E

Effectiveness   The extent to which a specific intervention, when used under ordinary circumstances, does what it is intended to do. Clinical trials that assess effectiveness are sometimes called pragmatic or management trials. See also intention-to-treat.

Efficacy   The extent to which an intervention produces a beneficial result under ideal conditions. Clinical trials that assess efficacy are sometimes called explanatory trials and are restricted to participants who fully co-operate.

EMBASE   Excerpta Medica electronic database. A major European database of medical and health research.

Epidural anaesthesia   Anaesthesia produced by injection of a local anaesthetic into the peridural space of the spinal cord.

Estimate of effect   The observed relationship between an intervention and an outcome expressed as, for example, a number needed to treat (NNT) to benefit, OR, risk difference, risk ratio, standardised mean difference, or weighted mean difference. (Also called treatment effect.)

Evidence-based medicine   The conscientious, explicit, and judicious use of current best evidence in making decisions about the care of individual patients. The practice of evidence-based medicine means integrating individual clinical expertise with the best available external clinical evidence from systematic research.

Evidence-based medicine does not mean "cook-book" medicine, or the unthinking use of guidelines. It does imply that evidence should be reasonably readily available in an easily understood and useable form.

F

Fixed-effect model   (In meta-analysis:) A model that calculates a pooled effect estimate using the assumption that all observed variation between studies is caused by the play of chance. Studies are assumed to be measuring the same overall effect. An alternative model is the random-effects model.

Forest plot   A graphical representation of the individual results of each study included in a meta-analysis together with the combined meta-analysis result. The plot also allows readers to see the heterogeneity among the results of the studies. The results of individual studies are shown as squares centred on each study's point estimate. A horizontal line runs through each square to show each study's CI – usually, but not always, a 95% CI. The overall estimate from the meta-analysis and its CI are shown at the bottom, represented as a diamond. The centre of the diamond represents the pooled point estimate, and its horizontal tips represent the CI.

Funnel plot   A graphical display of some measure of study precision plotted against effect size that can be used to investigate whether there is a link between study size and treatment effect. One possible cause of an observed association is reporting bias.

G

Gold standard   The method, procedure, or measurement that is widely accepted as being the best available, against which new developments should be compared.

H

Handsearching, handsearcher   Handsearching within The Cochrane Collaboration refers to the planned searching of a journal page by page (i.e. by hand), including editorials, letters, etc., to identify all reports of RCTs and CCTs. All the identified trials, regardless of the topic, are sent to the US Cochrane Center, for inclusion in CENTRAL, and forwarding to the US National Library of Medicine (NLM) for re-tagging in MEDLINE. Trials that are within the scope of a CRG or Field go into their specialised register of trials. A handsearching manual is available through the US Cochrane Center. A journal handsearch registration form must be completed for each journal title and sent to the US Cochrane Center to avoid duplication of effort.

Heterogeneity   Used in a general sense to describe the variation in, or diversity of, participants, interventions, and measurement of outcomes across a set of studies, or the variation in internal validity of those studies.

Used specifically, as statistical heterogeneity, to describe the degree of variation in the effect estimates from a set of studies. Also used to indicate the presence of variability among studies beyond the amount expected due solely to the play of chance.

Hypothesis   An unproved theory that can be tested through research. To properly test a hypothesis, it should be pre-specified and clearly articulated, and the study to test it should be designed appropriately. See also null hypothesis.

Hypothesis test   A statistical procedure to determine whether to reject a null hypothesis on the basis of the observed data.

I

I^2 A measure used to quantify heterogeneity. It describes the percentage of the variability in effect estimates that is due to heterogeneity rather than sampling error (chance). A value greater than 50% may be considered to represent substantial heterogeneity.

Incidence   The number of new occurrences of something in a population over a particular period of time, for example the number of cases of a disease in a country over 1 year.

Independent   A description of two events, where knowing the outcome or value of one does not inform us about the outcome or value of the other. Formally, two events A and B are independent if the probability that A and B occur together is equal to the probability of A occurring multiplied by the probability of B occurring.

Independent variable   An exposure, risk factor, or other characteristic that is hypothesised to influence the dependent variable. In a clinical trial, the outcome (over which the investigator has no direct control) is the dependent variable, and the treatment arm is the independent variable. In an adjusted analysis, patient characteristics are included as additional independent variables. (Also called explanatory variable.)

Intention-to-treat analysis   A strategy for analysing data from a RCT. All participants are included in the arm to which they were allocated, whether or not they received (or completed) the intervention given to that arm. Intention-to-treat analysis prevents bias caused by the loss of participants, which may disrupt the baseline equivalence established by randomisation and which may reflect non-adherence to the protocol. The term is often misused in trial publications when some participants were excluded.

Interaction   The situation in which the effect of one independent variable on the outcome is affected by the value of a second independent variable. In a trial, a test of interaction examines whether the treatment effect varies across sub-groups of participants. See also factorial trial, sub-group analysis.

Interim analysis   Analysis comparing intervention groups at any time before the formal completion of a trial, usually before recruitment is complete. Often used with stopping rules so that a trial can be stopped if participants are being put at risk unnecessarily. Timing and frequency of interim analyses should be specified in the protocol.

Intervention group   A group of participants in a study receiving a particular health care intervention. Parallel group trials include at least two intervention groups.

L

Local Anaesthesia   Loss of sensation in a limited (and often superficial) area especially from the effect of a local anaesthetic.

Logistic regression   A form of regression analysis that models an individual's odds of disease or some other outcome as a function of a risk factor or intervention. It is widely used for dichotomous outcomes, in particular to carry out adjusted analysis. See also meta-regression.

M

Malignant hyperthermia   A rare inherited condition characterised by a rapid, extreme, and often fatal rise in body temperature following the administration of general anaesthesia.

Mean   An average value, calculated by adding all the observations and dividing by the number of observations. (Also called arithmetic mean.)

Median   The value of the observation that comes half way when the observations are ranked in order.

MEDLINE   An electronic database produced by the US NLM. It indexes millions of articles in selected journals, available through most medical libraries, and can be accessed on the Internet.

MeSH (medical subject headings)   Terms used by the US NLM to index articles in Index Medicus and MEDLINE. The MeSH system has a tree structure in which broad subject terms branch into a series of progressively narrower subject terms.

Meta-analysis   A meta-analysis is where we pool all the information we have from a number of different (but similar) studies. It should not be about adding small piles of rubbish together to make a big pile of rubbish. It is only worth doing when individual trials are themselves of sufficient quality and validity. What meta-analysis does is to give enough size to have the power to see the result clearly, without the noise of the random play of chance.

Any meta-analysis must have enough events to make sense. Combining small, poor, trials, with few events will mislead.

The use of statistical techniques in a systematic review to integrate the results of included studies.

Morbidity   Illness or harm.

Mortality   Death.

Multivariate analysis   Measuring the impact of more than one variable at a time while analysing a set of data, for example looking at the impact of age, sex, and occupation on a particular outcome. Performed using regression analysis.

N

Narcotic   A drug (as opium) that in moderate doses dulls the senses, relieves pain, and induces profound sleep but in excessive doses causes stupor, coma, or convulsions; a drug (as marijuana or lysergic acid diethylamine, LSD) subject to restriction similar to that of addictive narcotics whether in fact physiologically addictive and narcotic or not.

Non-randomised study   Any quantitative study estimating the effectiveness of an intervention (harm or benefit) that does not use randomisation to allocate units to comparison groups (including studies where allocation occurs in the course of usual treatment decisions or peoples choices, i.e. studies usually called observational). To avoid ambiguity, the term should be substantiated using a description of the type of question being addressed. For example, a "non-randomised intervention study" is typically a comparative study of an experimental intervention against some control intervention (or no intervention) that is not a RCT. There are many possible types of non-randomised intervention study, including cohort studies, case–control studies, controlled before-and-after studies, interrupted-time-series studies, and controlled trials that do not use appropriate randomisation strategies (sometimes called quasi-randomised studies).

Normal distribution   A statistical distribution with known properties commonly used as the basis of models to analyse continuous data. Key assumptions in such analyses are that the data are symmetrically distributed about a mean value, and the shape of the distribution can be described using the mean and standard deviation.

Null hypothesis   The statistical hypothesis that one variable (e.g. which treatment a study participant was allocated to receive) has no association with another variable or set of variables (e.g. whether or not a study participant died), or that two or more population distributions do not differ from one another. In simplest terms, the null hypothesis states that the factor of interest (e.g. treatment) has no impact on outcome (e.g. risk of death).

Number needed to harm (NNH)   This is calculated in the same way as for NNT, but used to describe adverse events. For number needed to harm (NNH), large numbers are good, because they mean that adverse events are rare. Small values for NNH are bad, because they mean adverse events are common.

Number needed to treat (NNT)   The inverse of the absolute risk reduction or increase and the number of patients that need to be treated for one to benefit compared with a control. The ideal NNT is 1, where everyone has improved with treatment and no one has with control. The higher the NNT, the less effective is the treatment. But the value of an NNT is not just numeric. For instance, NNTs of 2–5 are indicative of effective therapies, like analgesics for acute pain. NNTs of about 1 might be seen by treating sensitive bacterial infections with antibiotics, while an NNT of 40 or more might be useful, as when using aspirin after a heart attack.

O

Observational study   A study in which the investigators do not seek to intervene, and simply observe the course of events. Changes or differences in one characteristic (e.g. whether or not people received the intervention of interest) are studied in relation to changes or differences in other characteristic(s) (e.g. whether or not they died), without action by the investigator. There is a greater risk of selection bias than in experimental studies. See also RCT. (Also called non-experimental study.)

Odds   A way of expressing the chance of an event, calculated by dividing the number of individuals in a sample who experienced the event by the number for whom it did not occur. For example, if in a sample of 100, 20 people died and 80 people survived the odds of death are 20/80 = 1/4, 0.25 or 1:4.

Odds ratio (OR)   The ratio of the odds of an event in one group to the odds of an event in another group. In studies of treatment effect, the odds in the treatment group are usually divided by the odds in the control group. An OR of one indicates no difference between comparison groups. For undesirable outcomes an OR that is less than one indicates that the intervention was effective in reducing the risk of that outcome. When the risk is small, ORs are very similar to risk ratios. (Also called OR.)

Opiate   A preparation (as morphine, heroin, and codeine) containing or derived from opium and tending to induce sleep and to alleviate pain; a synthetic drug capable of producing or sustaining addiction similar to that characteristic of morphine and cocaine; a narcotic or opioid peptide.

Original study   See primary study.

Outcome   A component of a participant's clinical and functional status after an intervention has been applied, that is used to assess the effectiveness of an intervention. See also primary outcome, secondary outcome, surrogate outcome.

P

Participant   An individual who is studied in a trial, often but not necessarily a patient.

Peer review   A refereeing process for checking the quality and importance of reports of research. An article submitted for publication in a peer-reviewed journal is reviewed by other experts in the area.

Performance bias   Systematic differences between intervention groups in care provided apart from the intervention being evaluated. For example, if participants know they are in the control group, they may be more likely to use other forms of care. If care providers are aware of the group a particular participant is in, they might act differently. Blinding of study participants (both the recipients and providers of care) is used to protect against performance bias.

Perioperative   Relating to, occurring in, or being the period around the time of a surgical operation (the pre-, intra- and postoperative period).

Per protocol analysis   An analysis of the subset of participants from a RCT who complied with the protocol sufficiently to ensure that their data would be likely to exhibit the effect of treatment. This subset may be defined after considering exposure to treatment, availability of measurements, and absence of major protocol violations. The per protocol analysis strategy may be subject to bias as the reasons for non-compliance may be related to treatment. See also intention-to-treat analysis.

Peto method   A way of combining ORs that has become widely used in meta-analysis. It is especially used to analyse trials with time to event outcomes. The calculations are straightforward and understandable, but this method produces biased results in some circumstances. It is a fixed-effect model.

Placebo   An inactive substance or procedure administered to a participant, usually to compare its effects with those of a real drug or other intervention, but sometimes for the psychological benefit to the participant through a belief that s/he is receiving treatment. Placebos are used in clinical trials to blind people to their treatment allocation. Placebos should be indistinguishable from the active intervention to ensure adequate blinding.

Power   The probability of rejecting the null hypothesis when a specific alternative hypothesis is true. The power of a hypothesis test is one minus the probability of Type II error. In clinical trials, power is the probability that a trial will detect, as statistically significant, an intervention effect of a specified size. If a clinical trial had a power of 0.80 (or 80%), and assuming that the pre-specified treatment effect truly existed, then if the trial was repeated 100 times, it would find a statistically significant treatment effect in 80 of them. Ideally we want a test to have high power, close to maximum of one (or 100%). For a given size of effect, studies with more participants have greater power. Studies with a given number of participants have more power to detect large effects than small effect. (Also called statistical power.)

Prevalence   The proportion of a population having a particular condition or characteristic: for example the percentage of people in a city with a particular disease, or who smoke.

Primary outcome   The outcome of greatest importance.

Prospective study   In evaluations of the effects of health care interventions, a study in which people are identified according to current risk status or exposure, and followed forwards through time to observe outcome. RCTs are always prospective studies. Cohort studies are commonly either prospective or retrospective, whereas case–control studies are usually retrospective. In epidemiology, "prospective study is sometimes misused as a synonym for cohort study". See also retrospective study.

Protocol   The plan or set of steps to be followed in a study. A protocol for a systematic review should describe the rationale for the review, the objectives, and the methods that will be used to locate, select, and critically appraise studies, and to collect and analyse data from the included studies.

PubMed   A free access Internet version of MEDLINE also including records from before 1966 (old MEDLINE), some very recent records and some other life science journals.

p-value   The probability (ranging from zero to one) that the results observed in a study (or results more extreme) could have occurred by chance if in reality the null hypothesis was true. In a meta-analysis, the P-value for the overall effect assesses the overall statistical significance of the difference between the intervention groups, whilst the P-value for the heterogeneity statistic assesses the statistical significance of differences between the effects observed in each study.

Q

Quasi-random allocation   Methods of allocating people to a trial that are not random, but were intended to produce similar groups when used to allocate participants. Quasi-random methods include: allocation by the person's date of birth, by the day of the week or month of the year, by a person's medical record number, or just allocating every alternate person. In practice, these methods of allocation are relatively easy to manipulate, introducing selection bias.

R

Random allocation   A method that uses the play of chance to assign participants to comparison groups in a trial, for example by using a random numbers table or a computer-generated random sequence. Random allocation implies that each individual or unit being entered into a trial has the same chance of receiving each of the possible interventions. It also implies that the probability that an individual will receive a particular intervention is independent of the probability that any other individual will receive the same intervention. See also quasi-random allocation, randomisation.

Random-effects model   Statistical models in which both within-study sampling error (variance) and between-studies variation are included in the assessment of the uncertainty (CI) of the results of a meta-analysis. See also fixed-effect model. When there is heterogeneity among the results of the included studies beyond chance, random-effects models will give wider CIs than fixed-effect models.

Random error   Error due to the play of chance. CIs and *P*-values allow for the existence of random error, but not systematic errors (bias).

Randomisation   The process of randomly allocating participants into one of the arms of a controlled trial. There are two components to randomisation: the generation of a random sequence, and its implementation, ideally in a way so that those entering participants into a study are not aware of the sequence (concealment of allocation).

Randomised controlled trial (RCT)   An experiment in which investigators randomly allocate eligible participants into an intervention group (arm), each of which receives one or more of the interventions that are being compared. The results are assessed by comparing outcomes between the arms. (Also called randomised clinical trial, RCT).

Reference Manager   A software package designed to manage bibliographic references. Sometimes confusingly referred to as RefMan.

Regression analysis   A statistical modelling technique used to estimate or predict the influence of one or more independent variables on a dependent variable, for example the effect of age, sex, and educational level on the prevalence of a disease. Logistic regression and meta-regression are types of regression analysis.

Relative risk reduction   The proportional reduction in risk in one treatment group compared to another. It is one minus the risk ratio. If the risk ratio is 0.25, then the relative risk reduction is $1 - 0.25 = 0.75$, or 75%.

Reliability   The degree to which results obtained by a measurement procedure can be replicated. Lack of reliability can arise from divergences between observers or measurement instruments, measurement error, or instability in the attribute being measured.

Retrospective study   A study in which the outcomes have occurred to the participants before the study commenced. Case–control studies are usually retrospective, cohort studies sometimes are, RCTs never are. See also prospective study.

Review   A systematic review.

A review article in the medical literature, which summarises a number of different studies and may draw conclusions about a particular intervention. Review articles are often not systematic. Review articles are also sometimes called overviews.

Risk   The proportion of participants experiencing the event of interest. Thus, if out of 100 participants the event (e.g. a stroke) is observed in 32, the risk is 0.32. The control group risk is the risk amongst the control group. The risk is sometimes referred to as the event rate, and the control group risk as the CER. However, these latter terms confuse risk with rate. Statistical texts in particular are happy to discuss risk of beneficial effects as well as adverse events.

S

Safety   Refers to serious adverse reactions, such as those that threaten life, require or prolong hospitalisation, result in permanent disability, or cause birth defects. Indirect adverse effects, such as traffic accidents, violence, and damaging consequences of mood change, can also be serious. These adverse effects may occur at various times during a long or a short period of treatment and may be relatively infrequent. They may or may not be detected in trials (depending on participant numbers, intensity of monitoring, and length of follow up), and data on such adverse effects may be available only from non-randomised studies.

Search strategy   The methods used by a CRG to identify trials within the CRGs scope. This includes handsearching relevant journals, searching electronic databases, contacting drug companies, other forms of personal contact, and checking reference lists. CRGs must describe their search strategy in detail in the CRGs module. Authors can refer to the CRGs search strategy when preparing a Cochrane Review, and if necessary supplement this with a description of their own additional searches.

The methods used by a reviewer to locate relevant studies, including the use of a CRG's trials register.

The combination of terms used to identify studies in an electronic database such as MEDLINE.

Secondary outcome   An outcome used to evaluate additional effects of the intervention deemed a priori as being less important than the primary outcomes.

Sedative   Tending to calm, moderate, or tranquillise nervousness or excitement.

Selection bias   Systematic differences between comparison groups in prognosis or responsiveness to treatment. Random allocation with adequate concealment of allocation protects against selection bias. Other means of selecting who receives the intervention are more prone to bias because decisions may be related to prognosis or responsiveness to treatment.

A systematic error in reviews due to how studies are selected for inclusion. Reporting bias is an example of this.

A systematic difference in characteristics between those who are selected for study and those who are not. This affects external validity but not internal validity.

Sensitivity analysis An analysis used to determine how sensitive the results of a study or systematic review are to changes in how it was done. Sensitivity analyses are used to assess how robust the results are to uncertain decisions or assumptions about the data and the methods that were used.

Sequential trial A randomised trial in which the data are analysed after each participant's results become available, and the trial continues until a clear benefit is seen in favour of one of the comparison groups, or it is unlikely that any difference will emerge. The main advantage of sequential trials is that they are usually shorter than fixed size trials when there is a large difference in the effectiveness of the interventions being compared. Their use is restricted to conditions where the outcome of interest is known relatively quickly. In a group sequential trial, a limited number of interim analyses of the data are carried out at pre-specified times during recruitment and follow up, say 3–6 times in all.

Side effect One type of adverse effect. It is any unintended effect of a pharmaceutical product that occurs at doses normally used for therapeutic purposes in man and is related to the pharmacological properties of the drug. While some side effects may be harmful (and can thus be considered adverse effects), there are also side effects that are beneficial.

Specificity (In screening/diagnostic tests:) A measure of a test's ability to correctly identify people who do not have the disease. It is the proportion of people without the target disease who are correctly identified by the test. It is the complement of the false positive rate (FPR = 1 − specificity). It is calculated as follows: Specificity = Number without disease who have a negative test/Number without disease.

(In trial searching:) There is no equivalent concept in trial searching, as we do not know the total number of irrelevant articles in existence. The concept of precision is usually used instead.

Spinal anaesthesia Anaesthesia produced by injection of an anaesthetic into the subarachnoid space of the spine.

Standard deviation A measure of the spread or dispersion of a set of observations, calculated as the average difference from the mean value in the sample.

Standard error The standard deviation of the sampling distribution of a statistic. Measurements taken from a sample of the population will vary from sample to sample. The standard error is a measure of the variation in the sample statistic over all possible samples of the same size. The standard error decreases as the sample size increases.

Statistically significant   A result that is unlikely to have happened by chance. The usual threshold for this judgement is that the results, or more extreme results, would occur by chance with a probability of less than 0.05 if the null hypothesis was true. Statistical tests produce a *P*-value used to assess this.

Sub-group analysis   An analysis in which the intervention effect is evaluated in a defined subset of the participants in a trial, or in complementary subsets, such as by sex or in age categories. Trial sizes are generally too small for sub-group analyses to have adequate statistical power. Comparison of sub-groups should be by test of interaction rather than by comparison of *P*-values. Sub-group analyses are also subject to the multiple comparisons problem. See also multiple comparisons.

Surrogate endpoints   Outcome measures that are not of direct practical importance but are believed to reflect outcomes that are important; for example, blood pressure is not directly important to patients but it is sometimes used as an outcome in clinical trials because it is a risk factor for stroke and heart attacks. Surrogate endpoints are often physiological or biochemical markers that can be relatively quickly and easily measured, and that are taken as being predictive of important clinical outcomes. They are often used when observation of clinical outcomes requires long follow-up.

T

t-test   A statistical hypothesis test derived from the t-distribution. It is used to compare continuous data in two groups. (Also called Students t-test.)

Type I error   A conclusion that a treatment works, when it actually does not work. The risk of a Type I error is often called alpha. In a statistical test, it describes the chance of rejecting the null hypothesis when it is in fact true. (Also called false positive.)

Type II error   A conclusion that there is no evidence that a treatment works, when it actually does work. The risk of a Type II error is often called beta. In a statistical test, it describes the chance of not rejecting the null hypothesis when it is in fact false. The risk of a Type II error decreases as the number of participants in a study increases. (Also called false negative.)

U

Utility   In economic and decision analysis, the value given to an outcome, usually expressed as being between zero and one (e.g. death typically has a utility value of zero and a full healthy life has a value of one).

V

Validity   The degree to which a result (of a measurement or study) is likely to be true and free of bias (systematic errors). Validity has several other meanings, usually accompanied by a qualifying word or phrase; for example, in the context of measurement, expressions such as construct validity, content validity, and criterion validity are used. See also external validity, internal validity.

Variable   A factor that differs among and between groups of people. Variables include patient characteristics such as age, sex, and smoking, or measurements such as blood pressure or depression score. There can also be treatment or condition variables, for example in a childbirth study, the length of time someone was in labour, and outcome variables. The set of values of a variable in a population or sample is known as a distribution.

Variance   A measure of the variation shown by a set of observations, equal to the square of the standard deviation. It is defined as the sum of the squares of deviations from the mean, divided by the number of observations minus one.

Index